"This compelling understanding of chronic pelvic pain syndromes offers a new and pioneering approach to its alleviation."

Frank Werblin, Ph.D.
Professor of Neuroscience
University of California, Berkeley

"It is important for the patient to learn all he can about his disease especially if he has prostatitis/chronic pelvic pain syndrome. That is difficult because doctors seldom agree on the cause, cure or treatment. The information contained in *A Headache in the Pelvis* will be essential for these patients."

Mike Hennenfent
President of The Prostatitis Foundation

"This book is something different something not seen before in the field of prostatitis/chronic pelvic pain. This book will take you to a place you have never been before within prostatitis/chronic pelvic pain syndrome. The relaxation techniques, exercise, and *Trigger Point Release* all are outlined and explained in great detail. Examples used to explain various points are truly excellent and enlightening. Pick up this book and you will be taken into a world of relaxation calm and above all a way to possibly ease your symptoms. The authors have created a new portal into the condition and offer you through the book just what they do to help sufferers get better. Lay back relax and you will not be able to put this book down. To suddenly be aware of your pelvic pain in the ways outlined in this book is a truly enlightening experience. This time last year we could not have dreamed it possible to see a book like this on the book shelf.

One of the authors of this book tells you about his own 22-year struggle (which he won) with chronic pelvic pain syndrome (*A Headache in the Pelvis*) so it's from a sufferers perspective at times you will often say to yourself YES I feel like that when reading this book and smile simply because you will feel one thing; the authors understand my problem. Every UK urologist should read this book. If you can afford it you may wish to buy your Doctor a copy."

The British Prostatitis Support Association

"I suffered from prostatitis/chronic pelvic pain syndrome for three years and my life became absolutely miserable. I received four different diagnoses from four urologists, tried over twenty prescription medications, vitamins, and herbs, and underwent several very uncomfortable and expensive procedures, all of which did hardly anything to help my symptoms which had slowly been increasing in intensity over time (sound familiar?) Eventually I met one of the authors of this book, David Wise, and he taught me the techniques described in the book. Slowly I began to heal myself, without any medication. Six months later my symptoms were diminished significantly and nine months later I felt I was healed. It is now 2-1/2 years after I first started to practice these methods and I feel that I have been freed of this horrific condition.

I cannot recommend this book highly enough for those who are still suffering. There are many schools of thought regarding this syndrome and I studied all of them obsessively at one time. I feel very strongly however that over the coming years the ideas in this book will eclipse the other models of this disease and come to be recognized as the most powerful methods for dealing with it as more and more people are seen to have solid and long-lasting benefits. Mine is not the last testimonial you will see. I should say however that it is not a simple or quick solution and it requires a lot of devotion, but chances are the end-result will be your freedom. Best of luck, do not abandon hope until you have given these methods your most sincere effort."

Reader review on Amazon

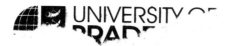
Comments about
A Headache in the Pelvis

"This is the book to read before you contemplate surgery, drugs or resign yourself to continue to suffer with chronic pelvic pain."

Erik Peper, Ph.D.
Professor and Director
Institute for Holistic Healing Studies
California State University, San Francisco
Past President, Biofeedback Society of America
Author of Make Health Happen

"*A Headache in the Pelvis* is a lamp in the dark human suffering of chronic pelvic pain. This book is a precious document that will help many people."

Robert Blum, M.D.
Director, North Bay Pain Center
Former Chief, Department of Neurosurgery
Marin General Hospital
Marin County, California

"Many pelvic pain patients go from doctor to doctor, specialist to specialist without improvement, often feeling abandoned. A majority of patients with chronic pelvic pain do not respond to conventional therapies (antibiotics and anti-inflammatory drugs) leaving a huge void. Drs. Wise and Anderson offer a therapeutic option that can bring relief to many."

Bart Gershbein, M.D.
Clinical Instructor
Department of Urology
University of California School of Medicine
San Francisco, California

"*A Headache in the Pelvis* is a very important contribution to understanding and treating pelvic pain. It is also an illuminating discussion of the relationship of mental and physical interaction in the production of disease, and an approach to a truly comprehensive treatment of illness that has relevance to a whole range of contemporary morbidities."

Donald L. Fink, M.D.
Professor Emeritus
University of California, San Francisco
School of Medicine

"The work described here by Drs. Wise and Anderson is at the forefront of the understanding and treatment of chronic pelvic pain syndromes like prostatitis. Their approach sees the big picture of these disorders and breaks new ground in our understanding of the subtlety of the mind-body continuum."

A.S. Hadland, M.D.
Former Director Integrative Medicine
Pain Management Service
Kaiser Permanente

"*A Headache in the Pelvis* is a book which casts an entirely new light upon the serious problem of chronic pelvic pain, and introduces a treatment that offers hope and relief to the many who suffer from it. It is surely "must read" for all who must deal with this debilitating problem as well as all who attempt to treat it."

Martin F. Schwartz, Ph.D.
Research Associate Professor
Department of Surgery
NYU School of Medicine

A Headache in the Pelvis:

A new understanding and treatment

for chronic pelvic pain syndromes

David Wise, Ph.D.   Rodney U. Anderson, M.D.

A Headache in the Pelvis:
A new understanding and treatment
for prostatitis and chronic pelvic pain syndromes

Copyright © 2010 David Wise, Ph.D. and Rodney U. Anderson, M.D.

National Center for Pelvic Pain Research
P.O. Box 54
Occidental, CA 95465
Toll Free 866-874-2225
Fax 707-874-2335

Cover Design by
Bob Lee Hickson

Publisher's Cataloging-in-Publication Data

Wise, David Thomas, 1945-
    A headache in the pelvis : a new understanding and treatment for prostatitis and chronic pelvic pain syndromes / David Wise, Rodney U. Anderson. – 6th ed. – Occidental, CA : National Center for Pelvic Pain Research, c2008.
    p. ; cm.
ISBN: 978-0-9727755-5-7
Previous ed. 2008.
1.   Pelvic pain. 2. Pelvic pain–Treatment. 3. Pelvis–Diseases.
4.   Prostatitis—Treatment. I. Anderson, Rodney U. II. Title.
RC946 .W55 2010
617.5/5—dc22 2010   2010925908

2 4 6 8 9 7 5 3 1

Sixth Edition

Sixth Edition

2010

Dedication

This book is dedicated to the many brave men and women who suffer daily from chronic pelvic pain and dysfunction.

Table of Contents

Preface to the first edition

As someone who suffered for twenty-two years with pelvic pain and dysfunction, I conducted a very long and personal research into the subject of this book. Today, I am grateful to have been symptom-free for years.

During the first several years of no pain, I was reluctant to be very public about it. This reluctance was born out of some kind of superstition in me that if I told my story, somehow the blessing of having no more pain would be taken away. I was also hesitant to share the very personal information related to my pelvic pain in a public forum.

Over the years, as I treated others with pelvic pain at Stanford and watched many of them improve, the kind of real improvement like my own that I rarely saw with any other treatment, I became more confident that the method that I used for my own recovery was substantial and should be communicated to people who were suffering as I had. My desire to help those with nowhere to turn, who were suffering as I had, overcame my embarrassment about sharing things most people don't share with others.

I joined with Dr. Rodney Anderson, the renowned neurologist at Stanford University Medical School, who has been the court of last resort for many people with pelvic pain. Dr. Anderson and I have worked together for eight years in developing the protocol I brought to Stanford. This book is the result of our collaboration.

When I see patients who describe the misery they are in because they are hurting constantly, I understand. For years, I hurt constantly. More times than I can remember I would wake up in the middle of the night weeping because my pain was so great and I saw no solution for it.

The doctors whom I saw were in the dark about my condition and no one that I knew, except one friend with whom I lost touch, had any idea of what I was going through. There was no Internet at that time, no support groups, and little access to any information on my condition. I would go to the medical library at a local hospital, or the medical library at the University of California Medical Center, and pore over old medical journals looking for some kind of clue that might help me. Then, through some serendipity, I found something that worked. Below I share with the reader a little bit of my journey.

When I was 28 years old, I remember sitting in my new office and feeling an uncomfortable sensation in my rectum. The feeling was as if a golf ball was lodged up inside and I could not get it out. No matter how I moved, what exercise I did or diet I tried, this feeling persisted. Along with rectal pain, I found the need to urinate frequently. To my dismay, my bladder never felt quite empty after urination. Intercourse sometimes was uncomfortable and often seemed to exacerbate my symptoms.

I went to see an urologist who gave me both good and bad news. The good news was that he couldn't find anything wrong. There was no infection, no growth or abnormality in the prostate or surrounding area. The bad news was that he couldn't find anything wrong and therefore couldn't help me. He called what I had "prostatosis," which meant, I believed at the time, the discomfort and urinary frequency and urgency that I felt somehow came from the prostate gland, but the prostate gland was normal.

I was lucky to find a kindly doctor. I say I was lucky after seeing many patients, some of whom saw doctors who did invasive procedures, surgeries and put them on courses of antibiotics and medications for years that didn't help. The doctor whom I found was wise enough to recognize that he didn't know what was going on with me and didn't offer any heroic measures despite my suffering.

I would see this doctor regularly, sometimes every three or six months. He would do a prostate exam, extract prostatic fluid, go into another room where he looked at the fluid under a microscope, and then come back into the little examining room I was in and say "It is clear–no infection." I would ask him "Is there anything new being tried, any new research?" He would reply: "No, not now, but I think this gets better as you get older and there is less sexual activity."

His comments were reassuring to me, especially the comment that I would get better. He was however incorrect in telling me that the condition gets better with age, even though I still appreciate this inaccurate statement. I noticed that the more anxious I was, the worse my symptoms got. Being someone who tends toward anxiety, I think I would have had a more difficult time without this doctor's kindly but inaccurate assurance.

I tried everything. I started out with the regular medical treatments of antibiotics, which did not help me. I experimented with diet, cutting out alcohol, coffee and spicy foods on the advice of the physician I was seeing. There was no benefit. Someone told me that certain reflexology pressure points near the ankle could help. I pressed those pressure points to the point of great pain for many months hoping for some relief. I read somewhere that zinc deficiency could cause my problem, and so I took zinc supplements regularly. I tried many sessions of acupuncture, psychotherapy, guided imagery visualization, hands on healing and prayer. All made no difference to my condition.

There were some things that helped a little and then stopped helping. Warm baths sometimes took the edge off of my pain. Occasionally, prostate massage temporarily reduced the symptoms but only for a few hours. Eventually when I would return to the doctor, prostate massage failed to have any effect.

The truth is, as I look at it now, nothing really helped in any lasting way. While there was almost always an underlying sense of discomfort, when flare-ups would occur, often after sex, they would last for months and months. Many patients have asked me how I lived with these symptoms for twenty-two years. As I reflect now, there was no magic to it. When times were bad, I muddled through. The cost to my quality of life was very high. When my symptoms were bad, I found myself distracted and I withdrew inwardly from social situations and my loved ones. Miraculously, I never took off work, even though I very much understand how someone would. In the language of current day America, "You do what you gotta do."

My symptoms waxed and waned, though never really went away. After years of having symptoms, I found myself in the fortunate position of not having to work. I had dreamed about this for many years and somehow it became a reality.

The effect of my newfound freedom on my pelvic pain was not what I expected. It never occurred to me that my anxiety would increase. In fact, my symptoms got much worse. More than that, their severity became constant and I found no relief day or night. I well remember lying in bed during a heavy rain storm. Being in a warm bed and hearing the rain on the roof had been one of my pleasures, but during this time there was no pleasure because I could find no escape from the constant aching that I felt.

In my desperation, I began making phone calls to doctors and researchers around the world whose names I took from the medical literature. It was from this desperate search that I discovered a way to eventually stop my symptoms.

After several months of using the protocol described in this book, I occasionally did not feel the need to go to the bathroom for four or five hours. This felt amazing to me. As time went on, I would notice that I was pain-free for brief periods. These periods gradually increased. Later, weeks passed when I had no symptoms.

To my dismay, there were still many flare-ups and my symptoms would return full-blown. The flare-ups, however, lasted a fraction of the time than they used to. I was getting better. Imperceptibly, my regular state became one of no pelvic pain or dysfunction.

I felt normal. I was grateful beyond words for the feeling that everything inside was working right. The joy of feeling normal in my bladder was beyond my ability to communicate. Feeling normal is a peculiar way to describe how I felt because it really doesn't communicate the ease and pleasure I felt about something that most people never even notice and simply take for granted. And aside from close friends being happy that I was feeling good, my sense was that no one really understood how it felt inside me to simply feel normal.

It took over two years for all of the symptoms to go away. To this day, I continue to use the relaxation protocol and I believe it has been essential in my remaining well.

We hope this book brings some clarity and direction to many who suffer from pelvic pain. It is written for those who have no familiarity with medical terminology or research and we include neither footnotes nor a bibliography, although we include a simplified review of literature.

David Wise, Ph.D.
Sebastopol, California
March 2003

*****

Many years ago I had the privilege and pleasure of being mentored by one of the giants of American Urology. Dr. Thomas A. Stamey, Chairman of the Department of Urology at Stanford University, introduced me as a resident in training to the problems that men endured with chronic prostatitis. More importantly, he introduced me to a way of evaluating patients with meticulous detail, being curious and mindful of every nuance of symptom and finding. He reiterated continuously the importance of paying attention to detail and being a "thinking" urologist as opposed to mindlessly throwing pills at or cutting your way through a problem. He also showed me through his clinical research methods that it was much better to study a few patients thoroughly than a lot of patients superficially.

Dr. Stamey taught me to look through the microscope and see what human inflammatory cells looked like in the prostatic fluid of men suffering with prostatitis. He got quite excited to demonstrate fat-laden macrophages that exhibited a Maltese-cross appearance under polarized light. He showed me how to carefully segregate the urine specimens from the prostatic fluid to prove whether a patient had true bacterial colonization of the prostate or some contaminant. His publication with our other colleague, Dr. Edwin Meares, still stands as the pivotal work to define prostatic infection.

Unfortunately, no matter how much we have studied this problem of chronic prostatitis and chronic pelvic pain syndrome, in both men and women, three decades later we still do not understand why it happens and how to prevent it. Fortunately my partner Dr. David Wise, a perceptive psychologist, came along and described his experience and discoveries in abating his symptoms after having dealt with his condition for many years. Since that time I have been impressed that this approach helps many more people than pharmaceutical agents or surgery.

This small book is our attempt to convey to the patients suffering from chronic pelvic pain syndromes our genuine concern for their well-being and to describe our experience with an alternative approach to improve or resolve their symptoms. At the same time we attempt to help clarify and explain the controversies and medical investigations ongoing to elucidate the biologic basis of these complaints.

Rodney U. Anderson, M.D., FACS
Stanford, California
March 2003

Preface to the second edition

In a little more than half a year we have sold out of the first hardbound edition of our book. The response to our book has been well beyond our expectations. Our book has been ordered from almost every state in the Union and many countries on every continent in the world. The emails we have gotten have brought home how the problem we describe is not limited to national boundary, culture, or race. The people who suffer from chronic pelvic pain syndromes all undergo the same kinds of symptoms and suffer the same kinds of pain, dysfunction, and anguish.

Most of the letters we have received express their appreciation for having received a new way of understanding and treating certain kinds of chronic pelvic pain. Indeed readers often report that their symptoms tend to reduce after simply reading our book. This may be because the simple reassurance that what they have is not life-threatening can frequently lead to alleviation of symptoms on a short-term basis.

In this new edition, we have included a number of additions. We have updated our research review with the latest important research findings. We have added a chapter that includes a number of reports from patients who have undergone our treatment and who continue to practice our protocol. We have added more stretches that have proven useful. We have included a section describing Respiratory Sinus Arrhythmia breathing that is used preliminary to *Paradoxical Relaxation*. Importantly, we have published this edition as a paperback for a significantly lower cost.

David Wise, Ph.D.
Rodney U. Anderson, M.D., FACS
September 2003

Preface to the third edition

Our book continues to be received with great enthusiasm by many who suffer from chronic pelvic pain. We continue to receive correspondence from people in many different countries who express their gratitude at the possibilities that our book opens up.

This third edition is a significant edition because we have included an extensive written and graphic presentation of our physical therapy protocol. We have updated the section on research to include the latest studies on pelvic pain. We have included a section about what we believe are the common origins of chronic pelvic pain and other disorders including hemorrhoids, anal fissures and constipation, and the possible use of the *Wise-Anderson Protocol* for these difficulties. A more extensive discussion of biofeedback is also included as well as an expanded explanation of the technique of *Paradoxical Relaxation*.

During the time of our second edition, we began offering treatment for pelvic pain in the form of a 6-day, 30 hour intensive clinic in which both *Paradoxical Relaxation* and physical therapy are offered on site in California. This format has proved to be the most effective one we have used. We have also begun a new website, www.pelvicpainhelp. com which contains much information about different aspects of our work. We are more enthusiastic about our work than we ever have been in the past and there is slow but growing interest on the part of the medical community.

We have recently submitted an analysis of our experience and outcomes in over 100 men who have used our protocol to a medical journal. Because of the policies of the journal we are not at liberty to publish that information at this time, but we are very pleased with the results and look forward to releasing that information soon.

David Wise, Ph.D.
Rodney U. Anderson, M.D., FACS
February 2004

Preface to the fourth edition

We are very happy to be able to present the 4th edition of *A Headache in the Pelvis*. This edition is a major one. Since the publication of the 3rd edition, we have presented our results at the American Urological Association and the National Institutes of Health meetings on pelvic pain. We have published two articles in the Journal of Urology on the results of our treatment. We have conducted approximately thirty 6-day intensive clinics in which we continue to grow and learn regarding how to more and more effectively train patients in our protocol.

What strongly stands out about this edition is the focus on female pelvic pain included in a separate chapter. We discuss interstitial cystitis in detail, the relationship and likely connections between anxiety, nervous system arousal and bladder inflammation. We present what we believe to be the most comprehensive illustrated discussion of external and internal trigger points relating to female pelvic pain as well as expand the number of illustrations of the very important anterior levator ani trigger points and the trigger points of the quadratus lumborum. Importantly, we present our observations on the proper degree of pressure in doing trigger point release and the very important subject of hyperirritability and how it must be treated.

We have attempted to further simplify our language and make the often difficult and technical discussion of our research and treatment on pelvic pain understandable to the lay person. With this in mind we have expanded our research chapter to include the most recent relevant research. We have expanded the discussion of *Paradoxical Relaxation* and the subtle aspects of this practice that makes a qualitative difference in the results of this method. We have introduced the idea that pelvic pain is part of having a knotted up insides that cause pelvic pain in particular, and the experience of not being able to feel peaceful and enjoy life in general.

Finally, we have included more stories of patients in their own words who have recently undergone our protocol. We hope that this edition offers further help for those seeking help for pelvic pain.

David Wise, Ph.D.
Rodney U. Anderson, M.D., FACS
November 2006

Preface to the fifth edition

As we approach this 5th edition of our book we are happy to report that many men and women suffering from chronic pelvic pain syndromes have taken our concepts and suggestions to heart and have made significant progress in conquering their disorder. While no book alone can solve everyone's issues with chronic pain we are encouraged by the endorsements from most patients who have read it.

We are enormously fortunate to be able to treat patients every month in our 6-day immersion clinic, a format new to the treatment of pelvic pain syndromes. Our clinic format has afforded us an abundance of precious experience in treating so many patients every month with the same problem in an intensive setting. This edition reflects our new insights and the changes and improvements in method we have made in our ongoing treatment of patients since the publication of our last edition.

Specifically, this edition adds a section on advice to partners and loved ones of people with pelvic pain, practical advice on minimizing the risk of pelvic pain during childbirth, an expanded discussion of the possible use of a modified *Wise-Anderson Protocol* for anal fissures, irritable bowel syndrome, constipation and other anorectal disorders, further clarification for the layman with prostatitis on the confusing names used in this disorder, discussion of the effect of food and drink on interstitial cystitis, further discussion of anxiety as the breeding ground for pelvic pain, the central practice of attention training in relaxing the pelvic floor, the use of RSA breathing during *Trigger Point Release*, further insights in the practice of *Paradoxical Relaxation*, new drawings illustrating *Wise-Anderson Protocol* physical therapy self-treatment, the first time explanation of post-bowel movement pain associated with pelvic pain, updating of the literature on the medical science being conducted to help those individuals suffering from pelvic pain around the world, and more.

David Wise, Ph.D.
Rodney U. Anderson, M.D., FACS
May 2008

Preface to the sixth edition

This 6th edition of our book represents our continued study and understanding of muscle related pelvic pain and dysfunction. We develop and grow in our understanding and in our treatment because we have the ongoing privilege of seeing a stream of patients with pelvic pain participating in our monthly 6-day immersion clinics. Each month, this experience of treating the different shades and varieties of pelvic pain in individuals who come to see us from around the world confirms, deepens, refines and clarifies for us how to most effectively help our patients. Since the last publication of this book, we have published an article in the Journal of Urology, for the first time documenting with clinical data the relationship between the location of trigger points in and around the pelvic floor and the location and kinds of complaints of patients suffering from this disorder. More and more, we appreciate the necessity of empowering our patients to do all of their treatment themselves. Since the publication of our book, we have given our internal trigger point wand to over 200 patients who have demonstrated the possibility of significantly reducing the sensitivity of internal trigger points and areas of pelvic floor tissue restriction and pain themselves, in the comfort of their own homes—areas that heretofore have been inaccessible for self treatment. We discuss our wand in this edition. We have revised our section on female pelvic pain, included stories from female patients, updated the section on the medical science of pelvic pain with the most current information, presented an explanation of the possible biological basis of pelvic pain syndromes in discussing it as a 'tail-pulled-between-the-legs' syndrome, presented a hypothesis on why a group of men develop pelvic pain after an anxiety producing sexual encounter, and discussed the relationship between compulsive sexual activity, pornography and pelvic pain. We have included an essay explaining the location and function of the pelvic floor in the most simplified way. We continue to be intensely interested and excited in our work with pelvic pain and are grateful that interest in our work continues to grow throughout the world.

David Wise, Ph.D.
Rodney U. Anderson, M.D., FACS
May 2010

The *Wise-Anderson Protocol* and the *Stanford Protocol*

In the middle 1990's, David Wise, a psychologist in California who recovered from chronic pelvic pain syndrome he suffered from for many years, contacted Rodney Anderson, a professor of Urology at Stanford Medical School and one of the experts at Stanford in pelvic pain. Dr. Wise shared the method he used to resolve his pelvic pain with Dr. Anderson, who ran the chronic pelvic pain clinic in the department of Urology at Stanford University Medical Center. After this meeting, Dr. Wise began working as a Visiting Research Scholar with Dr. Anderson at Stanford University Medical Center in the Department of Urology with patients with pelvic pain. For 8 years Rodney Anderson and David Wise pioneered the development of the treatment that David Wise used for his own recovery. The treatment at Stanford was done patient by patient, on an individual basis in a conventional medical form.

During these early years, this protocol was presented at meetings for prostatitis researchers at the National Institutes of Health and other scientific meetings. In 2003, Dr. Wise and Dr. Anderson published the first edition of *A Headache in the Pelvis* describing the protocol that they developed at Stanford over the past 8 years. In the first edition of *A Headache in the Pelvis*, this protocol was called the *Wise-Anderson Protocol*. As the protocol became more widely disseminated, those on the internet dubbed it the *Stanford Protocol*. In the subsequent editions of this book, the *Wise- Anderson Protocol* has been referred to as the *Stanford Protocol* because the term continued to be so widely used on the internet. In this edition we have gone back to using the original term *Wise-Anderson Protocol*. The *Wise-Anderson Protocol* and the *Stanford Protocol* for pelvic pain are one and the same.

In 2003 Dr. Wise left Stanford and began doing the protocol he and Dr. Anderson developed at Stanford in a 6-day immersion clinic in Sonoma county in California. Patients often come from far away to learn the *Wise-Anderson Protocol* in the intensive clinics and be trained to be able to do the protocol on a daily basis without the assistance of professionals. Competence in self treatment has turned out to be the most effective way the protocol can be used. The 6-day immersion clinics that have continued to be offered on a monthly basis since 2003 up to the present, are not affiliated with Stanford. Dr. Anderson has continued to evaluate many patients at Stanford and refer them to the immersion clinic when they are appropriate candidates. From 2003 to the present, Rodney Anderson, David Wise and Tim Sawyer have actively and enthusiastically collaborated in research on patients seen in the immersion clinics, held now in Santa Rosa, California. Since 2003, Anderson, Wise and Sawyer have published articles in the Journal of Urology on data from patients they have collaboratively seen and treated. Dr. Wise has been a plenary speaker at the National Institutes of Health in 2005, presenting research on the *Wise-Anderson Protocol,* and recently presented the protocol at the International Continence Society. Dr. Anderson has presented research on this protocol at meetings of the American Urological Association and other professional meetings. Recently, Anderson, Sawyer and Wise have published a pioneering article in the Journal of Urology showing the relationship of trigger point location and symptoms in patients with pelvic pain using the clinical data from the immersion clinics held in Santa Rosa. Currently Anderson, Wise and Sawyer are preparing an article on the effectiveness of a new internal trigger point wand for the self treatment of internal trigger points. This is discussed in the current edition.

Acknowledgments

We wish to express our gratitude to the following individuals who have helped and inspired us in the writing of this book:
Elaine Orenberg Anderson, Harold Wise, Marilyn Freedman, Erik Peper, John Moses, Ruth Dreier, Tiaga Liner, Frank Werblin, Jeanette Potts, Ragi Doggweiler, Jennifer Tien, Pat Lachman, Claudia Fiori, Hilary Garcia, Helene Korn, Amanita Rosenbush, Dan Poynter, Suzanne Pregerson, Sara Siebert-Sawyer, Dara Gaethe, Susan Page, Steve Hadland, Anneke Vanderveen, Robert Moldwin, Walter Blum, Ramana Maharshi, Jean Klein, Jane Kramer, Mitch Feldman, Kathy Harris, Rick Harvey, Allaudin Mathieu, Larry Rabon, Nathan Segal, Joseph Segal, Clair Sutton, Lindy Woodard, Bart Gershbein, June Wise, Shera Wise Silver, Ted Silver, Benjamin Silver, Leo Silver, Fay Nathanson, Lawrence Nathanson, Brian Nathanson, Richard Gevirtz, Byron Katie, Mary Kenney, Harry Kenney, Steve Wall, Jerome Weiss, Annmarie Cosby, Donald Fink, Daniel Fink, Judith Klinman, Zepporah Glass, Cinnamon Wise, Helen Wise, Symon Wise, Francine Shapiro, Frederick Perls, Jim Simkin, Martin Schwartz, Judith Schwartz, Alan Leveton, Ann Armstrong, Ann Dreyfuss, Leo Zeff, Walter Kaufmann, Milton Rosenberg, Edmund Jacobson, Helene Morcos, Richard Miller, Ann Miller, Larry Bloomberg, Ed Sampson, Phil Curcuruto, Howard Glazer, Nadia Nurhussein, Rhonda Kotarinos, Ellen Vandenberg, Judith Goleman, Rick Larue, Dawn Larue, Donna Spitzer, Daniel Goleman, Diana Schlaufler, Patricia Speier, Marlene Cohen, Susan Todd, Cheri Quincy, Joel Alter, Alan Dreyfuss, John Adair, Larry Todd, Stephanie Rosencrans and Cynthia Frank. Special thanks tot Marilyn Freedman for her help with the sections on pelvic pain and childbirth and anorectal disorders. We express our deep appreciation for the seminal work of Dr. Edmund Jacobson in *Progressive Relaxation* and to Drs. Janet Travell and David Simons for their work in trigger point release. We are particularly indebted to Tim Sawyer, P.T., for his great skill, talent and experience in *Trigger Point Release* related to pelvic pain, who has been our senior consultant in physical therapy in our work at Stanford and the architect of the *Wise-Anderson Protocol* physical therapy methodology..

CHAPTER 1

DEFINITIONS AND CATEGORIES

Millions of men and women suffer from pelvic pain, discomfort, or dysfunction. These disorders, which can be called chronic pelvic pain syndromes (CPPS), usually include one or a number of symptoms including *rectal, genital, or abdominal discomfort or pain, increased discomfort or pain sitting down, discomfort or pain during or after sexual activity, and often urinary frequency, urgency and hesitancy.* Historically, these conditions have been given many different names.

As a result, they have been thought to have numerous causes. In the majority of cases, doctors can find little or no physical basis for the symptoms and most or all tests usually come back normal. In this book, we will demonstrate that there is a simple physical basis for the symptoms and that the seemingly wide array and variability of the symptoms are simply idiosyncratic expressions of the same underlying problem in both men and women. A treatment protocol has been developed, called the *Wise-Anderson Protocol*. We no longer treat the symptoms; instead we treat what triggers those symptoms. Our approach substantially reduces or abates symptoms in a large majority of qualifying patients who undertake our full protocol as we have demonstrated in our published research.

In this book we will use the terms, *a headache in the pelvis, chronic pelvic pain syndrome(s), chronic pelvic pain, pelvic pain,* and *CPPS* synonymously to refer to all the conditions discussed.

Traditional names and diagnostic categories

In Men

- Prostatitis (National Institutes of Health categories)
  I Acute bacterial prostatitis
  II Chronic bacterial prostatitis
  IIIA CPPS nonbacterial inflammatory prostatitis
  IIIB CPPS nonbacterial non-inflammatory prostatitis
  IV Asymptomatic inflammatory prostatitis
- Orchalgia and/or epididymitis
- Proctalgia fugax

In Women

- Urethral syndrome
- Vulvodynia (vulvar vestibulitis)

In Both Men and Women

- Interstitial cystitis
- Levator ani syndrome
- Pudendal nerve entrapment syndrome

What is common in the different names

The central notion in this book is that there is a *common factor that unites the different names: that there is a common effective treatment for many of them; and that the body and the mind are intimately involved in the cause and the treatment.*

For many years, chronic pelvic pain syndromes have posed an enigma to the medical community. Nonbacterial prostatitis, for example, has routinely been confused with acute or chronic bacterial prostatitis even though an accurate and easy method for diagnosis has been available for years. At the same time, nonbacterial prostatitis, which makes up the overwhelming number of cases of prostatitis, tends to be regarded by doctors as a kind of wastebasket diagnosis for pelvic symptoms that the doctor does not understand or know how to treat. Gross pathology, as measured by the latest medical instruments, has not been able to explain the degree of suffering caused by these disorders.

Doctors often tell patients with chronic pelvic pain syndromes that they can find little or nothing to account for their symptoms

What we are proposing in this book is that these conditions are rather like a headache, except the location of the headache is in the pelvis. Hence *A Headache in the Pelvis* is our title. A further implication from the title is that these disorders are problems of chronic muscle tension, which is often the basis of headaches. If chronic pelvic pain syndromes are, in fact, a headache in the pelvis, then treatment needs to be radically different from what has traditionally been followed.

A Headache in the Pelvis is the name we are giving to chronic pelvic pain syndromes where no gross pathology has been found. These syndromes often include pain and dysfunction related to urination, defecation, and sexual activity. This discomfort or pain and dysfunction occur in both men and women. One person may experience only one symptom while another may experience all symptoms. Sometimes symptoms inexplicably vary from day to day or week to week. Symptoms vary, as do their anatomical locations, yet we propose that the trigger for these symptoms is the same and a common effective treatment may exist for all of them.

Not something you talk about at a party

Even though many people suffer from *a headache in the pelvis*, most of them feel alone in their difficulty. The genital, urinary, and defecation areas of the body are considered private and are often very difficult to talk about, even with close friends or relatives. Basically, most people want the areas of the genitals and rectum to work, but don't want to know much about them or to have to pay any attention to them.

These areas of the body are not treated with much respect. This is a truth that is reflected in how we word profanities. What do we call people at whom we are angry? Usually terms related to defecation or procreation are used in a derogatory way. Indeed, these are terms of denigration. In our culture, the genitals and rectum are shrouded in shame and guilt. As we discuss later, the genitals and rectum are areas that are often psychologically and energetically disowned by people. Being rejected in some way, it is not uncommon for people to try to distance themselves from these body parts by tightening against them. The healing of the abused pelvis, as Steven Levine has stated eloquently, in part involves bringing the genitals and rectum "back into the heart." This means changing one's attitude from shame, guilt, and rejection to compassion and appreciation.

People's aversion toward these areas can be so strong they will often go to the doctor only when the symptoms are marked. Sometimes they dismiss these symptoms as aging or as normal aches and pains that have to be tolerated. Sometimes people will endure symptoms for long periods of time, if they can bear them, because they are afraid that if they seek a diagnosis, it will be one that they really don't want to hear. They prefer not to know. Given the embarrassment about these areas, the anxiety over what symptoms can lead to, and the poor treatment record of the medical profession, it is not surprising that sufferers of chronic pelvic pain syndromes often feel isolated.

The confusion of names

An old parable to explain a current confusion

Once upon a time, ten blind men, each with a cane, went for a walk along a road that skirted a jungle. Soon they came upon an elephant, and each one found himself at a different place in relationship to the animal. One blind man touching the elephant's leg remarked, "Oh, this creature is like a tree trunk." Another, who was positioned under the elephant's stomach, pushed up and said, "Oh no. This creature is like a soft ceiling, with nothing else around on the sides." A third positioned at the tail, pulled on it and said, "No, this creature is like a rope connected to a tree." Another, touching the trunk of the elephant, said, "No, this creature is like a large, soft pipe." Yet another, reaching and touching the elephant's tusk, said, "No, this creature is like a curved spear stuck into rock."

On and on they argued. What was this creature they had come upon? Finally, a fellow traveler came by and heard the argument. Noticing right away they were blind, he said, "No, you're all correct, and you're wrong, because this is an elephant and each one of you is only touching one part, thinking that each part constitutes the whole."

For reasons about which we can only speculate, up to the time we wrote this book, the manifestations of chronic pelvic pain syndromes have been perceived by blind men. This is not to disparage the sincere physicians and researchers who grapple with these conditions. It is, however, in the nature of the specialization of medicine, that physicians only see a problem through the lenses of their own field, and depending upon the specialist you see, the condition may be called by a different name.

What might be called *prostatitis* by a urologist might be called *coccygodynia* or *pudendal nerve compression syndrome* by a colorectal surgeon. Other names used by specialists to describe the same condition are *chronic genital pain, prostatodynia, essential anorectal pain, idiopathic pelvic pain, pelvic floor dysfunction, pelvic floor myalgia, levator ani syndrome, spastic piriformis syndrome*, and others.

Similarly, what might be called *vulvar vestibulitis, lichen sclerosis, lichen planas,* or *lichen simplex chronicus* by a dermatologist might be called a yeast infection by a gynecologist, or an anxiety disorder by a psychiatrist. If you go to three doctors for chronic pelvic pain, it is easily possible you can get two or three different diagnoses.

One important reason for this "blindness around seeing the whole elephant" is the lack of communication among the many medical specialties. If they all spoke to each other and shared information, they might realize they often are talking about the same condition. It is the hope of the authors of this book that we can bring eyes to bear on this problem that have a broader scope. We aspire to see the whole elephant.

General Symptoms of Chronic Pelvic Pain Syndrome in Men

Intermittent or constant discomfort or pain

Many sufferers of pelvic pain typically say that they don't feel pain but discomfort, soreness, fullness, aching, burning or some other disagreeable sensation. Most people rarely feel a sharp searing pain. It is usually more like a nagging ache, soreness, burning or tightness. Of course it is often out and out pain.

For both sexes, all of the symptoms described below can either be intermittent or constant, diurnal or nocturnal (daytime or nighttime), during sitting or standing and often more profound during periods of stress. Symptoms can involve discomfort or pain and no urinary or sexual dysfunction, discomfort or pain and urinary symptoms with no sexual symptoms or all three. One of the perplexing aspects is the variable cycles of intensity.

In men, chronic pelvic pain includes *discomfort or pain in the rectum* or *perineum*, between the scrotum and anus. Patients report that it feels as if there was a "golf ball" there. Often symptoms include *increased discomfort or pain when sitting.* Many men experience discomfort in the area above the pubic bone in and around the area of the bladder, called *suprapubic discomfort or pain. Discomfort or pain in the groin* is typical and can be experienced unilaterally or bilaterally (on one side or both sides). Discomfort or pain in the testicles called *orchalgia* is not uncommon. *Discomfort or pain in the penis* is often felt at the penile tip or in the urethra. Sometimes there is *coccygeal discomfort or pain* (in or around the tailbone), or *discomfort or pain in the lower back* or, not uncommonly, *thigh discomfort or pain* in the back, side, or front of the thigh, either on one side or both.

Intermittent or constant urinary symptoms in men

Disturbances in urination are often associated with pelvic pain. Commonly with pelvic pain, men experience something called *dysuria,* which is pain, discomfort or burning when urinating. They sometimes complain of a *reduced urinary stream, frequency of urination* (in which they have to urinate every half hour to two hours), *urgency of urination* (in which they feel they can't wait to urinate once the urge arises), and/or *nocturia* (a need to urinate frequently at night).

Intermittent or constant sexual dysfunction in men

Increased discomfort or pain during or after ejaculation is very often associated with pelvic pain. Commonly, men complain of a *reduced libido* or desire for sex and sometimes erectile dysfunction (occasional or frequent inability to attain or maintain an erection), reduced ejaculate, softer erections, and reduced sexual pleasure. Some men observe a reduction in ejaculate. Often the discomfort or pain related to ejaculation acts as a deterrent to sexual desire.

Intermittent or constant psychological symptoms in men

Almost universally, men experience *anxiety* and various levels of low spirits or *depression.* They have the sense that "there's something wrong inside me that isn't going away." It is not unusual for men to complain of *dysphoria*—to have a reduced interest in participating in life and in interpersonal relationships. Some degree of withdrawal from social situations occurs and self-esteem often suffers.

General Symptoms of Chronic Pelvic Pain Syndrome in Women
(for more detail on female pelvic pain, see Chapter 7)

Intermittent or constant discomfort or pain in women

In women, the symptoms described can be either intermittent or constant. As with men, women can experience discomfort or pain or related dysfunction more during the night or during the day, more in the morning or in the afternoon, more during or not during their menstrual cycle, and often more during periods of stress.

Location of discomfort or pain in women

Women can experience genital discomfort or pain in the form of *vaginal/vulvar discomfort or pain* (pain at the opening of the vagina or deep inside). In certain conditions, women experience *coccygeal discomfort or pain* (at the tailbone) and *rectal discomfort or pain* (at the opening or inside the rectum). In other conditions, women, like men, report *suprapubic discomfort or pain* (right above the pubic bone, in and around the area of the bladder), *groin discomfort or pain, and discomfort or pain when sitting.* Some women complain of discomfort or pain in the sub-pubic region and *pain in the clitoris.*

Intermittent or constant urinary symptoms in women

Urinary symptoms may coexist with many conditions of pelvic pain. Women can experience *urinary frequency, urinary urgency, even urinary urge incontinence, dysuria, reduced urinary stream, and incomplete bladder emptying.*

Intermittent or constant sexual dysfunction in women

Because there is often *vaginal pain* at the opening or inside the vagina, *dyspareunia* (pain during or after intercourse) is almost always present. In more severe cases, particularly with women who have *vulvar vestibulitis*, there is an *inability to have intercourse*. This may be their only complaint.

Pelvic pain or discomfort usually puts life on hold: intermittent or constant psychological symptoms

Given the nature of the symptoms of these conditions, it is easy to understand why feelings of *anxiety* and *depression* so often accompany pelvic pain. Because of the part of the body that is involved, and the severe impact on the ability to be sexual, an *impairment of intimate relationships* occurs with many women. Women may lose their zest for living. Generally, the more pronounced and constant the symptoms, the more severe the dysphoria. Naturally, the self-esteem of many women who suffer from these conditions tends to be low.

A Headache in the Pelvis in Men

In the following section, we will introduce the name that has been traditionally used for a certain pelvic pain syndrome, followed by a simple explanation of what the name means. We will then summarize the symptoms that are traditionally included under this name, the number of people affected by the condition, the traditional treatments used, and how helpful or unhelpful they are. Following this, we will discuss in more detail the symptoms and the condition in general.

Prostatitis

Category I – Acute Bacterial Prostatitis

Description

Acute Bacterial Prostatitis is quite clear both in its diagnosis and in its treatment. Infection and inflammation are evident and traditional treatments work well. We do offer the idea that chronic pelvic tension may be its initiating cause.

It can occur at any age and manifest with symptoms such as fever, chills, pain, and urinary dysfunction. Positive findings involving the presence of white blood cells in the urine as well as pathogenic bacteria confirm this diagnosis. Acute bacterial prostatitis develops relatively quickly and is often associated with a feeling of being sick. Newer antibiotics produce good results. It is important to have this condition treated quickly because of the risk of the spread of bacteria into the bloodstream, retention of urine, and potential abscess formation. Chronic bacterial prostatitis can develop from acute bacterial prostatitis that is poorly treated. Antibiotic therapy should be extended to 28 days to assure eradication of the infection.

Symptoms

- Fever and chills
- Prostate pain
- Dysuria
- Lower back pain
- Perineal pain (pain between the anus and scrotum)
- Difficulty urinating
- Urinary retention

Because of retention of urine due to swelling of the prostate gland, a catheter may be inserted into the penis to allow for proper flow of urine. While this catheter may increase the risk of prostatic abscess or infection in the gland, catheterization is an important part of therapy when there is urinary retention. Some men with acute urinary retention may be better served with a small plastic catheter inserted directly into the bladder through the skin of the suprapubic area.

Factors associated with onset

- Migration of bacteria up the urethra
- Unprotected anal intercourse
- Immune disorders
- Urinary retention or instrumentation

Prevalence

- Relatively rare (approximately 5% of reported diagnoses of prostatitis)

Tests for Diagnosis

- Urinalysis (microscopic inspection)
- Culture of urine (important and often neglected by physicians)

Traditional treatments used

- Antibiotics (muscle injection of aminoglycosides or penicillin, oral fluoroquinolones)

Success of traditional treatment

- The most successfully treated type of prostatitis

Category II – Chronic Bacterial Prostatitis

Description

Chronic Bacterial Prostatitis represents a more difficult condition than acute bacterial prostatitis. Most chronic bacterial prostatitis develops because of inadequately treated acute prostatitis. Men who have recurrent bacterial colonization of the urethra because of poor hygiene, poor sexual practices, or a need to instrument the urethra may have bacterial colonization and infection. Men who have strictures or scar tissue in the urethra that narrow the tube restricting urinary flow may be prone to developing recurrent bacterial infection. Often there is no bacterial growth in the bladder and one can be completely asymptomatic between episodes of acute flare-up, at which time the bacteria grow, spread, and begin to infect the bladder. This is a hallmark of chronic bacterial prostatitis. Men are usually free of symptoms between episodes.

Symptoms (may be intermittent or constant)

- Urinary frequency (need to urinate more than every two hours)
- Dysuria (pain or burning during urination)
- Recurring urinary tract dysfunction with poor flow, hesitancy, and nocturia (frequent voiding at night). These symptoms also mimic enlargement of the prostate gland.
- Symptoms are intermittent depending on the bacterial burden. In an individual, repeated episodes tend to be associated with the same bacteria.

Factors associated with onset

- Inadequately treated acute bacterial prostatitis
- Calculi or stones in the prostate
- Uncircumcised, with poor hygiene
- Partial urinary retention

Prevalence

- Relatively rare (approximately 5% of all men who have prostatitis)

Tests for diagnosis

- Localized urinary and prostate fluid cultures are very important but often neglected by physicians
- Positive bacterial localization from prostate during periods with no symptoms

Traditional treatments used

- Fluoroquinolone antibiotics have proven to be the most effective, usually requiring a minimum of six weeks of therapy
- Nitrofurantoin can suppress flare-ups of infection but does not eradicate the organism
- Occasionally, because of enlargement of the prostate with age and the occurrence of multiple stones in

the prostate, a patient may benefit from transurethral resection of the recurrently infected tissue

Success of traditional treatment

- Antibiotics are usually effective for acute flare-ups
- Eradicating recurrent episodes is difficult. Antibiotics used for this condition may become less effective over time because the bacteria may mutate and become resistant

Category III – Chronic Nonbacterial Prostatitis
(sometimes with inflammation IIIA, or without inflammation IIIB)

Description

Chronic Nonbacterial Prostatitis represents by far the largest number of cases of men diagnosed with prostatitis. It has been estimated that this category involves 90-95% of all cases diagnosed as "prostatitis." In terms of numbers in the United States, this condition affects tens of millions of men at some time in their lives. Recent research has increasingly pointed out that conventional ideas and treatments for nonbacterial prostatitis have simply failed to both explain and treat the problem. Traditional approaches have treated this kind of prostatitis as an infection, although in recent years, doctors have acknowledged their befuddlement about the cause and cure of this condition. In 1995, the National Institutes of Health, in a consensus conference on prostatitis, acknowledged that the terms *chronic nonbacterial prostatitis* and *prostadodynia* neither explained nor were even related to the symptoms. A new name was then adopted for this condition: *chronic pelvic pain syndrome (CPPS)*. In changing the name of the most common disorder seen by urologists, there was the clear implication that the prostate may not be the cause of this disorder.

Studies have shown that men undergo severe impairment in their self-esteem and their ability to enjoy life in general because the pain and urinary dysfunction is so profoundly intimate and intrusive. The effect on a person's life with nonbacterial prostatitis has been likened to the effects of having a heart attack, having chest pain (angina), or active Crohn's disease (bleeding/inflammation of the bowel). If nonbacterial prostatitis moves from a mild and intermittent phase to a chronic phase, sufferers tend to live lives of quiet desperation. Having no one to talk to about their problem, usually knowing no one else who has it, and receiving no help from the doctor in its management or cure, they often suffer depression and anxiety.

Symptoms (may be intermittent or constant and include one or more of the following)

- Discomfort/aching/pain in the rectum (often described as a "golf ball" in the rectum)
- Sitting triggers or exacerbates discomfort/pain/symptoms
- Pain or discomfort during or after ejaculation
- Reduced libido (reduced interest in sex)
- Urinary frequency (more than every two hours)
- Urinary urgency (hard to hold urination once urge occurs)
- Discomfort/pain in the penis (commonly at the tip or shaft)
- Ache/pain/sensitivity of testicles
- Suprapubic discomfort or pain (above the pubic bone)
- Perineal discomfort or pain (between the scrotum and anus)
- Coccygeal pain or discomfort (in and around the tailbone)
- Low back discomfort or pain (on one side or both)
- Groin discomfort or pain (on one side or both)
- Dysuria (pain or burning during urination)
- Nocturia (frequent urination at night)
- Reduced urinary stream
- Sense of incomplete urinating
- Hesitancy before or during urination
- Anxiety about having sex
- Discomfort or relief after a bowel movement
- Anxiety in general
- Depression
- Social withdrawal and impairment of intimate relations
- Impairment of self-esteem

Nonbacterial prostatitis is a condition that produces much suffering. There are no curative drugs or effective surgical procedures. *We reiterate several times in this book that we have never seen surgery be helpful for this condition as it usually complicates the condition and sometimes makes it worse. Antibiotics are also not useful here.* Experimental treatments have been attempted and have also failed. These treatments include acupuncture, reflexology (foot acupressure), nerve decompression therapy, magnetotherapy (magnets inside the rectum), broccoli, optical-quantum-generator radiation therapy, rectally-administered ultrasound, bee pollen, corticosteroids, mud therapy, intrarectal electrical stimulation, saw palmetto (herb), and zinc (mineral).

What is often more troubling to men who have this condition than their actual physical symptoms, is the depression and discouragement that comes from their helpless and catastrophic thinking. Many doctors are less than enthusiastic to treat nonbacterial prostatitis because they know that they have very little to offer the patient. This often leads patients to feel that no doctor gives them any time or consideration when they seek help for this problem.

Furthermore, it is common to see high levels of anxiety in men with nonbacterial prostatitis because of their fear that their symptoms indicate they have cancer or some undiagnosed catastrophic disease.

The desperation of men with this condition leads some of them to find doctors who do heroic and unwarranted kinds of interventions. In our clinic we have seen patients who have had resection or removal of prostate tissue or years of antibiotics, all in the service of "doing something" about the problem.

Factors associated with onset (may include one or more of the following)

- High periods of stress
- Weight lifting
- Pelvic surgery

- Anxiety-producing sexual encounter
- Trauma to the pelvis
- Bacterial prostatitis
- Compulsive sexual activity or masturbation
- Prolonged sitting at work
- Extensive bicycle riding

Prevalence

- It has been estimated that up to 50% of all men at some time in their lives (in U.S., tens of millions) suffer from this condition.

Tests for diagnosis

- Absence of significant bacteria as determined by culturing and counting load from the prostatic secretion. This requires laboratory bacterial culture
- Microscopic analysis of prostatic fluid to determine the presence of white blood cells or inflammation. This category may involve inflammation or be completely without inflammation
- Analysis of urinary, bladder and pelvic floor behavior utilizing physiologic testing (urodynamics) such as urine flow rate, retention of urine, measurement of bladder pressure, and nerve activity
- Digital rectal examination and prostate serum enzyme to rule out cancer or other abnormalities of the prostate
- Transrectal ultrasound (TRUS) may be beneficial to evaluate the image of the prostate and sperm storage organs (seminal vesicles), but most importantly to perform prostate biopsies in the event of abnormal blood tests or palpation

Traditional treatments used

- Antibiotics almost always given whether or not there is a sign of infection
- Prostate massage
- Adrenal nerve blocking agents (alpha blockers) to relax the smooth muscle of the prostate and bladder neck

- Low dose antidepressants (low doses of Elavil®)
- Muscle relaxants/tranquilizers (antidepressants such as Prozac® or Paxil®)

Success of traditional treatment

- Antibiotics generally not useful
- Prostate massage occasionally gives symptomatic relief, but is of limited effect
- Alpha blockers (Hytrin®, Cardura®, Flomax®) sometimes give limited symptomatic relief but may have high levels of adverse side effects
- Muscle relaxants/tranquilizers, especially benzodiazepines such as Valium®, offer some temporary reduction in pain but because of side effects and tendency towards dependence, are not useful as a main-line treatment

Category IV– Asymptomatic Prostatitis

Description

Asymptomatic Prostatitis can be thought of as a 'sleeper condition' in that a man will not recognize he has it because there are no subjective symptoms. Usually it is discovered when a man sees a doctor who finds evidence of inflammation through either a biopsy or examination of prostatic fluid under a microscope. This is a significant condition because there is evidence that inflammation of the prostatic fluid or semen may cause a rise in the PSA level (prostate specific antigen), which is routinely screened now in men over 50 and thought to be an indicator of possible prostate cancer. When men eliminate infection through antibiotic treatment, the PSA level returns to normal, and the concern about cancer is removed. Diagnosing this condition therefore eliminates the need for further testing for prostate cancer including prostate biopsy. PSA also usually rises in proportion to enlargement of the prostate gland.

Symptoms *(may be intermittent or constant)*

- No subjective symptoms for patient
- Increased level of white cells in prostatic fluid or semen
- PSA often elevated (prostate specific antigen that sometimes indicates prostate cancer when elevated)

Factors associated with onset

- Unknown

Prevalence *(number of people)*

- Number unknown. This condition is poorly understood, and is usually only detectable through PSA screening or prostatic fluid analysis

Tests for diagnosis

- Elevated PSA
- Indications of inflammation in the prostatic fluid/semen

Traditional treatments used

- Four weeks of antibiotics

Success of traditional treatment

- Unknown

A Headache in the Pelvis in Women
(see also Chapter 7)

Vulvodynia (Vulvar Vestibulitis, Dysesthetic Vulvodynia)

Vulvar vestibulitis is a syndrome that is marked by pain at the opening of the vagina when touched. There are women who have vulvodynia who only have pain when the vulva is touched and at no other time. As a result, many women who suffer from this simple kind of vulvodynia have pain during intercourse or simply cannot have intercourse. Many cannot wear tight clothing or engage in any activities that put pressure on the opening of the vagina.

The other kind of vulvodynia is called dysesthetic vulvodynia. This is a more challenging condition because it involves chronic pain and a sense of burning in the vulva whether the vulva is touched or not. Dr. Howard Glazer, the psychologist who discovered the usefulness of biofeedback for this condition, has found that simple vulvar vestibulitis syndrome is associated with abnormally high tension in the muscles of the pelvic floor. Dysesthetic vulvodynia, on the other hand, seems to be connected with pelvic floor muscle weakness.

Symptoms (may be intermittent or constant and women may have one or more of the following symptoms)

- Pain when the opening of the vagina is touched
- Pain during intercourse
- Erythema (redness of tissue at the bottom of the opening of the vagina)
- Chronic pain (dysesthetic vulvodynia)

Women with vulvodynia often end up seeing a number of doctors before they receive the correct diagnosis. Gynecologists have often confused vulvodynia with a yeast infection. They then prescribe treatments for a yeast infection which aggravate rather than help the condition. In a way, this is not unlike the man who sees the urologist for pelvic pain and is reflexively given antibiotics.

Dermatologists are also consulted for this problem and have had little to offer. Patients sometimes go to a dermatologist because vulvodynia appears to be a problem involving the skin, but treatments of the skin have rarely proven helpful.

As has happened with many conditions for which the cause is unclear, numerous alternative and fringe treatments have emerged. Modifications of diet (including elimination of foods with oxalates, chocolate and caffeine), acupuncture, reflexology (foot acupressure), and analgesic creams are among some of the treatments offered for this problem. Neither the traditional treatments nor the alternative/ fringe treatments have offered much help.

Factors associated with onset (may include one or more of the following)

- Chronic yeast infections and the use of antifungal agents sometimes associated with onset
- Often no obvious associated factors
- Higher incidence is associated with sexual trauma (rape, sexual abuse)

Prevalence

- Approximately 16% of women at sometime in their lives

Tests for diagnosis

- Patients report intermittent or constant pain and/or burning at the opening of the vagina upon touch.
- Severe tenderness to a cotton swab that brushes over the opening of the vagina
- Dyspareunia (pain during intercourse)

Traditional treatments used

- Surgery
- Topical estrogen creams
- Psychotherapy

Success of traditional treatment

- Surgery is controversial with very inconsistent results

- Topical creams have little effect upon symptoms
- Psychotherapy is also used, but is generally
  not useful in reducing symptoms

Urethral Syndrome

Urethral syndrome is another condition that affects women and has not been well understood or treated. Women with urethral syndrome often complain of one or several of the following symptoms: dysuria, a sense of straining in order to urinate, urinary frequency, urinary urgency, hesitating at the commencement of and during urination, incontinence, and urethral or suprapubic pain. The symptoms can be either intermittent or constant, and they tend to wax and wane and can be stressed related.

Symptoms (may be intermittent or constant)

- Dysuria (pain during urination)
- Urinary frequency (the need to urinate
  with abnormal frequency)
- Urinary urgency (an urgent need to urinate
  with little ability to postpone urination)
- Hesitation during urination
- Incontinence (the inability to hold in urine)
- Suprapubic pain (pain above the pubic bone)

While urethral syndrome tends to resolve itself without treatment after a period of time, there are women who seem to have this problem chronically. Sometimes alleviation of symptoms occurs after dilation of the urethra using a thin metal rod, although there is considerable controversy about this method in medical circles. When this procedure does not help and the physician is unable to detect any obvious physical problem, the woman who suffers from urethral syndrome often has to deal with her exasperated doctor who may label her condition as a psychiatric one. Psychotherapy, as with almost all conditions of pelvic pain, tends not to be helpful in its resolution.

Factors associated with onset

- Unknown

Prevalence

- Unknown

Tests for diagnosis

- Patients report of urinary frequency, urgency, hesitancy, incontinence
- Suprapubic pain (pain above the pubic bone)

Traditional treatments used

- Antibiotics
- Urethral dilation (inserting a metal rod into the urethra with the intention of stretching it)

Success of traditional treatment

- Antibiotics tend not to be helpful
- Urethral dilation does help some women

A Headache in the Pelvis in Both Men and Women

Interstitial Cystitis and Painful Bladder Syndrome
(see expanded discussion in Chapter 7)

Interstitial cystitis (IC) has been a controversial diagnosis. Some doctors even believe it does not exist as a separate entity. Other doctors are clear about the existence of IC as a separate and distinct disorder caused by inflammation of the bladder.

Common symptoms of IC include suprapubic pain and perineal pain. Dyspareunia is often reported by women who have this problem. Some foods, such as those considered spicy, as well as alcohol and caffeine, seem to exacerbate symptoms. Urinary frequency and burning discomfort in the urethra are present in almost all cases of IC. We have seen patients who have had to urinate as often as four times an hour, day and night.

The frequency of urination plays havoc with routine activities. Sufferers have to go to the bathroom very frequently during work, when they're attending a conference or a concert, and during the myriad of other activities that require one to be able to comfortably hold urine for reasonable periods of time. Urinary frequency often seriously disturbs sleep.

People with IC tend to report a history of urinary tract infections. In IC, however, the inflammation of the bladder that is believed to be the cause of the symptoms of IC is not the same as the inflammation that one finds with an ordinary urinary tract infection that can be treated with antibiotics.

Interstitial cystitis used to be thought of as a "woman's disorder." Today, while most cases of IC affect women, men have been diagnosed with it as well. The estimate is that out of the approximately one million people who are affected by IC in the United States, 88% of the sufferers are women, and 12% are men. However, these estimates represent only the 20% of sufferers who have been diagnosed.

People with IC often have other problems. It has been observed that some women with IC also may have fibromyalgia and vulvar vestibulitis as well. IC tends to be more prevalent among Jews and less common among African-Americans. There may be associated bowel discomfort sometimes diagnosed as irritable bowel syndrome as is often the case with most of the conditions of pelvic pain that we discuss.

While no treatments at this time are curative, a number of treatments do exist that can sometimes reduce symptoms. One treatment, about which there is not universal agreement, is also thought to be diagnostic, although its diagnostic accuracy has been called into question in recent years as well. This is cystoscopy under anesthesia with bladder hydrodistention. This means that one is put under general or regional (spinal) anesthesia, and a tube is inserted into the bladder with a video camera assisting the view and allowing pictures of the lining of the bladder after the bladder is pumped full of water. If the tissue or urothelial lining tends to break and bleed after releasing the pressure, it is suggestive of a chronic inflammation. This procedure alone, however, sometimes alleviates the symptoms for a while after the procedure pain has passed.

In a study that throws some question on this standard test for IC, however, women who had no symptoms of IC underwent cystoscopy under anesthesia with hydrodistention of the bladder. A considerable number had bleeding in their bladders when dilated in the same way as women who complained of IC-like symptoms. These women, however, reported having no pain and no symptoms. This observation has cast some doubt on the standard procedure to diagnose IC. If there are people who have sensitive and fragile bladders but complain of no symptoms whatsoever, the question arises as to whether the sensitive and fragile bladder is in fact the cause of the suffering of IC. There is evidence that half of the people with IC symptoms spontaneously get better with no treatment at all. Furthermore, research in Scandinavia revealed that the source of IC pain was not found in the bladder, but mostly in the muscles of the pelvic floor. We discuss IC more extensively in Chapter 7.

Symptoms (may be intermittent or constant)

- Urinary frequency (the need to urinate more than once every two hours)
- Pain during urination (as well as before or after urination)
- Suprapubic pain (pain above the pubic bone), presumed to be bladder pain
- Some patients report dietary sensitivity (spicy foods, alcohol, chocolate, caffeine) while others do not

- Fragile bladder wall (as seen in cystoscopy under anesthesia)
- Perineal pain (pain between the scrotum and rectum in men, and between the vagina and rectum in women) and penile pain in men
- Dyspareunia in women (pain during and after sexual intercourse)

Factors associated with onset (may include one or both of the following)

- Occasionally acute bladder infection
- Usually factors seem to be unknown

Prevalence

- Approximately one million people in the United States (90% women, 10% men)

History for diagnosis

- Patients report of urinary frequency (the need to go to the bathroom very frequently or more than once every two hours on a regular basis)
- Patients report of urinary urgency (the subjective sense of an urgent need to urinate)
- Patients report of increase of symptoms with spicy foods, alcohol, chocolate, and caffeine
- Ulceration, mucosal tearing, glomerulations (microhemorrhage with distention) in several places in the bladder
- Hypersensitivity to a potassium solution put in the bladder

Traditional treatments used

- Elmiron® (pentosan polysulfate, a medicine partially secreted in the urine to assist coating the bladder surface)
- Elavil® (amitriptyline, an antidepressant to suppress the pain fiber response)

- Antihistamines to combat mast cells that secrete stimulating biochemicals (histamines)
- Bladder instillations that infuse medication like DMSO (a solvent-type product derived from wood) directly into the bladder—may be accompanied with cortisone and heparin
- Bladder stretching (pumping water directly into the bladder to stretch it)
- Modifications in diet involving elimination of foods that seem to increase symptoms

Success of traditional treatment

- Most treatments help some people some of the time
- Self-help efforts like diet modification and smoking cessation tend to reduce symptoms
- No procedure thought to cure

Levator Ani Syndrome/Spasm

In the 1950's the term *levator ani syndrome* was used to describe a disorder that involves a high degree of pain in the rectal area. Both men and women can suffer on either an intermittent or constant basis. When sufferers are in constant pain, sitting can make it worse. For those with intermittent pain, it can be set off by sitting, standing, or lying down. Some patients sometimes also complain of constipation. It is estimated that the majority of these patients are women, and that this condition seems to affect people at midlife.

When a digital-rectal examination is performed, pain is elicited by pressing on a small area within the levator ani muscle. When the doctor sweeps his finger from back to front along the muscle, it feels like a tight band. Often, though not always, the tenderness is on one side.

Levator ani syndrome is rarely associated with urinary or ejaculatory symptoms. While proctologists (doctors who specialize in disorders of the colon and rectum) naturally tend to see patients with levator ani syndrome, gastrointestinal doctors, urologists, and physical therapists also see such patients.

In recent years, a small group of physicians have diagnosed what has been called levator ani syndrome as pudendal nerve compression syndrome. This controversial viewpoint theorizes that the source of rectal pain derives from the compression of the pudendal nerve. Nerve blocks and surgery to presumably decompress the pudendal nerve are advocated by these physicians. The results of these treatments of nerve blockade and surgery have been very mixed. There is little published research that documents the efficacy of such procedures and, perhaps more important, little or no research that documents what appears to be the risks of surgery. These risks may include the destabilization of the pelvis as the result of cutting the sacrotuberous and sacrospinal ligaments as well other symptoms some patients have reported to us that were not present before this surgery that they underwent.

It is not uncommon for patients with levator ani syndrome to see many doctors and travel great distances in the hope of relief. A number of different approaches have been used for this problem. Some doctors have attributed the condition to poor posture and have educated the patient on how to sit in a less stressful way, although poor posture as a cause of levator ani syndrome remains speculative. In the middle of the 1930's, a series of studies reported success in digitally massaging the tight levator ani muscle. Later in the 1950's and 1960's, others also reported some degree of success in doing this.

Electrical stimulation (inserting a steel probe in the rectum and running an electrical current into the rectal muscles) has been used by a number of physicians with mixed results.

Biofeedback, in which a probe is inserted into the rectum and hooked to a sensitive machine that feeds back to the patient slight degrees of tension in the external muscles of the anal sphincter, has also been used with mixed results.

Symptoms (may be intermittent or constant)

- Intermittent or constant rectal pain
- Absence of abnormal physical findings

Factors associated with onset (may include one or more of the following)

- Constipation in some patients
- Increased level of tension at the opening of the anus
- Reduced strength of the external anal muscles

Prevalence (number of people)

- Majority are female
- Absolute numbers unknown

Tests for diagnosis

- Patients report of rectal pain
- Pain elicited when pressing levator ani muscle in rectum
- Absence of urinary symptoms
- Absence of ejaculatory or post-ejaculatory discomfort

Traditional treatments used

- Reassurance to patient that no life-threatening illness is found
- Electrical stimulation sometimes used
- Ultrasound sometimes used
- Biofeedback sometimes used
- Hot baths
- Tranquilizers, muscle relaxants
- Anti-inflammatory medications

Success of traditional treatment

- Reassurance to patient that no life-threatening illness is found is useful and relieving but not curative

- Electrical stimulation sometimes used with varying degrees of usefulness
- Ultrasound sometimes used with results unclear
- Biofeedback sometimes used with mixed results
- Hot baths often temporarily reduce symptoms
- Tranquilizers and muscle relaxants like Valium, have been reported to temporarily reduce symptoms
- Anti-inflammatory medications have unclear results

Proctalgia Fugax

There are individuals who experience episodic, severe localized pain in the rectum lasting from a few seconds to even 10-20 minutes or more. This pain/spasm is called proctalgia fugax. Episodes of proctalgia fugax often occur at night and it is our theory that they are associated with stressful dreams in which an already tight pelvic floor contracts in response to the dream. Occasionally this kind of pain accompanies orgasm and again, the pleasure spasm of orgasm, when occurring in a very tight pelvic floor, can trigger these episodes of intense pain. Some patients are very frightened by these episodes and live in fear about when they may reoccur. We believe anxiety exacerbates the pain of the episodes.

This is a harmless condition although it can be painful to the point that some patients have reported that they approached passing out because of the pain. Because it is of such short duration, by the time any medication is taken for it, the episode has passed.

We consider this to be a condition in which chronic tension in the pelvis creates a situation in which strong increased tension is felt, deriving from anxiety, orgasm or other factors, and acts as a kind of off-on switch that throws the muscles of the anal sphincter rectum and pelvic floor into spasm or charley horse. Because of the benign and short-termed episodic nature of this condition, most patients often don't even seek medical help for it. Knowing it is harmless and not panicking when it occurs helps to reduce its pain. Warm baths or gentle massage using a gloved lubricated finger in the anal canal, taught by a professional who understands this kind of intervention, is sometimes is helpful. When it is sufficiently bothersome, and the sufferer is sufficiently motivated, our protocol can help to reduce or resolve the frequency and intensity of these episodes by rehabilitating a chronically contracted pelvis.

The assumptions underlying the conventional medical understanding

As we will discuss, one of the most important factors in the treatment of any condition is your understanding of what it is in the first place. In the next chapter, we will present the existing conventional ideas of chronic pelvic pain syndromes while making explicit the often unspoken assumptions upon which they rest.

CHAPTER 2

THE OLD MODELS AND TREATMENTS

*"It's not a good idea to do open heart surgery
if the problem is heartburn."*
Anonymous

*"The answer to an unsolved problem is rarely
found in the field designated to study it."*
Martin Schwartz, Ph.D.

The way you see a problem is the key to solving it

In the nineteenth century, Ignaz Semmelweiss, a Hungarian physician, sought to discover the cause of what in his day was called *puerperal fever,* a horrific malady that took the lives of many young pregnant women and the children they bore. While this scourge was known throughout the history of medicine, its occurrence was relatively uncommon. This usually rare malady reached epidemic proportions in the European hospitals of the seventeenth, eighteenth and nineteenth centuries. Indeed, the "fever," that was a streptococcal infection, would now be considered the result of unconscionably bad hygiene. It occurred almost exclusively in the crowded hospitals of the urban areas of Europe.

The physicians in the large hospitals of France, Germany, England, and Ireland could not figure out why so many women died of the puerperal fever. A number of theories explaining the fever were popular at the time. They included the beliefs that it came from a discharge of the uterus, from the accumulation of milk inside the body of the mother, from gastric biliousness, from the emotions of fear and shame, from an increase in fibrin in the bloodstream of the mother and from influences of the weather. Considering what we understand about hygiene and infections now, these ideas seem preposterous, but they were part of the accepted lore explaining the deaths from the fever.

Semmelweiss painstakingly investigated the illness. Several clues pointed him toward viewing the fever as an infection caused by poor hygiene. He noticed that women, who gave birth outside the hospital, usually because they were giving birth to illegitimate children, rarely got the fever. He concluded that the problem was to be found within the hospital itself.

Secondly, Semmelweiss noticed that a close friend of his, whose work included dissecting cadavers during anatomy classes, became sick and died after he cut himself with the knife that he was using to dissect a cadaver. His symptoms appeared identical to those of women who had died of the *fever*. From this and other evidence, Semmelweiss concluded that unwashed particles from the dissection of cadavers and from surgery on infected patients were entering the bodies of the pregnant women.

With this understanding, Semmelweiss devised a protocol for doctors and other caregivers. It involved making the environment as clean as possible for the delivering mother. This included always washing the hands with a mixture of lime juice and chlorine as an antiseptic.

While it is hard for us to understand how people could object to such a protocol, one that simply insisted upon cleanliness and frequent hand washing in and around the hospital, Semmelweiss in fact came up against great opposition. There were vicious attacks upon his proposals, attacks which brought about much suffering in his life.

Among his detractors was his immediate boss and supervisor, a Dr. Klein, who blocked and hampered him at every turn. Klein was not the only one. Semmelweiss had to deal with many opponents, even though the efficacy of his efforts appeared indisputable.

As we examine Semmelweiss's situation now, it appears that his supervisor, Dr. Klein, may have been threatened by Semmelweiss's vigorous campaign to reform the hygienic habits in the hospital. Klein may have felt that Semmelweiss was indicting him for the deaths of women who contracted puerperal fever.

In his biography of Semmelweiss, Frank Slaughter observes that *when a new idea is introduced, it is usually first met with rejection and repudiation by forces in medicine that are invested in maintaining the old way.* Only after time passes and the efficacy of the new idea is established, is the advance accepted.

Medical knowledge and treatment is always a work in progress. The world of pelvic pain research and treatment is no different. Some practitioners are invested in a certain way of looking at this problem, and they resist any change, especially if the new methodology fails to depend upon their expertise and/or does not benefit them economically.

If we are in hot water long enough, we forget we are hot and wet

As we see in the case of Semmelweiss, it is difficult to dislodge old assumptions. People often don't even know they have them. *When frogs are placed in warm water and the temperature is gradually increased to the boiling point, the frogs remain in the water and boil to death. On the other hand when a frog is immediately placed in hot water, it immediately jumps out.* Most of us are 'swimming' in the old ways of thinking and don't even know we are wet.

Our way of thinking defines a problem and it dictates the kind of solutions that are possible. In the Middle Ages, for example, the concept of disease was that it was caused by four humors being out of balance. Consequently, it would make sense to treat disease with blood letting, purging, and vomiting, since it was believed that such maneuvers purged and rebalanced the system. We gradually discovered over time that this way of thinking is not based on fact and that it severely limited the effectiveness of treating illness. Our concepts of disease and medicine have evolved, and new and more efficacious approaches have been the result.

Changing our ideas of disease alters the way we treat it. On an individual level, *your notions about what is wrong with you determine what you will do to help yourself.* In modern times we have discarded the idea that illness is caused by humors. None of us would consider bloodletting or purging to improve our health. It is equally important, however, to be clear today about the thoughts and assumptions we hold about pelvic pain that motivate our choice of treatment.

Does the old way of thinking empower the patient or stimulate fear and helplessness

Fifty years ago, two gastroenterologists who did research at a medical center near New York conducted an experiment to show the effect of one's mental picture of a bodily condition on the condition itself. These researchers did rectal examinations of naïve male subjects. Looking up the rectum of a subject, one of the two doctors present would casually say to the other within earshot of the subject, that something looked cancerous inside the rectum. The other doctor would agree and then they would observe what happened in the subject's colon. The researchers reported that commonly the colon of the subject would go into an immediate spasm. As soon as the doctors reassured the subject that he was healthy and did not have cancer, the spastic colon immediately released. This experiment illustrated how a catastrophic idea about your health can have an immediate and profound physical effect.

Negative and catastrophic thinking palpably increase discomfort or pain in those diagnosed with pelvic pain. Many of the men we see with prostatitis are, at some level, worried they have cancer or some other life-threatening disease. It is not uncommon for patients with pelvic pain to walk around for many years carrying catastrophic thoughts relating to their pain that, as we will discuss later, exacerbate their pain and impoverish the quality of their lives. *The reassurance that what they have is not life-threatening can even alleviate their symptoms on a short-term basis.*

The power of trust, reassurance and the placebo effect

A placebo is commonly thought of as a sugar pill, essentially a substance with no known medically active ingredient. It is thought that the power of the placebo derives from the patient's belief that the pill will help. It is this trust that the substance will make everything okay that is the key ingredient in the placebo's power.

However, in addition, most placebo medication is given during randomized controlled trials and participating in the trial adds a huge amount of "placebo effect." It is a form of behavioral conditioning.

When you talk about the placebo effect, you are talking about the effect of feeling with complete certainty that "you are going to be completely okay, everything is fine, it will all be taken care of, don't worry, or fret at all, forces larger than you love you and will make sure you are safe, sound, and happy." The placebo effect = everything-is-going-to-be-okay effect. The placebo effect is the great antidote to anxiety and fear. The placebo, with regard to our condition, returns us to being carefree as children are carefree. No anti-anxiety drug can equal the power of the real placebo effect.

Some have suggested that the placebo effect is the highest form of body-mind healing. Indeed, combining the placebo effect with the use of effective methods can only enhance the methods. The power of placebo attests to the power of a *thought* reassuring someone that they are safe and everything will be okay. The power of placebo indirectly attests to the power of fear to disturb both body and mind because placebo simply acts to remove fear and doubt.

The communication of this thought also appears to be the chief ingredient in the power of a good doctor's bedside manner. In the presence of such a doctor, the patient's anxiety dissolves in the idea that all will be well again. This is not unlike a child's trust that his loving parents will take care of him.

If you are experiencing pelvic pain or discomfort now and the anxiety and contraction that usually comes with it, imagine that someone were to say to you, "We will take care of this. You will be completely healed and back to normal." Notice what effect this might have on your symptoms. Many people with pelvic pain experience a reduction or sometimes even an abatement in symptoms on a short-term basis as the result of trying something new that they think will help them. This is the placebo effect.

It is agreed among researchers in the field that there is a substantial placebo effect with *any* treatment for chronic pelvic pain. For example, antibiotics have become one of the reliable foundations of contemporary medical treatment. We all have a profound respect for antibiotics and their power. We believe however, that the short-term relief people with a nonbacterial condition obtain from antibiotics is primarily borrowed from this huge public confidence and in the case of pelvic pain, is a result of the placebo effect. In the second printing of our book, we reported on a published study that scientifically validates our long held position. *Ciprofloxin®, one of the most powerful of antibiotics, on a long-term basis proves to be only as effective as a placebo for nonbacterial prostatitis.*

The power of placebo is not small. A dramatic example occurred with a man who suffered from pelvic pain for ten years. He reported he entered a doctor's office in a great deal of pain. The doctor, whom the patient described as kindly and confident, felt this patient's prostate gland and said "Your prostate is completely normal. Our test revealed no evidence of anything wrong. You are completely healthy down there. Go out with your wife and have a night on the town and celebrate your good fortune." The man reported he left the doctor's office with no pain. Moreover, he remained pain-free for months, even though it gradually returned. There is no known medicine that can alleviate pelvic pain for months. This illustrates that the placebo effect and the trust that everything will be okay, on a short-term basis, has the ability to loosen the knot of chronic tension and anxiety that binds the contents of the pelvis.

The letting go of tension and anxiety afforded by a placebo is analogous to the letting go that is the focus of our treatment. However, placebos only work as long as the person either consciously or unconsciously believes the problem has been solved. The difference between our treatment and a placebo is critical. As we shall discuss, we actively assist our patients in restoring their *ability* to voluntarily relax the pelvis. This centrally includes the entire self-administered physical therapy component of our protocol, as well as the relaxation and cognitive therapy component, all aimed at helping a patient to reduce anxiety and the thinking associated with chronic pelvic tension.

In our culture, the doctor is thought to understand the true reality of the patient's mental and physical state. Typically, patients with pelvic pain adopt the doctor's viewpoint of their condition and they adopt the implications of the diagnosis as well. The doctor's diagnosis can add to a sense of fear and foreboding that patients already carry with them. For example, a doctor's suggestion that prostatitis may be an autoimmune disorder, a suggestion that is simply theory with little data to support it, can easily scare patients who are already confused. Many doctors lose sight of how much their ideas communicate to patients. An offhand comment that a doctor makes to a patient can either haunt or relieve a patient for years.

A Stanford psychiatrist found that women with breast cancer who participated in support groups lived significantly longer than those who did not. This was startling information and demonstrated the profound positive impact of social/psychological factors in creating disease on the one hand and extending life and well-being on the other.

How you name what is wrong with you can hurt you or help you

If the positive thought of knowing that there is a place to share your deepest feelings can enhance both the quality and length of life, as was the case in the Stanford study, so too can adverse thoughts injure us. A number of researchers have found that the *diagnosis* of cancer itself can traumatize individuals. Studies have shown that some people who have been diagnosed with cancer subsequently exhibit signs of post-traumatic stress disorder. These signs do not derive from the physical presence of cancer but from the terror that the diagnosis triggers.

It is not difficult to understand why the diagnosis of cancer is a traumatic event. Imagine what it would mean to your life if a doctor told you that you had cancer. Your life would invariably change as the shock of the diagnosis settled in. Even if it was untrue and the doctor had made a mistake in his diagnosis, the diagnosis alone would shake you to your foundation. *What you call what is wrong with you can clearly hurt you or help you.*

Before we see patients, we ask them to fill out a form in which they score their pain and urinary dysfunction levels. In the past, this sheet was titled "Chronic Pelvic Pain Symptom Score" and its purpose was to establish the person's experience of his or her condition. When we first developed the form, no attention was given to the effect of the title on the patient. In light of our discussion, we saw that patients had to confront the term *chronic pelvic pain* and identify themselves as chronic sufferers every time they came into the clinic.

The term *chronic* means ongoing and continual, and implies that the condition will not go away. We came to realize that the title of the form might be sending a message to our patients that their condition would never go away. While our patients' discomfort or pain may have been chronic in the past, we could not say with certainty that their pain, discomfort or dysfunction would not go away in the future. We changed the name of the sheet to "Pelvic Pain Symptom Score."

We saw that *a diagnosis almost always implies a prognosis.* Why would any caring doctor want to use a diagnosis that sentenced someone to a depressing future when such a negative outcome is in no way a certainty? Our title, *A Headache in the Pelvis*, reflects our compassionate interest in discussing these difficult conditions in a credible way that does not condemn people to such dismal future outcomes. Indeed, our title reflects our optimism for the possibility of a successful resolution of the problem.

Limitations of the Old Model

When you view your body as a machine

When we see a doctor, the nurse often puts us in a small, windowless room where we wait on an examining table or sit on a chair. We busy ourselves, often nervously, reading a magazine until we hear the door open and the doctor enters. He talks to us for a few minutes, perhaps examines our body, and then gives us a piece of paper, which we take to the pharmacy. When all goes well, and after a few pills, the complaint is resolved.

We take for granted that the doctor usually does not talk to us about our thoughts, feelings, home situation, sex life, or spiritual practices. We assume it is normal for the doctor to be interested only in the specific problem for which we are in the office, a problem with our body. Furthermore, we take for granted that the actual time spent with the doctor will probably be a few minutes or less.

We know that modern medicine typically looks at the body as a machine. However, the implications of that view are profound and far-reaching. If the body is a machine, it is a thing, an object, a piece of meat. The body, in some profound way, is not considered to be conscious, to have any intelligence, or to be something to which one has to listen carefully.

When the body is seen as a machine, one searches for the defective part to be fixed. An illustration of this is found in the treatment of vulvar vestibulitis. Doctors observe redness at the bottom of the vagina, which the woman reports as tender. For some physicians, the solution to this problem has been to surgically remove this red and irritated tissue. In our experience, the results have largely been ineffective.

In our practice, we have seen patients whose prostates have been removed, whose pelvic muscles have been surgically severed, whose bladders have been removed, whose testicles have been removed, whose pelvic nerves have been dissected and whose pelvic stabilizing ligaments have been severed—all in the service of getting rid of the part of the body/machine that is thought to be the source of the problem. The patients we have seen who have undergone such medical care have most often not been helped by such interventions, and more often have had to endure greater suffering, not only from the original source but from the surgical interventions.

The rest of the person, including his or her way of thinking, his emotional state, his lifestyle, values and importantly, what causes fear and anxiety—things that are not measurable—tend to have only secondary importance in the doctor's office. When the doctor examines the patient and can find no part of the body that appears to be causing the problem, the doctor often concludes that the problem is mental. To the patients we have seen, this kind of diagnosis has been invalidating and depressing and the treatments they have undergone for the so-called 'mental' condition have routinely failed to help their problem.

In treating your painful pelvic floor from the current body-as-a-machine perspective, it is as if the doctor were saying to your pelvic floor: "You must have been invaded by bacteria or are inflamed for some reason. I am going to use drugs or do surgery to get rid of this bacteria or inflammation. Your pain is something that shouldn't be there. It is not informative. It shouldn't be considered or listened to, but just gotten rid of. It is not saying anything. Your pain and dysfunction has no relation to how your owner is thinking, feeling, working, being in relationship, or generally living his or her life and I have neither the time for nor the interest in how you may be connected to the larger picture of your owner's life. Considering the larger picture of your owner's life and how that might help you is a foreign idea to me. I am simply interested in silencing you. If I do that, I have been successful in my work."

When the doctor brings this viewpoint to the suffering of someone with a chronic pelvic pain syndrome, the patient often adopts the following kind of view of his or her own pelvic floor:

"I feel your discomfort, burning, pain, tightness, soreness, or rawness and I am afraid of you. The doctor wants to get rid of you but can't. He doesn't seem to know what's wrong with you. Whatever I try to do does not get rid of you. You might mean terrible things. You may mean that I can never have health, happiness, joy, love, relationship, parenting, and fulfillment in my life. You shouldn't be here. You are a mistake, an error and a defect in me. You have nothing to say to me. You are bad. Whenever I feel you, I feel afraid and discouraged. I want to get as far away from you as possible. I hate you and want to get rid of you."

Your body wants to heal

The old medical model views the body as composed of modular parts that can be replaced or repaired when defective. This modular model seems to dismiss the notion that the body has intelligence and consciousness and that it can heal itself.

Dr. Dean Ornish pioneered a treatment that derives from a dynamic and functional way of understanding the body. He offered a treatment for individuals with heart disease, which put them on a low-fat diet, taught them yoga, and provided them with group support. He discovered that, following this multifaceted regimen, the blocked state of their arteries reversed.

Dr. Ornish demonstrated the truth that *the body has the intrinsic capability of regenerating and healing itself under the right conditions.*

By intrinsic, we mean that this ability for regeneration and self-healing is part of the very nature of the body. In the healing process, the challenge is to learn how to provide the best environment for healing to occur.

Nowhere is the dynamic and intelligent nature of the body more visible than in the effects of exercise. Sit in a chair without moving for three or four weeks and your muscles atrophy. Your heart muscle will actually diminish in size because the requirement for pumping blood has been reduced. Those who have been bed-ridden for a prolonged period know all too well the effect of no exercise on muscle tone and strength and general well-being.

All of us have observed that when we cut ourselves, clean the wound, and put a band-aid over it, a miracle occurs. In a number of days, the cut is healed. Most of us take this miracle for granted and simply expect this stunning intelligence of the body to do its own healing. If a car that was damaged in a car accident could gradually fix a dent or scrape all by itself we would be stunned and regard this event as a miracle.

We know the cut does not need our conscious effort or direction to heal. The healing is intrinsic, natural, and in the very nature of tissue. There is however, a condition necessary for the healing to occur. *One must give the cut an environment within which it can heal.* Pick at it, allow dirt and bacteria to enter it, and it won't heal. The key is to understand what the requirement for healing is and make it a reality. This is obvious for some conditions and not so obvious for other conditions. In the past, when human beings did not understand that microbes that were invisible to the eye could enter a wound and infect it, they often failed to make the kind of environment needed for their healing.

Healing is a word that is seldom used in the discussion or treatment of chronic pelvic pain syndromes. The word 'heal' comes from the Old English *healen* which means "to make whole, sound and well." At the time of the second printing of this book, in the National Library of

Medicine, in over 5000 medical research studies on the chronic pelvic pain syndromes discussed in this book, the word healing occurs only 11 times. The current thinking by researchers in this area does not seem to be focused on making the pelvis whole, sound and well. In our book, we are proposing that to treat pelvic pain and dysfunction one must first understand what the pelvis needs to become whole, sound and well. *We are proposing that the key to healing, in general, and the resolution of certain kinds of pelvic pain and dysfunction in particular, involves learning skills that will free the healing forces in the body.*

Appreciate the intelligence of your body; see your symptoms as your body trying to talk to you in the form of pain and dysfunction

When you appreciate the intelligence of your body and see your symptoms as your body trying to talk to you, you take a different viewpoint from the one resulting from the conventional medical model. From this viewpoint, it is as if you are saying to your pelvic floor, "I feel your burning, pain, tightness, soreness, or rawness and it doesn't feel good to me and I know it doesn't feel good to you. I know you want to feel better and be out of pain. I know you are happiest when you function properly. I know that you wouldn't be complaining this way without a reason. I know you want to heal, to be whole, sound and well. I want to understand what you are saying to me in your pain and dysfunction and listen to how I can help you. I want to regard you like my own child who does not feel well, who can't speak to tell me what is wrong, and who needs my compassion, love, unconditional presence, and help. I don't want to separate myself from you but instead I want to stay close to you as a loving parent would stay close to his or her unhappy child. I am here for you without condition and will do whatever I can to lovingly make an inner home for you so that you can get better. I care about you."

Such a viewpoint brings about joining and not separation between you and your pelvic floor. It brings an attitude of peace and understanding to your pain and dysfunction. It does not wage a war. Such an attitude relaxes and does not tighten. It sees the sore contracted area of the pelvis as an inarticulate friend in need and not an enemy. It brings love and not hate, integration and not separation, compassion, understanding and not fear.

A man who recovered from pelvic pain by using our protocol reported an experience that illustrates how bodily symptoms represent a language the body is using. Here is his story.

"I did not have any problem with my teeth for quite a while. I was brushing regularly and my dentist told me my gums reflected the good care I was taking of them. One day, out of the blue, I noticed that my upper molar was exquisitely tender. I was dismayed. I thought that I was doing such a good job with my teeth. Whenever I would go to the dentist, it would always cost many hundreds of dollars. I dreaded the pain, the expense, and the time in having to go yet again. I was also anxious about what it might mean about the strength of my teeth given that this pain was happening in the midst of the best care I could give myself.

Discouraged, I picked up the phone and dialed my dentist's office. The receptionist quizzed me as to what the problem was and where the location of the pain was, and suggested that I come in for the dentist to check my teeth. In the middle of making this appointment, I poked around the painful area of the tooth and felt a little piece of toothpick lodged there. I told the secretary to hold the line as I dislodged the end of a toothpick that was stuck in between the teeth.

To my amazement the pain suddenly stopped. Incredulous, I asked the secretary if a piece of toothpick lodged in between teeth could cause pain and she answered yes. I told her that I had just dislodged this piece of toothpick and that I was going to cancel the appointment I had just made because perhaps I had found and solved the problem.

I realized that the pain in my tooth was the only way the tooth had to tell me there was something wrong. The pain was not arbitrary or vindictive. It was simply the language of my body. I realized that I usually don't listen to my body's language, especially when there is pain. I usually get frightened by this kind of bodily communication and run to ask someone to reassure me that I am okay.

The suddenness with which the pain stopped brought home to me the intelligence and sincerity of my body. It was telling me that something was stuck in my tooth that needed to be removed. I felt like apologizing to my tooth for my distrust of the pain, and for not understanding that the pain was my friend and not my enemy."

In our view, pelvic pain is no different from the tooth pain described above. It represents the pelvis trying to talk to us and tell us that something needs correction. *The purpose of the pelvic pain we treat is to notify us that something needs attention so it can heal.*

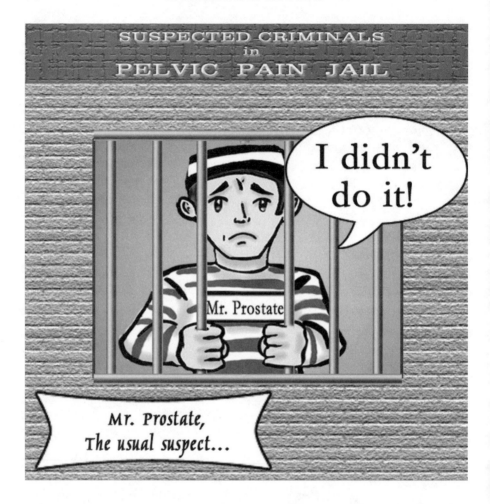

As we discuss throughout this book, 95% of men who are diagnosed with prostatitis have no infection in their prostate gland. Dr. Jeannette Potts originally presented the idea of representing a prostate behind bars in the way we present such a cartoon above to emphasize that the prostate has gotten a 'bum rap' and that the source of the pain with men diagnosed with prostatitis is almost always the chronically tightened pelvic floor and not the prostate. Below we present the old, and in our view erroneous idea that any of the symptoms of pelvic pain and urinary dysfunction in men is automatically prostate related.

The old way of treating prostatitis

There are some readers of our book who mistakenly think that the *Wise-Anderson Protocol* is primarily for men. In fact, muscle related pelvic pain is an equal opportunity employer and does not make distinctions between gender or age. As we discuss later, the *Wise-Anderson Protocol* is equally effective for pelvic pain of neuromuscular origin, in both men and women. Because we developed this protocol at Stanford University in the Department of Urology, the large majority of patients we saw included men who were diagnosed with prostatitis. This diagnosis represents a very large group suffering from pelvic pain and urinary dysfunction. Given the large group of people diagnosed with prostatitis, we will discuss this particular grouping of individuals with pelvic pain in this section.

Ninety five percent (95%) of what is called prostatitis is not prostatitis: the confusion about what prostatitis is and isn't

Most men diagnosed with prostatitis do not understand the confusion among doctors about what is and is not prostatitis. In fact, many doctors do not understand this confusion either. We hope to clarify these misunderstandings in this section.

First of all, we want to be very clear that most cases of pelvic pain diagnosed as 'prostatitis' are not prostatitis: *that the overwhelming majority of diagnoses of prostatitis do not appear to be caused by any known problem of the prostate gland.* Nevertheless most urologists have continued to use the term prostatitis and treat complaints of pelvic pain and urinary dysfunction as if they were caused by an infection or inflammation of the prostate. If you were given the diagnosis of prostatitis by your doctor, you might feel confused and ask, "Well, what does it mean that I've been diagnosed with prostatitis?" As we will discuss further in this book, most men diagnosed with prostatitis don't have a problem with their prostate gland. *The past decades of treating the prostate in such men has shown that in approximately*

95% of men with symptoms, treating their prostate gland for infection or inflammation doesn't help them.

Historically, the conventional medical viewpoint has tended to explain most cases of pelvic pain and related urinary dysfunction as an infection and/or inflammation of the prostate gland. Indeed, that's what the name prostatitis indicates, namely, an "itis" of the prostate. The conventional advice of many urologists to men they diagnose as having prostatitis related to increasing sexual activity derives from the idea that there is inflammation or infection in the prostate gland and more frequent ejaculation will empty it of these noxious critters.

When a man comes into the physician's office and complains about pelvic/urinary/rectal/genital pain and/or urinary symptoms like frequency, urgency, dysuria (pain during urination), sitting pain or ejaculatory discomfort, where there is no evidence of structural disease, the doctor typically treats the patient as if the cause of the problem is an infected or inflamed prostate gland and routinely gives antibiotics. If you type in 'prostatitis' in a search on the Internet today, this misinformation comes right up, from a large number of sources, on the screen.

Prostatitis, which means an infection or inflammation of the prostate gland, is often diagnosed without the doctor doing any tests at all to establish the validity of such a diagnosis. As we have seen in a study of physicians in Wisconsin, a large majority of doctors view prostatitis as an inflammation or bacterial infection, and almost all prescribe antibiotics as a treatment. Most urologists know from their own experience that antibiotic treatment for prostatitis without evidence of infection routinely fails to help the patient's symptoms and yet almost 100% of the cases of this kind of prostatitis receive antibiotics. We are always troubled to hear this routine diagnosis and antibiotic treatment in the patients who come to see us, when the patient's doctor made no attempt to establish the presence of infection.

Let us be clear. *We do not consider it a good practice of medicine to be giving antibiotics for symptoms of pelvic pain without verifying the presence of infection in the prostatic fluid.* We always check for evidence of infection and inflammation in the prostatic fluid with men who complain of pelvic pain and urinary dysfunction. As we will discuss, antibiotics can have serious side-effects, especially taken long-term. And we have had more than a few men suffer the consequences of inappropriate long-term antibiotic treatment.

We want to emphasize that the antibiotic treatment of *bacterial prostatitis* has been an achievement of modern medicine. If you have bacterial prostatitis, antibiotics are a very good treatment—certainly the only treatment. *Viewing all conditions of pelvic pain and dysfunction in men, however, as acute or chronic bacterial prostatitis is an error in therapeutic judgment. Despite the clear scientific evidence to the contrary and almost every urologist's clinical experience of the ineffectiveness of antibiotics for nonbacterial prostatitis, it is amazing that giving antibiotics routinely for nonbacterial prostatitis is the common practice. This is very important to understand, particularly if you have been diagnosed with prostatitis and it has not been determined whether infection or inflammation is present.* We would consider it quite appropriate for a patient diagnosed with prostatitis to ask his doctor if there is clear evidence of bacteria, should the doctor prescribe antibiotics.

It is not difficult to determine whether the prostatic fluid is inflamed or infected. This is how it is done. The urologist does a prostate massage, expels some fluid which comes out of the penis and then puts the fluid on a microscope slide where he examines it microscopically. Alternatively, the sediment of an immediate post-massage specimen of urine can be examined.

When there is infection or inflammation, white cells are visible through the microscope and their numbers are counted in a conventional way per high-powered field, referred to as 'x' number of white cells per high-powered field. A few white cells are not uncommon in the prostatic fluid of normal men and in some studies men who have no symptoms have more white cells in their prostatic fluid than men who are symptomatic. Studies have shown that in the prostate fluid of men whose prostates show no evidence of infection, inflammation in the form of white cells in the fluid can come and go. *Most important, in these men there is no evidence that inflammation has any relationship to symptoms.* It is most likely that the symptoms of what is variously called abacterial prostatitis, non-bacterial prostatitis, prostatodynia, pelvic floor dysfunction or chronic pelvic pain syndrome are *not* caused by inflammation.

When there are large numbers of white cells, it is appropriate to send the prostatic fluid specimen to a laboratory to be cultured to see if any bacteria grow. If there are bacteria that grow in culture, then a diagnosis of bacterial prostatitis is appropriate, and antibiotics are an appropriate treatment. Some bacteria are problematic and some are not. Some bacteria require longer incubation times to identify and some require elaborate culturing techniques to identify accurately.

Urologists are trained rigorously in the skills of the surgeon. The narrow focus on a part of the body that is defective and needing surgical intervention or drugs is also, in large part, the focus of these doctors. Furthermore, many surgically-trained doctors scoff at the intimation that prostatitis-like pelvic pain involves the relationship between the body and the mind and that both body and mind need to be addressed in treatment. Issues that appear to be non-medical ones, like anxiety, negative and catastrophic thinking, sexual activity, work environment and interpersonal relationships are, in fact, very significant in diagnosing and treating certain pelvic pain disorders. Unfortunately, these issues are ones that most urologists rarely consider. These are areas that are messy, difficult to treat and do not fit into the medical model and the neat, 15-minute slot in which most patients are evaluated and treated.

The system of reimbursing the doctor for his services contributes powerfully to the way the patient is treated. Several doctors have confided in us that their prostatitis patients are the most difficult, complain the most, and are the patients for whom insurance companies reimburse the least. Indeed, in the minds of most physicians, there is little financial incentive to explore what else might be going on in the life of the person who has prostatitis or in the relationship between his mind and his body. It is important for us to say, that there are caring and sensitive physicians who do look more deeply into the situation of the patient with pelvic pain, despite the lack of financial incentive to do so. We believe however that the current system that does not pay for physicians to take the time to listen to what is going on in their pelvic pain patient's life, is one of the reasons why so many of our patients complain about how badly treated and how ignored they feel by the physicians to whom they have gone for help.

Drug companies and resistance to changing medical thinking

Pharmaceutical and medical equipment companies, who happen to comprise a significant source of funding for medical research in America, obviously tend not to favor supporting alternative non-drug or non-surgical treatments for pelvic pain. The focus of their research efforts lies in developing new drugs and medical equipment, the sale of which will allow their companies to financially prosper. This economic reality supports the continued use of the traditional methods of treatment and perpetuates the paradigm that only drugs or surgical procedures are the answer to chronic pelvic pain disorders.

New forces for change

Dr. Lawrence True, a pathologist at the University of Washington Medical School, was part of a team that took multiple biopsies of the prostates of 97 men who complained of pelvic pain and symptoms of prostatitis. He found that in 95% of the cases, there was no evidence of clinically significant infection or inflammation. Furthermore, he found there was no correlation between evidence of inflammation or infection in the prostatic fluid and any inflammation or infection in the tissue of the prostate. He concluded that the evidence suggested that researchers look elsewhere to determine the cause of prostatitis symptoms.

In our experience at Stanford, we found that symptoms were most severe with prostatitis patients who had *no evidence of infection or significant inflammation.*

The growing demand for answers: the power of the Internet

When we published the first edition of this book in 2003, the Internet had become a major force for change in many areas, including traditional thinking about prostatitis and chronic pelvic pain syndromes. Prior to the Internet, it was common for a man with prostatitis to see a urologist, be given antibiotics that failed to help, and then fade away out of medical view to simply suffer with his symptoms.

With the advent of the Internet and the simplicity for ordinary people to do medical research about their condition, increasingly men or women suffering from pelvic pain, who receive no help from their doctor, go to the Internet for help. This is now true for all medical conditions. The popularity of websites offering medical information is a testimony to this. The ability to search on the Internet for solutions to problems that a patient's doctor has not prescribed or mentioned represents a profoundly important change in medicine. Increasingly, the doctor has ceased to have the last word.

The rise of patient advocate organizations

The Internet has made it possible for sufferers to form support groups. No matter how obscure the medical condition, one can go easily onto the "net" and find an appropriate group.

The information accessible on some pelvic pain related websites is not confined to traditional viewpoints held by most doctors. Viewpoints that patients would never have heard about ten years ago now coexist along with the traditional ideas. It has been suggested that the webmaster may ultimately be more influential in medicine than the doctor by democratizing the exposure of different viewpoints that otherwise would not have been made available to patients.

The word 'prostatitis' is searched many thousands of times per month. When you consider that it takes an educated and sophisticated individual to do a search on the Internet and even to spell the word "prostatitis" correctly, it is not unreasonable to assume that the real size of the population of sufferers exceeds this number. As the Internet grows, and as it becomes more commonplace for ordinary people to have access to it, we will likely see the power of these organizations increase.

Examining the limitations of the old way of thinking about chronic pelvic pain syndromes

When we examine the old ideas, the limitations become obvious. When doctors train to become specialists, the assumptions underlying the old way of thinking about chronic pelvic pain syndromes are rarely discussed. The doctors-in-training adopt these assumptions as a way of becoming members of the specialist's club. Below we ask a series of pointed questions about the old way of looking at and treating chronic pelvic pain syndromes. These questions relate to the issue of whether the old ideas about chronic pelvic pain syndromes see the body as a machine, and whether they see "non-medical matters" such as any relationship between body and mind, lifestyle, intimate relations, work environment, sexual behavior, spiritual life, patient responsibility, and the healing of pelvic pain.

The body as a machine

Does the medical viewpoint regard the body as a machine and symptoms as a sign that the parts need to be replaced or repaired? Is the body viewed as an unintelligent object and the disorder compartmentalized, simply requiring that the problematic part be fixed?

Acute bacterial prostatitis

- Yes

Chronic bacterial prostatitis

- Yes

Chronic nonbacterial prostatitis, with or without evidence of inflammation

- Yes

Asymptomatic inflammatory prostatitis

- Yes

Proctalgia fugax

- Yes

Interstitial cystitis

- Yes

Levator ani syndrome

- Traditionally, the syndrome involves rectal pain with unknown origin

Vulvodynia (vulvar vestibulitis)

- Yes

Urethral syndrome

- Yes

Body and mind

Does the medical viewpoint include a connection between body and mind? Is the condition seen as some event related to a person's mental and emotional life? Is the patient prone to anxiety and catastrophic thinking?

Acute bacterial prostatitis

- No

Chronic bacterial prostatitis

- No

Chronic nonbacterial prostatitis, with or without evidence of inflammation

- No

Asymptomatic inflammatory prostatitis

- No

Proctalgia fugax

- No

Interstitial cystitis

- No

Levator ani syndrome

- No

Vulvodynia (vulvar vestibulitis)

- No

Urethral syndrome

- No

Lifestyle

Does the medical thinking take into account any connection between the condition and the patient's lifestyle? By lifestyle, we refer to whether someone is living alone or with others and whether they have a support system.

Acute bacterial prostatitis

- No

Chronic bacterial prostatitis

- No

Chronic nonbacterial prostatitis, with or without evidence of inflammation

- No

Asymptomatic inflammatory prostatitis

- No

Proctalgia fugax

- No

Interstitial cystitis

- No connection to lifestyle except for diet

Levator ani syndrome

- No

Vulvodynia (vulvar vestibulitis)

- No

Urethral syndrome

- No

Intimate relationships

Does the medical thinking see any relationship between the patient's conditions and his or her intimate relationships? Is he or she married, and if so, what is the state and quality of their relationships? What is the relationship with family? Does he or she have friends? Does he or she feel connected to others or isolated?

Acute bacterial prostatitis

- No

Chronic bacterial prostatitis

- No

Chronic nonbacterial prostatitis, with or without evidence of inflammation

- No

Asymptomatic inflammatory prostatitis

- No

Proctalgia fugax

- No

Interstitial cystitis

- No

Levator ani syndrome

- No

Vulvodynia (vulvar vestibulitis)

- No

Urethral syndrome

- No

Work environment

Does the medical thinking see any relationship between a person's work and condition? How does patient feel about his work? Is it a pressure cooker requiring 100 hours per week or an easy job? Does he or she have a boss with whom the patient gets along or does he or she feel oppressed by the boss? Is the job sedentary or active?

Acute bacterial prostatitis

- No

Chronic bacterial prostatitis

- No

Chronic nonbacterial prostatitis, with or without evidence of inflammation

- No

Asymptomatic bacterial prostatitis

- No

Proctalgia fugax

- No

Interstitial cystitis

- No

Levator ani syndrome

- No

Vulvodynia (vulvar vestibulitis)

- No

Urethral syndrome

- No

Sexual behavior

Does this viewpoint see any relationship between a person's sexual life and practices and the condition of the pelvis? Is he or she sexually active? Does the patient masturbate and if so how frequently? What goes on during sex in terms of a person's level of relaxation or tension? Is sexual activity compulsive?

Acute bacterial prostatitis

- No

Chronic bacterial prostatitis

- No

Chronic nonbacterial prostatitis, with or without evidence of inflammation

- No

Asymptomatic bacterial prostatitis

- No

Proctalgia fugax

- No

Interstitial cystitis

- A person with IC often has pain during sex when symptomatic

Levator ani syndrome

- No

Vulvodynia (vulvar vestibulitis)

- No

Urethral syndrome

- No

Spiritual life

Does this way of thinking see any relationship between a person's spiritual life and the condition of his or her pelvis? Does the patient have a spiritual interest or spiritual practice? Is there any comfort or distress in his life as a result of his or her spiritual beliefs or practice?

Acute bacterial prostatitis

- No

Chronic bacterial prostatitis

- No

Chronic nonbacterial prostatitis, with or without evidence of inflammation

- No

Asymptomatic bacterial prostatitis

- No

Proctalgia fugax

- No

Interstitial cystitis

- No

Levator ani syndrome

- No

Vulvodynia (vulvar vestibulitis)

- No

Urethral syndrome

- No

Patient responsibility

Does the physician assume the sole responsibility for the patient's healing or does he view the patient equally responsible?

Acute bacterial prostatitis

- Only insofar as patient must take medication

Chronic bacterial prostatitis

- No

Chronic nonbacterial prostatitis, with or without evidence of inflammation

- Only insofar as the patient must take medication

Asymptomatic inflammatory prostatitis

- Only insofar as the patient must take medication

Proctalgia fugax

- No

Interstitial cystitis

- Traditional model sees management of diet sometimes helpful for symptom relief

Levator ani syndrome

- No

Vulvodynia (vulvar vestibulitis)

- No

Urethral syndrome

- No

Empowerment or fear and helplessness

Does the viewpoint itself empower the patient, imply, or specifically state measures that can be taken to resolve the condition, or does the perspective leave the patient feeling afraid and helpless?

Acute bacterial prostatitis

- Empowers patient because antibiotics usually stop the symptoms

Chronic inflammatory prostatitis

- Both empowers and encourages helplessness.
- Empowers if antibiotic stops symptoms.

- Encourages helplessness if episodes reoccur.

Chronic nonbacterial prostatitis, with or without evidence of inflammation

- Tends to create fear and helplessness because therapy is ineffective; the model does not correspond with most patients' experience

Asymptomatic inflammatory prostatitis

- Empowers

Proctalgia fugax

- Empowers

Interstitial cystitis

- Viewpoint in part tends to encourage fear and helplessness in that no cure is offered

Levator ani syndrome

- Encourages fear and helplessness, as the traditional approach does   not understand the condition and there is no agreement upon effective treatment

Vulvodynia (vulvar vestibulitis)

- Encourages fear and helplessness, as there is no effective cure

Urethral syndrome

- Encourages fear and helplessness, as there is no effective cure

Cause

What is the essential element (according to the conventional medical thinking) that causes the condition?

Acute bacterial prostatitis

- A bacterium

Chronic bacterial prostatitis

- A bacterium

Chronic nonbacterial prostatitis, with or without evidence of inflammation

- Immune disease

Asymptomatic inflammatory prostatitis

- A bacterium

Proctalgia fugax

- Muscle spasm

Interstitial cystitis

- Probably immune disorder

Levator ani syndrome

- Unknown

Vulvodynia (vulvar vestibulitis)

- Unknown

Urethral syndrome

- Unknown

Cure

What is the essential element (according to the conventional medical thinking) that brings about resolution or cure of the condition?

Acute bacterial prostatitis

- An antibiotic

Chronic bacterial prostatitis

- An antibiotic

Chronic nonbacterial prostatitis, with or without evidence of inflammation

- An antibiotic, anti-inflammatory agent, alpha nerve blocker

Asymptomatic inflammatory prostatitis

- An antibiotic

Proctalgia fugax

- Unknown

Interstitial cystitis

- Traditional treatments can sometimes alleviate symptoms, but no cure is offered

Levator ani syndrome

- None

Vulvodynia (vulvar vestibulitis)

- None

Urethral syndrome

- Stretching the urethra

Treatments

What are the treatments that are used in the conventional model?

Acute bacterial prostatitis

- Oral antibiotics

Chronic bacterial prostatitis

- Oral antibiotics

Chronic nonbacterial prostatitis, with or without evidence of inflammation

- Oral antibiotics
- Prostate massage
- Sitz baths
- Dietary recommendations – avoiding alcohol and caffeine
- Zinc tablets
- Recommendations to increase frequency of ejaculations
- Alpha blockers (Hytrin®, Cardura®, Flomax®)
- Antidepressants (Elavil®)
- Muscle relaxants (Valium®)

- Non-steroidal anti-inflammatory agents

Asymptomatic inflammatory prostatitis

- Oral antibiotics

Proctalgia fugax

- None

Interstitial cystitis

- Elmiron® (a medication which attempts to help restore a competent surface mucosa to the lining of the bladder)

- DMSO bladder instillation (infusing DMSO and other substances in the bladder to alleviate inflammation)

- Bladder behavior modification (bladder drill)

- The patient is asked to increase the time between urinations in order to stretch the bladder

- Immune therapy using tuberculosis vaccine in the bladder (BCG)

- Antidepressants (Elavil®)

- Antihistamines

- Electrical stimulation neuromodulation

Levator ani syndrome

- Electrical stimulation

- Ultrasound treatment

- Hot baths

Vulvodynia (vulvar vestibulitis)

- Surgery in certain cases

- Topical estrogen creams

- Low oxalate diet

Urethral syndrome

- Urethral dilation that includes inserting a metal rod in the urethra and stretching it

Efficacy

How effective are the treatments used within the conventional model?

Acute bacterial prostatitis

- Very effective

Chronic bacterial prostatitis

- 70%-80% are symptom-free after effective antibiotic therapy

Chronic nonbacterial prostatitis, with or without evidence of inflammation

- All traditional treatments are largely ineffective

- Antibiotics that permeate the prostate are not effective

- Dietary modifications are not effective when bladder is not involved

- Prostate massage can give occasional temporary symptomatic relief

- Zinc tablets and saw palmetto berry are not effective

- Increased ejaculations are not effective

- Alpha blockers sometimes provide relief, often have distressing side effects, and are not curative

Asymptomatic inflammatory prostatitis

- Unknown

Proctalgia fugax

- Not effective

Interstitial cystitis

- Traditional treatments sometimes alleviate symptoms

Levator ani syndrome

- Levator ani syndrome is not seen to have a known cause or cure in traditional practice

- Generally a low level of efficacy with conventional treatments

Vulvodynia (vulvar vestibulitis)

- Surgery sometimes claims good results with certain kinds of vulvar pain, while other times surgery is claimed to have bad results with more symptoms

- Topical estrogen creams have reported minimal effects

- Psychotherapy has reported minimal effects

- Generally a low level of efficacy with conventional treatments

Urethral syndrome

- Urethral dilation is sometimes effective but remains a controversial treatment

.

CHAPTER 3

A NEW UNDERSTANDING OF CHRONIC PELVIC PAIN SYNDROMES LEADS TO AN EFFECTIVE THERAPY

Summary of Our Understanding

We have identified a group of chronic pelvic pain syndromes that we believe are associated with the overuse of the human instinct to protect the genitals, rectum, and contents of the pelvis from injury or pain by chronically contracting the pelvic muscles. This tendency becomes exaggerated in predisposed individuals and over time results in chronic pelvic pain and dysfunction. The state of chronic constriction creates pain-referring trigger points, spasm and chronic hypertonicity, reduced blood flow, and an inhospitable environment for the nerves, blood vessels, and structures throughout the pelvic basin. This results in a cycle of tension, anxiety, and pain, which has previously been unrecognized and untreated.

Understanding this tension, anxiety, and pain cycle has allowed us to create an effective treatment. Our program aims to break the cycle by rehabilitating the shortened pelvic muscles and connective tissue supporting the pelvic organs while simultaneously using a specific methodology to modify the tendency to tighten the muscles of the pelvic floor under stress.

It is our belief that most cases of chronic pelvic pain syndromes begin with a person's habit of focusing tension in the muscles of the pelvis. This tendency sets the stage for the disorder. What triggers the symptoms can be a major stress or several minor stresses occurring simultaneously. The stressors can be psychological or physical. Once set off, anxiety and protective bracing fuel pain and dysfunction and a self-feeding cycle begins that seems to have a life of its own.

The reason that chronic pain and dysfunction resist a simple mechanical fix is that they tend to emerge from a life-long habit of focusing tension in the pelvic muscles. It is necessary to rehabilitate the pelvic muscles in conjunction with changing the predisposition to pelvic tensing. In order to make our understanding clear, we offer the allegory below, followed by a step-by-step analysis of the story.

An Allegory

Once upon a time, there was a land called the pelvic floor upon which the whole world depended for its survival and pleasure. The pelvic floor provided vital services for the world including filtering and eliminating wastes, providing sexual pleasure, and helping to structurally support the world in its various activities. The land of the pelvic floor performed these services best when its citizens lived a life of balance between work and rest.

It came to pass that the world went through a period of strife, and the citizens of the pelvic floor were required to work more and more. Night shifts became commonplace. In some parts of the land, citizens were required to work twenty-four hours a day, seven days a week, with no rest.

Soon the pelvic floor citizens were completely exhausted and very unhappy. They had stopped doing their jobs well. Their normal processing of wastes was no longer done efficiently, and they became unable to give pleasure to the world. Their cries of distress were increasingly heard.

Painful protests from the pelvic floor were made, along with demands for a return to balance between rest and work. The world, however, did not seem to understand what the pelvic floor was trying to say.

So the world hired a consultant who suspected the source of the problem to be foreign troublemakers and recommended sending in legions of anti-troublemakers. The troublemakers, however, could not be found and the problem continued.

The world became desperate and decided to hire a new consultant who saw the problem differently. The new consultant said, "If you want to solve this problem, you cannot simply have an idea of what the problem is without getting down into the trenches of the problem. To know the problem and its solution you must get to know it intimately and face-to-face. You must go to the land of the pelvic floor and listen to its complaints." The world replied, "We don't know how to talk to or understand the pelvic floor. We have never had a conversation with it." The consultant answered, "I know the language of the pelvic floor and will teach you how to understand what it is trying to tell you."

After meetings with the pelvic floor and the consultant, the world finally understood that its contribution to the problem was the demand it made for the pelvic floor to work constantly. So the world decided to change this. However, while the world agreed in principle to stop demanding constant work, it often forgot this agreement and lapsed back into its old habit of making unreasonable work demands. The consultant had to remind the world over and over to stop forcing the pelvic floor to work constantly. This was not easy for the world to learn.

After a while, the world said to the consultant, "Your method seems to be working much of the time but why is everything not completely back to normal?" The consultant replied, "Both you and the land of the pelvic floor are used to the unhappy state of affairs. If you are not reminded, you will continue to force the citizens of the pelvic floor to work without rest."

The world, however, was not the only perpetuator of the problem. The pelvic floor had also gotten used to the misery of constant work and had forgotten how to rest even when the world allowed it.

Therefore, a curriculum was set up for the pelvic floor as well. The people of the pelvic floor went to special clinics where they learned to stretch the contracted posture that they developed due to their constant work. This stretching and their lessons in learning not to fall back into the old habits enabled them to relearn how to relax and rest as they used to do.

As the world and the pelvic floor learned to coexist in a balance of work and rest, the land of the pelvic floor became a happy place again.

The dummies guide to the pelvic floor

Let's start with a very basic question many people with pelvic pain have—What and where is the pelvic floor? For someone who has never had pelvic pain or even for people that have had pelvic pain for a long time, the pelvic floor is some mysterious place that is not clear.

If you think of the pelvis as a cereal bowl, the term pelvic floor refers to a group of muscles that can be thought of as the bottom of the cereal bowl. Tighten up the muscles you would use to interrupt urination, and you are tightening the muscles of your pelvic floor. When you tighten up your pelvic muscles you often also tighten the abdomen, the diaphragm, the inner thighs and your sides.

In some muscle stretching and strengthening practices, these muscles make up part of what are called the core muscles. They're required for posture, supporting the back to keep you straight and to keep you upright when your arms and legs move outward. If these muscles didn't exist to form a solid muscular girdle, you'd raise your arms or put your legs up and you'd fall over. It can be said that these muscles stabilize you during movement and hold the internal organs in place. Without these muscles you couldn't walk, move or lift anything. These muscles have to keep the center of the body stable for all different activities in life.

Generally speaking, the core muscles can't be seen in the way the biceps or calves can. You can tighten your pelvic muscles and most people would never notice it. They are hidden from view but play an essential role in life. Keeping them strong and healthy is the task of stretching and strengthening programs, like yoga and pilates. These core muscles are places we sometimes tighten up when we're stressed. Having pelvic pain generally means being knotted up in these muscles. Resolving pelvic pain means dissolving a tightened up inner core.

The three functions of the pelvic floor: support, opening and closing the different orifices, and managing the symphony of sexual activity

Here we will briefly discuss the functions of the pelvic floor. Don't be overwhelmed reading this. We want to stay with the big picture of what the pelvic floor is, how pelvic pain can occur, and how to help it.

The pelvic muscles make it possible to control when you urinate and/ or defecate. If you think about the pelvic floor muscles as a hammock connected to the pelvic bones, three very important structures pass through this hammock. These structures include: the vagina in women (whose muscles control childbirth and accommodate the penis during sexual intercourse), the urethra, which is the muscular tube connecting the bladder and providing passage of urine (and in men controlling the closing of the urethra and providing the passage of sperm during sexual activity through strong, rhythmic contractions) and the anorectal tube that provides the passage of stool. The pelvic muscles allow for the voluntary control of both urination and defecation, and when you cough, there is an involuntary contraction of the pelvic floor muscles to prevent urine or stool from leaking out as a result of the inner force in the core that would cause this kind of leakage.

Generally speaking, people who have no pelvic pain, have pelvic muscles that tighten up and then they relax. For people who do have pelvic pain, who's way of expressing their anxiety is to tighten up the pelvis strongly and for a long time, or for people who have had some kind of injury and pain that has caused the pelvic muscles to reflexively tighten against the pain, the pelvic muscles don't relax well after contraction. They stay in a tight state or spasm and when the pelvic muscles don't relax, all kinds of weird symptoms occur, symptoms that you can't know firsthand unless your pelvis has been tight for a long time.

Because the pelvic muscles are involved in so many complex and essential activities, chronically tightening up the pelvic muscles can create havoc in the interaction and communication between these muscles during vital activities. We all intuitively know this, although we may not know why. If anyone asked you to voluntarily tighten up the pelvic muscles that you would have to use to interrupt urination, for an hour, probably in the whole world, no one would volunteer. Without knowing why, we intuitively know we don't want to go there. We don't want to tighten the pelvic muscles up for any extended period of time. People with pelvic pain often have chronically tightened up the pelvic muscles for years.

The pelvic floor as a cereal bowl

Think of the pelvic floor as a kind of cereal bowl made up of two parts. There are the bones of the pelvis which are relatively rigid and there are the muscles attached to the bones that make up the bottom of the bowl. If the pelvis only had a bony structure and you put cereal and milk in it, they would all spill out. One of the important functions of the pelvic floor bowl is of holding up the inner organs.

So don't be intimidated by the complexity of what we will now describe, because it's complex for everybody and it's amazing for everybody. Just because you studied the physiology and function, doesn't mean that you necessarily have any better understanding of it. The pelvic floor is still an amazing thing and all you can do is stand back and say, "this is amazing, how this whole thing works." For our purposes here, we want to describe what the pelvis does, the amazing things it does and how easy it is to create the problem of pelvic pain in it.

How to think about self treatment and the rehabilitation of your own pelvic muscles if you have muscle related pelvic pain

Tension in the muscles in the bottom of the cereal bowl is connected to the legs, abdomen, side and back of the body. In other words, areas of pelvic restriction and places of trigger points referring into the pelvic muscles are found in the lower abdomen, buttocks, inner thighs and places where non-pelvic muscles attach to the pelvic bones. Therefore, pelvic rehabilitation requires internal and external trigger point release, loosening of muscle constriction and stretching both inside and outside the pelvic floor, and in many of the muscles immediately connected to the pelvis.

Not confusing pelvic strengthening with pelvic relaxation

Among the problems that can occur with the pelvic floor muscles, two prominent ones are weak pelvic muscles and chronically tightened pelvic muscles. Many practitioners confuse treating chronically tight pelvic muscles in the same way you would treat weak pelvic muscles. Elsewhere in our book we state that we are opposed to this because Kegel exercises were originally meant to help women with weak pelvic muscles, and often had urinary incontinence, strengthen them or cure their incontinence. Kegel exercises are meant to strengthen the muscle that connects the pubic bone to the sacrum, through which the urethra passes. Kegel exercises are in our view the very best and not harmful treatment for most cases of urinary incontinence. Chronically tightened pelvic muscles, however, do not benefit from tightening them up more, such as with Kegel exercises. It's important to understand that weak pelvic muscles and chronically tight and painful pelvic muscles are different problems requiring different solutions.

Rehabilitating your painful pelvic muscles with your hands, with your stretching, and with your mind

When someone has muscle related pelvic pain, the muscles on the bottom of the pelvic cereal bowl are typically painful, tense, shortened and contain knots of exquisite tenderness called trigger points; areas of restriction and spasm. These muscles can cause havoc with urination, defecation, orgasm, sexual arousal, and sitting. The goal of the protocol we developed at Stanford is to restore these muscles to a loose, flexible, and comfortable state.

Pelvic pain and dysfunction associated with overused and chronically tensed pelvic musculature

In our allegory, the world stands for you, the conscious person, who makes decisions and sends commands to your body. You send these commands, often out of habit. They feel normal and familiar to you.

The land of the pelvic floor is your pelvis and the contents of your pelvis including the structures that are involved in urination, defecation, sexual activity, and physical movement. These functions and their myriad of biochemical, nervous, and mechanical processes go on, often without requiring your awareness, will, conscious effort, or attention.

We see in the allegory that the problem begins when the world demands that the pelvic floor work on a constant basis. Normally, the pelvic floor muscles are dynamic, working and resting throughout the day. Even though they tighten, they have the ability to relax. The relaxed state allows for proper oxygenation, nutrition, management of wastes and rejuvenation of tissue.

The pelvic floor muscles are not meant to be chronically contracted. When muscles are chronically tensed, they tend to shorten, knot up, and eventually accommodate, so that the posture of a shortened state of the muscles feels uncomfortable but normal.

People who have pelvic pain syndromes tend to habitually focus tension in the pelvic muscles as a response to stress, anxiety, trauma, or pain. In our allegory, we allude to this by saying that the continual strife of the world prompted it to make the pelvic floor work too much.

When the pelvic muscles work too much they become painful. In all of the patients that our protocol is able to help, stretching or pushing on at least some muscles of the pelvic floor or muscles outside the pelvic floor but related to it, cause pain or recreate symptoms. Our patients are often surprised when we tell them that these trigger points on a person without pelvic pain won't hurt when pressed. In fact, as someone's pelvic pain reduces or resolves, areas in and around the pelvis that once hurt when pressed will stop hurting.

The tendency to focus tension in the pelvic muscles is not an accident. *Some have suggested that a person's inclination to focus tension in the pelvic muscles may begin with toilet training. The child is able to stop his parent's reaction to soiling by tightening his pelvic muscles. Over time, tightening the pelvis becomes a conditioned reaction to any situation in which anxiety arises.* This idea of focusing tension in the pelvic muscles as a result of early toilet training is simply an idea, and we do not propose that it should be taken as fact. It is however, a compelling explanation of how pelvic tension may well begin early in life in some of our patients. Other thoughtful investigators such as Tony Buffington, a veterinarian, also imply that neuroendocrine patterns may be formed early in life to create susceptibility to pain pathways.

Research has shown, and it is our clinical experience as well, that people with chronic pelvic pain syndrome tend to have elevated pelvic floor tension even when resting. The pain and dysfunction gets worse in the presence of stress. Many of our patients notice this relationship between stress and the severity in their symptoms. This observation leads to the heart of our understanding.

In our allegory, we see that the constant demand made upon the pelvic floor leads to a disruption in its ability to function. It is our view that, over time, a constant demand on the pelvic floor to tense and knot up, results in an environment that is inhospitable to the nerves, blood vessels, and structures within it. The pelvic floor is not made of steel and in certain individuals is quite disturbed by chronic tension.

It is our view that the person who has the kind of pelvic pain we discuss in this book has sore and irritated pelvic tissue. This tissue is not viewed by conventional medicine as pathological. We believe that this sore, shortened, contracted tissue is a very real physical condition.

People who have chronic pelvic pain feel this soreness and irritation acutely. It sometimes feels like a burning, aching, tight, tearing or a very sore area of what feels like raw tissue. When the doctor or physical therapist trained in *Trigger Point Release* feels the inside of the rectum or vagina, or related external pelvic floor tissue, in patients with chronic pelvic pain syndromes, he or she often reports feeling areas of restriction, tension and taut bands (trigger points) which, when touched, cause patients to jump with pain. Some professionals who work inside the pelvic floor of people with pelvic pain describe the tissue as *hard, restricted, tight, or rock-like*. Areas within the pelvic floor which have been subjected to years of continual contraction need time to heal even when the muscles are no longer under tension. When physical therapy is done properly, and the pelvic floor is regularly rested, what feels like hardened tissue often becomes soft, supple and pain free. This is the goal of our treatment.

In muscle related pelvic pain, the painful pelvis is like a continually contracted fist

Imagine tightening your fist as hard as you can for an hour. You notice that there are places of lighter color in your hand that result from squeezing the blood out of the blood vessels. Your hand will feel uncomfortable and you feel relieved to stop the squeezing.

Now imagine you maintain this clenched fist for a day. Now imagine you maintain this fist for a week. Now imagine a month of tightening your fist constantly twenty-four hours a day. Now imagine doing it for a year. Now imagine doing it for several years. This is one way to understand the state of the pelvic floor in people with pelvic pain.

Imagine, after several years, you stopped tightening your fist. Do you think the great discomfort and irritability of the tissues of your hand would immediately stop? Almost certainly not. It is not hard to imagine that you would want to rub your hand, massage it, take each finger, and stretch it out to relieve it from the contracted state it had been in. Nor would it be hard to imagine that, even after you stopped tightening your fist, your fist would still be sore. It would take some time, some pampering, and most importantly, no chronic retightening of the fist before your hand felt normal again.

Imagine continually tensing your pelvis

Chronically tightening your fist is one thing. Now imagine you were asked to tighten your pelvic muscles for 30 seconds as if you were stopping yourself from urinating. For most people, this pelvic tightening would not be the most pleasant thing to do, but it would be doable. Imagine you tightened up in the pelvis like this for a minute. It would still be doable. Now imagine you were asked to keep your pelvic muscles continually tensed for 30 minutes... now 1 hour... now 6 hours... now 12 hours... now 24 hours... now 1 week... now 1 month... now 1 year... now 2 years... now 5 years.

People who have never had pelvic pain would think it is crazy to be asked to contract their pelvic muscles for 30 minutes. The prospect of continual tightening of the pelvic muscles for a week, month, or year would be unthinkable and yet the research shows increased tone in the pelvic floor for many people with pelvic pain. Dealing with such a condition is the focus of our protocol.

In our allegory, the first consultant the world chose refers to the traditional physician who routinely assumes the presence of infection as the source of the difficulty (foreign troublemakers). But treating these troublemakers, or the presumed bacteria, has failed to resolve the problem of chronic pelvic pain syndromes. Recent research has shown antibiotics to be no more effective than a sugar pill or placebo. The second consultant who is called in refers to a clinician trained in our viewpoint and protocol. The clinician sees the problem emanating from within the individual. In our allegory the new consultant offers the solution we suggest, which is aimed at rehabilitating the chronically contracted posture of the tissues in the pelvic floor, as well as teaching the individual to cease the habitual and chronic pelvic tensing.

In our allegory, we make the point that 'the world' has lost communication with the pelvis. Most of our patients tend to be out of touch with what is going on in their pelvis. We offer a method to open communication with the pelvis to help bring about a healing of the sore and irritated pelvic tissues. We also aim to change a patient's attitude toward their pelvis.

Healing pelvic muscles by changing bad habits

If chronic tension and nervous system arousal result in an irritation of the pelvic floor that give rise to pain, then anything one does to reduce or eliminate the tension has the potential to eliminate the pain. *The restoration of the contracted tissues to a normal state of flexibility and relaxation has to be done repetitively.*

It is the repetitive application of our methods that gives the pelvic muscles a chance to return to their normal state. In later chapters, we introduce the methods used to accomplish this called *Paradoxical Relaxation* and *Trigger Point Release. Paradoxical Relaxation*, discussed in depth in this book, trains the patient to break the habit of chronically tensing the pelvic muscles and chronically maintaining an aroused and anxious nervous system. *Trigger Point Release* makes it possible for the pelvic muscles to become freed from pain. The physical therapy home self-treatment literally lengthens and softens the constricted pelvic tissue.

We tell our patients to expect ups and downs, and not to celebrate when symptoms reduce, or to despair when they flare-up. This is easy to say and not so easy to do when you are anxious and in pain, but it becomes easier with the practice of our protocol.

There are important reasons why chronic pelvic pain syndromes are misunderstood and why progress is slow. One reason is that the pelvic muscles are almost always active in the service of the normal functions in life. The pelvic muscles need a rest from their chronic contraction. There are two factors that make this difficult. The first is that you can't simply rest the pelvic muscles for any extended period of time unless you are restfully sleeping. They are needed to allow you to stand up, to hold in urine and stool, to walk, to lift—to do the things that allow you to be able to function normally. It is a delicate juggling act to deal with the need for rest and healing of this vital part of the body on the one hand, and the demand on the pelvic muscles to do the work required to function in life on the other.

The other factors that operate against the healing of the pelvic floor are the conditioned tendency of many of our patients to focus tension in it when under stress and the natural biological protective guarding that occurs when someone is having pelvic pain.

The tendency to tense the pelvis under stress is usually a deeply ingrained one, especially when this focus of tension has been practiced many times without awareness. Modifying this habit so that contracting the pelvic muscles under stress is *not* the default mode is no small enterprise. Changing this habit is one of the main foci of the method of *Paradoxical Relaxation.*

In our allegory, we show that while the intervention of the second consultant began helping the situation, the situation did not immediately go back to normal. The process of healing takes time and much self-treatment, especially inside an active pelvic floor.

Reassurance and emotional support
help pelvic pain syndromes

Harry Miller, M.D. from the Department of Urology at George Washington University reported on his successful treatment of many men who had prostatitis. Dr. Miller offered a kind of stress management therapy. He gave patients simple and kindly advice not unlike that of a grandmother to her grandson. Miller's approach reinforced the idea to his patients that there was a critical relationship between how they managed the stress in their life and their symptoms. In doing so, he helped most of his patients reduce their symptoms.

Dr. Miller's work focused on the person and not the prostate. He addressed the social and psychological context in which pelvic pain occurs. Similarly, the approach discussed in this book insists that prostatitis and related pelvic pain syndromes intimately involve a person's body and mind and are not limited to a sore part of the person's body independent of his mind and lifestyle.

What seems obvious may not be the problem:
the source of the disorder in interstitial
cystitis may not simply be the bladder

The focus of the problem in interstitial cystitis (IC), which we discuss later in Chapter 7, may not be limited to the bladder, but found in the muscles of the pelvic floor. Treatment protocols in traditional medicine have focused exclusively on the bladder.

Some compelling evidence throws doubt on this view that the bladder is the essential problem in IC. One study showed that when the pelvic muscles of patients with IC were palpated, the pelvic muscles appeared to be the source of the pain. The bladder was rarely found to be the most painful when touched. In a Finnish study, 25 of 31 women who were diagnosed with IC reported pain in the pelvic muscles and not in the bladder when the bladder and the pelvic floor were palpated.

Perhaps even more compelling is the experience we had with patients whose level of pain with IC prompted their physicians to remove their bladders. *Tellingly, bladder removal did not reduce their pain and instead created new problems.*

There is evidence suggesting that the source of the problem in many cases of IC may not be the bladder. Instead, the source may be the interaction of nerves, muscles, and blood vessels in the pelvic floor connecting to the bladder.

Pelvic muscle pain often coexists with bladder pain

Even when there is clear evidence of bladder inflammation or ulceration and the bladder itself is painful, the pelvic muscles are often chronically tight, painful, guarding against the bladder pain. Therefore, chronic tightening against the bladder pain can result in pelvic floor dysfunction.

It can be seen that these represent two different problems that must both be treated. That is to say, what is called pelvic floor dysfunction, often coexists with bladder-related symptoms.

Our multidisciplinary treatment protocol

Our multidisciplinary treatment team for the *Wise-Anderson Protocol* is comprised of a urologist, a psychologist, and a physical therapist. It is unusual for these specialties to cooperate closely in the way that we do in the *Wise-Anderson Protocol* and we consider it essential to our success. The urologist does the initial diagnosis and makes sure that the condition is appropriate for our protocol. His or her work involves an examination of the patient, the administration of various medical tests, and interpretation of the results. It is the physician's findings that rule out serious illness as a factor in the patient's symptoms. The physician or physical therapist examines and maps out the pelvic floor for trigger points and areas of restriction, then administers intrapelvic *Trigger Point Release* and trains patients to do this at home.

The psychologist's primary role in the treatment team is to train the patient in *Paradoxical Relaxation* for the purpose of profoundly relaxing the pelvic floor and helping the patient modify their habit of focusing tension in the pelvic floor under stress. The psychologist on our team teaches a method to help the patient modify the difficult and often ingrained habit of catastrophic and negative thinking that then becomes associated with the condition of pelvic pain and dysfunction. This method requires regular practice as the negative thinking arises during the course of a day. The method is simple and easily learned and applied, although the habit of catastrophic thinking tends to be very stubborn and requires great effort to change.

To facilitate continued *Trigger Point Release* therapy in the home setting, when possible, the willing spouse or partner is taught the method. It is important to note however a partner is not necessary for this protocol to be effective. The physical therapist teaches the patient to self administer the internal and external myofascial release and gives instructions for a home program of stretches, not unlike a home yoga program, except that these stretches are oriented toward the rehabilitation of the chronically tensed pelvic muscles.

Members of these different disciplines work well together, as they hold the same cross-disciplinary understanding of the problem being treated, as well as collaborating with each other on treatment.

The treatment is most likely to help when you reduce the stress in your life

John B., a 38 year-old small business owner, came to see us with pelvic pain and urinary dysfunction. Upon examining him, we determined that in fact, he had no problems of an organic nature. He had trigger points inside his pelvic floor that when palpated exactly recreated his symptoms.

Under normal circumstances, John was someone we would be very optimistic about being able to help, but it became clear he was not. He owned a car repair facility where he employed 45 people, and his business consumed his days from six in the morning until nine at night. His wife was unhappy because of his absence from their relationship. His children had behavioral and academic problems at school. He was also involved in a lawsuit with his brother-in-law with whom he had owned a previous business. He was in the middle of a major renovation of his house that left both he and his wife sleeping on a mattress on the floor.

John had no time for himself, let alone the time to do physical therapy self-treatment and daily relaxation to relax his pelvic floor. Under these circumstances, the program we offered would have been ineffective because he would not be able to do it properly in the face of the demands and stress calling for his attention. Only when John himself decided that his life would have to change, would our treatment have a chance to help him resolve his pelvic pain.

Effective treatment requires adherence to the complete program

Patients who seem to get the best results from our treatment are those who are clearly committed to earnestly practicing our approach. Usually these patients have suffered for a long time and have seen numerous doctors and explored many avenues. These patients often assume the attitude of, "I will do whatever it takes to get better" and have no problem following the protocol. *We tend to discourage patients who are skittish or unsure about doing our treatment. These are usually patients whose level of pain and dysfunction is minimal or who have been suffering for a short period of time and are still searching for some 'magic bullet' or easier way to resolve their problem.*

Calming down pelvic pain is like coaxing a kitten out of a tree

Calming down muscle related pelvic pain is like getting a frightened kitten out of a tree. Just like a kitten that has to be coaxed, soothed and calmed down before it will cooperate, so the pelvis has to be coaxed into calming down. Just like trying to rescue a terrified kitty caught in a tree, if you approach your painful pelvis without understanding it—if you approach it with anger, fear, resentment, impatience or uncertainty, it will pick up your attitude and be more resistant to your help. You can't reach a kitten caught up in a tree without appreciating its fear, trepidation and need for gentleness, love and consistency.

When people experience pain in their pelvis, they will go to the doctor with the idea that the doctor will give them a pill or do a procedure that will take the pain away. The boon of conventional medicine is in its ability to diagnose major pathologies, including cancer, as the source of the patient's pain and dysfunction. The presence of major pathology must be addressed and ruled out in the case of a patient's complaints of pelvic pain, and conventional medicine is unmatched at doing this. When no signs of major pathology have been found, as is the case with the vast majority of patients with pelvic pain, enormous sums are spent in the service of using drugs, procedures and surgeries to cure pelvic pain. Alas in vain. The tools of conventional medicine have failed to help the muscle related pelvic pain in men and women. This pelvic pain is variously known as chronic pelvic pain syndrome, pelvic floor dysfunction, prostatitis, levator ani syndrome, pelvic floor myalgia, among other diagnostic categories .

The way we think about fixing a broken arm or curing an infection unfortunately does not apply to fixing muscle related pelvic pain. In muscle related pelvic pain, the pelvis has usually been held tight, often for many years, and the muscles remain sore, contracted and painful in a self feeding cycle of tension, anxiety, pain and protective guarding. The contraction of the painful pelvis is usually part of a person's inner posture of self defense, and can react on hair trigger to anxiety.

Strangely, relaxing a painfully contracted pelvis can create problems for the unconscious inner defenses. "How do I defend myself if I cannot guard myself in my pelvis?" can be a major dilemma of the unconscious psychological defense system of the body. On the surface, this dilemma is irrational. Nevertheless, the unconscious defenses of the body are primitive, formed early in life, and not friendly to reason.

Typically, the pelvis has been tight for years, part of a default inner posture. This default inner posture remains in place despite all conventional and reasonable treatments. No drug has been able to fix this enormously distressing problem. The strangest solution is the surgical cutting of the anal sphincter by colorectal surgeons for patients with anal fissure in order to relax the tension of the anal sphincter. Just like there are no forceful or straight line strategies of getting a frightened cat out of a tree, there are no forceful or straight line strategies for relaxing the pelvis when one has pelvic pain.

A painful pelvis has to be coaxed out of its contraction

Healing muscle related pelvic pain has its own rules. Antibiotics, sedatives and muscles relaxants in the long term are of little use. Needles and knives often alienate the pelvis, create more suffering, and don't help you with the real problem, which is the ingrained habit of tightening up the pelvic floor. Even trigger point release that is not done in conjunction with relaxation, as well as a change in attitude toward the symptoms, at best, tends to be short lived.

Richard Gevirtz, David Hubbard and Ali Oliveira conducted a study on whiplash showing the relationship between the catastrophic stories people tell themselves about their muscle related injury, and the significantly increased physical pain they experience. It is best to change your attitude toward your pelvis because the fear, dread, anger, and withdrawal toward the pelvis which is typical in most people with chronic pelvic pain, can be a real contributor to the cycle that keeps the symptoms going.

The painful pelvis has to be coaxed into letting go. It is best to persuade your pelvis with firm and loving release of its chronically held tissue. It is best to change your attitude toward your pelvis to one of love and understanding—like the attitude of a devoted mother to her newborn child. The painful pelvis can come out of its dark contraction, with acceptance, kindness, consistency and devotion. If you have shame or judgment about your pelvis, it can help to give that up. If you get frightened by your symptoms, it helps to stop this fear reaction.

The pelvis responds to informed, firm, patient coaxing. It responds to gentle persuasion. It responds to devotion and confidence in what you are doing. It responds to you being able to relax your fear and anger. It responds to you being able to regularly calm down your nervous system, free yourself from the grip of ongoing states of anxiety and storms of catastrophic thinking. It responds to your confidence in knowing where to press and loosen, both inside and outside of your pelvis.

The painful pelvis can't be conned or coerced. The pelvis and the areas of the body around the pelvis must be lovingly and gently coaxed out of pain.

Chronic pelvic pain as a functional disorder

The closest that current medical paradigms come to understanding the nature of chronic pelvic pain syndromes, as we understand it, is using the concept of the functional somatic disorder. The concept of functional somatic disorder, or more simply, functional disorder, is a facile concept. And while researchers and medical practitioners nod with an apparent clear understanding of what functional disorders are, when examined closely, the concept of functional disorder is flawed and imprecise at best, and incorrect at worst.

When a researcher or doctor says that a condition is a functional disorder, he is usually saying that the source of the medical problem is not found in the physical structure but in the *functioning* of the structure. For instance, in the functional disorder of irritable bowel syndrome, the tissue of the bowel is not pathological or sick but it behaves in a way that does not permit proper colonic processing, giving rise to bloating, motility dysfunction like diarrhea or constipation, pain and discomfort. In current discussions of functional disorders, little more is said. The implication among many doctors is that the problem is psychiatric. This viewpoint is brought to bear on headache, non-cardiac chest pain which is usually esophageal reflux or esophageal spasm, low back pain, and TMD (temporal mandibular disorder) among other conditions.

We are proposing that the error in the concept of functional disorder is that it paints a picture of the physical component of the problem as basically unproblematic and not usefully addressed in treatment. A gastroenterologist will do a colonoscopy, and in the absence of ulceration, tumor or infection, will report to the patient that there is nothing wrong with the colon. Perhaps he might note that the colon might appear contracted, but this is not seen to be remarkable. Similarly, the neurologist will look at a CAT Scan (CT) of the brain and in the absence of tumor, bleeding or other gross pathology, will report that the findings were unremarkable.

What we are asserting here if we look at pelvic pain, for instance, is that there are disturbances in structure albeit not life-threatening or irreversible ones. While we believe that the physical findings of irritation, pain, increased muscle tension, trigger points and spasticity are not indicative of any life-threatening illness and are in fact reversible, these symptoms tend to be trivialized and overlooked by the urologist. Also, these symptoms usually cannot be imaged by contemporary imaging technology such as the CT or MRI. Neither does the doctor with his eye, his finger, or a blood test that he takes, find any significant physical basis, at least from his point of view, that accounts for the pain and dysfunction. *It is very common that our patients are told by their urologist that there is nothing wrong with them, or that they should consider their problem mental and seek psychiatric counseling.*

Often, our patients feel dismissed by their doctors. Some patients have reported the doctor did not believe their complaints. This dismissal and invalidation of a patient's symptoms on top of the huge distress of the symptoms, creates much unnecessary suffering in the lives of those dealing with pelvic pain.

In the kind of pelvic pain we describe in this book there are clearly problems with the structure of the soft pelvic tissue and adjacent areas relating to the pelvis. When you palpate the pelvic tissue of someone who has pelvic pain, the muscles tend to be very tight and chronically contracted. In the extreme, we have patients who can't tolerate the lightest touch of the opening of the anus or vagina and some in whom we cannot even insert a finger because the muscles of the opening of the orifice are so tightly held. This is in contrast to someone who doesn't have pelvic pain, who experiences no particular discomfort when a finger is inserted inside the pelvic floor and the tissue pressed. The tissue is soft, relaxed, and even with vigorous palpation there is no pain or discomfort.

Is there something physically going on in the patient with pelvic pain that is not going on in the person without pelvic symptoms? The answer is unequivocally yes. But in the current medical model, soreness, trigger points, tissue hyper-irritability, and chronic tension are more or less non-events. Furthermore, treating these non-events, from the conventional medical viewpoint, is not seen to produce any particular therapeutic benefit. So these areas remain untreated.

The point of this discussion is to make clear why our treatment intimately employs the skills of the psychologist, the physical therapist and the urologist. The *Wise-Anderson Protocol* must treat both the behavioral and physical components of pelvic pain. Both are real and treating one without the other in our experience doesn't really work. Furthermore, what is thought to be mental has real physical consequences as seen in the increased electrical activity in trigger points with increased anxiety that we see in the work of Gevirtz and Hubbard. People call up and ask whether we'll just do relaxation training in the absence of physical therapy or physical therapy in the absence of relaxation and we tell them that we don't believe it is effective to break up our protocol this way.

Renewed interest in pelvic pain as a functional disorder

The concept of a functional disorder is the closest that conventional medicine gets to understanding our perspective on pelvic pain. Below are excerpts from a recent essay in the Journal of Urology written by Dr. J. Quentin Clemens discussing pelvic pain as a functional disorder referring to a study we did at Stanford on the rise of salivary cortisol in pelvic pain patients. Following these excerpts is Dr. Wise's response.

"The term 'functional somatic syndrome' is used to describe a pattern of "persistent bodily complaints for which adequate examination does not reveal sufficiently explanatory structural or other specified pathology"... In recent years there has been a clear shift away from viewing these conditions as organ specific disorders... The outcomes of organ specific therapies directed at the prostate or bladder have been uniformly disappointing in relieving IC/PBS and CP/CPPS symptoms... An example of this conceptual shift is provided in this issue of the Journal by Anderson et al, who hypothesized that the development of urological pain symptoms, may be associated with hypothalamic-pituitary-adrenal (HPA) axis dysfunction... Compared with controls, men with CP/CPPA exhibited significantly increased awakening cortisol responses and multiple psychosocial abnormalities. Abnormalities in the HPA axis have been previously observed in IC/PBS... This report adds to the increasing evidence that stress reduction techniques should be incorporated into the management of these chronic and often debilitating symptoms... We desperately need a better understanding of the pathophysiology of the disorders so that effective prevention and treatment strategies can be developed. Hopefully the inclusion of expertise outside of urology will help us make progress in these areas.

(Dr. Wise's response to Dr. Clemens' essay)

In the March 2008 issue of the Journal of Urology, Dr. J. Quentin Clemens comments on Dr. Rodney Anderson's new study documenting the significant rise of salivary cortisol in patients with chronic pelvic pain syndromes. Dr. Clemens cites a number of studies showing the significant association between IC, prostatitis, stress, and what he refers to as hypothalamic-pituitary-adrenal (HPA) axis dysfunction (in my view, a complicated way of describing the tendency toward nervous excitability). He discusses Dr. Anderson's study in the context of prostatitis and IC-type symptoms as functional somatic syndromes and the common observation that people who have pelvic pain syndromes tend to have other functional somatic syndromes. Dr. Clemens concludes that, "We desperately need a better understanding

*of the pathophysiology of the disorders so that effective prevention
and treatment strategies can be developed."*

*As a researcher and co-developer of the Wise-Anderson Protocol for
pelvic pain I am writing to suggest that the issue in finding a new
understanding and treatment for pelvic pain syndromes in the direction
of what Dr. Clemens suggests does not lie in a dearth of data into the
pathophysiology of the disorders or in lack of research. I suggest that
the organ-specific paradigm (as opposed to a functional paradigm)
that urology continues to choose is strongly fueled by economics, and
not the lack of data, research or understanding into the functional
nature of the problem. This is why I suggest this problem has been
missed in the field of urology for so many years.*

*What would it mean for a urologist to change his paradigm of
prostatitis, for instance, and see it as a functional somatic syndrome
and not a prostate-specific disorder? It would mean that there would
not be the immediate conclusion that the symptoms of pelvic pain in
men meant there was an infection or inflammation of the prostate and
therefore antibiotics would not be used routinely without any evidence
to justify their use. It would mean that the urologist understood there
was a strong association with anxiety and emotional disturbance. It
might well mean that the urologist would shift the focus on searching
for a drug to treat prostatitis and become interested the success of the
Wise-Anderson Protocol in treating the hypertonicity of the muscles of
the pelvic floor and autonomic arousal which feeds this hypertonicity.
It might well mean that the urologist would have to learn how to
diagnose pelvic floor trigger points, and as we do in the Wise-Anderson
Protocol, instruct patients in self-treatment to reduce pelvic floor tone
and anxiety which feeds it.*

*So we have two paradigms facing off here. In one corner, is the paradigm
alluded to by Dr. Clemens and embodied in the Wise-Anderson
Protocol. Such a paradigm sees pelvic pain as the consequence of
mind-body interaction in the pelvic floor and is treated behaviorally
with patient self-treatment being the central ingredient. In the other
corner, we have the paradigm of conventional urology, that prostatitis*

and other pelvic pain syndromes are organ specific problems requiring conventional physical/pharmaceutical/surgical intervention.

In order for physicians to embrace what Dr. Clemens calls "the functional somatic syndrome paradigm" they must overcome formidable obstacles. The first and perhaps largest obstacle is an economic one. Insurance reimbursement pays a paltry amount to a urologist for treating psychogenic pelvic floor myofascial pain. The 15-minute office visit is the mainstay of a conventional medical practice and the kind of intervention required in the paradigm Dr. Clemens discusses would have great difficulty in effectively fitting into a 15-minute slot. Furthermore, effectively treating pelvic pain as a functional somatic syndrome is questionable economically given the pressing economic requirements of a urologic practice that often must produce $20,000 + per month just to meet overhead.

Furthermore, there is little support offered by pharmaceutical or medical equipment companies to support research into treatment that aims to eliminate patients using drugs or undergoing surgery as would be the case in any bona fida treatment of functional somatic syndromes. Additionally, philosophically and ideologically, many physicians who treat pelvic pain tend not to be interested in mind-body medicine for the treatment of urologic disorders.

For all of these reasons shifting paradigms in treating pelvic pain from organ specific to what Clemens calls "functional somatic syndromes" has little support and major disincentives at this time. Leroy Nyberg of NIH, in the May, 2006 edition of Best Life, was reported saying "it doesn't go over well when a big organization loses a disorder." So patients with pelvic pain are stuck between a rock and a hard place. They are seeing specialists who can't help them, but may be loathe to understand their problem from a viewpoint that can help them.

Patients who experience the benefit of our treatment frequently ask us why their doctors didn't tell them about our approach. On the Internet, the chat groups are often less than complimentary toward physicians whom patients have seen for pelvic pain and incredulous as to why many tend to remain closed to the experience of many patients who benefit from the kind of treatment we describe in this book. Often patients will buy our book to give to their doctors, only to have our book politely accepted and then put in the trash bin after the patient leaves. I think this all has to do with the conflict of paradigms discussed here and the disincentives with regard to the conceptual shift Dr. Clemens urges.

We find ourselves stuck in an age where most urologists still diagnose men who complain of myofascial pelvic pain as having "prostatitis" and who routinely give them antibiotics, often without even checking if there's an infection present in the prostate. The economic disincentives for changing paradigms about pelvic pain are huge. And let us be clear that the paradigm itself is the problem. While there are urologists who think outside of the box, no matter how many incentives or disincentives may be present, such a paradigm shift seeing pelvic pain as a neuromuscular disorder intimately associated with nervous system arousal does not seem to be on the horizon for most urologic practitioners.

And unfortunately, the pelvic pain patient is the biggest loser.

Being told your condition is all in your head

We would never say that pelvic pain is any less real than a broken bone. As we have discussed above, more than a few patients have told us that they have seen doctors who have told them that there is nothing wrong and that they should either live with their condition or go to a psychiatrist. This is naturally disturbing to a patient who is faced with his doctor telling him that his pain and dysfunction are somehow not real or treatable. If the doctor, for one hour, experienced what the pelvic pain patient experiences chronically, the doctor would not be so quick to tell the patient such things.

When a doctor tells you you'll just have to live with it—the *nocebo effect*

Elsewhere we discuss the *placebo effect* – the phenomenon that occurs when a patient believes in and is helped by a sugar pill. There is an opposite effect called the *nocebo effect*. The *nocebo effect* describes the negative effects of believing a sugar pill will hurt you. In Latin *placebo* means, "I shall please" and *nocebo* means, "I shall harm." So the *placebo* will help your symptoms (only if you believe it will) and the *nocebo* will hurt your symptoms (only if you believe it will). Your thought about the substance and not the substance itself, appear to be the causative factor. Just as the positive and optimistic attitude of a doctor can have a profound *placebo effect*, as we have discussed elsewhere, so can the negative, hope destroying comments of a doctor have a *nocebo effect*.

We are often distressed at the insensitivity of some doctors who bring about a *nocebo effect* in their patients by telling them that they will simply have to "live with their condition" and that nothing can be done about it. Numerous patients have reported to us how such a pronouncement on the part of their doctor brought about one of the blackest moments in their lives and one of the worst flare-ups in their symptoms. When a doctor gives a patient a life sentence of chronic pain, it is tantamount to the doctor putting himself in the position of being God, who can know the patient's future absolutely. Such a pronouncement is particularly egregious given the position of authority that the doctor has and the degree of trust most patients put in the doctor, particularly doctors who are supposed to be experts in an esoteric sub-specialty of medicine having to do with pelvic pain.

In truth, at the time of the printing of this book, most doctors have little understanding of muscle-related pelvic pain or how to treat it. In fact, the point of our book and this chapter is that conventional medical ideas about pelvic pain and its treatment are at best incomplete and at worst incorrect and potentially harmful. How can a doctor who has no real understanding about the nature of a problem or its amelioration tell anyone anything about his or her future?

Most doctors treating pelvic pain are caring and appreciate the effect of their words on their patients. For a moment, we are going to indulge in some psychological speculation about this small number of insensitive doctors who tell patients they're never going to get better. Here is a possible psychological profile of such doctors. We present this here to help patients who have been on the other side of this kind of physician in order to help them gain some perspective. Unfortunately, there are doctors who have little tolerance in believing that if they can't help someone, or do not understand the nature of someone's condition, that they think they are 'supposed' to understand and help

If this kind of doctor were to be forthright and caring, he would say, "I can't help you given the level of my skills, knowledge and healing tools. Just because I can't help you doesn't mean that someone else might not be able to help you and so, go forth and see if you can find someone else who might be able to help you."

Relationship between Irritable Bowel Syndrome and Pelvic Pain

In our practice, we have noticed that there is a high incidence of irritable bowel syndrome in patients who also have pelvic pain. Given the proximity of the colon and the pelvis, it makes sense that both may well be the result of a chronic abdominal/pelvic tension. While gastroenterology and urology make a distinction between the urogenital and gastrointestinal tract, the body has never heard of either specialty. Pelvic and gastrointestinal tightening often go hand in hand.

We will discuss later in this book how the use of the *Wise-Anderson Protocol* with some slight variations, has been helpful for some of our patients in reducing pain associated with irritable bowel syndrome, and in a few patients, with their distressing symptoms of esophageal reflux.

The concepts of symptom threshold and pelvic pain

When first facing pelvic pain, one faces what seems to be a monolithic, curtain of discomfort and distress that feels incomprehensible and overwhelming. Patients usually feel helpless in the face of pelvic pain because they know little or nothing about what they can do about their condition. Therefore, the concept of a threshold, and proximity to the threshold, is often a useful idea to help patients gain perspective on their progress.

We assess the effectiveness of our treatment by looking at the presence, intensity, and frequency of symptoms. Consider the following scheme. The symptom threshold is the point your pelvic tension/neuromuscular irritability reaches in order to produce discomfort/pain and dysfunction. You can locate your proximity to the threshold, above which you are symptomatic and below which you are not. When patients are able to see their symptoms from the viewpoint of their proximity to the symptom threshold, they can sometimes better understand their situation.

One's proximity to the symptom threshold

#4   CHRONICALLY SYMPTOMATIC

#3   SYMPTOMS WAX AND WANE WHEN
      SLIGHTLY ABOVE THRESHOLD

SYMPTOM THRESHOLD

#2   NO SYMPTOMS WHEN SLIGHTLY BELOW
      THRESHOLD; CAN BECOME SYMPTOMATIC
      AT THE SLIGHTEST STRESS

#1   NO SYMPTOMS

In the threshold schema, the person who is located in position #1 is well below the threshold, displays no symptoms, and can tolerate a great amount of tension/nervous system arousal in the pelvic floor without becoming symptomatic. Even when this person's pelvic tension goes over the threshold, the pelvic tissue is not irritated, and the pelvic floor muscles are flexible, and immediately drop below the threshold after the individual has stopped tensing. The person in this position has a normal, healthy pelvis.

The person situated in position #2 represents someone who likely will have pelvic pain but on an intermittent basis. It does not take great increases in pelvic tension/nervous system arousal level to throw them above the threshold where he or she will become symptomatic. The person at position #2, generally speaking, has a reduced level of flexibility in the pelvic floor and often does not relax as easily as someone in position #1 once the muscles are tensed over the level of the threshold. People with pelvic pain who are in position #2 are often bewildered at what brings on their symptoms. They conclude that there was nothing much that seemed to be associated with the onset of symptoms, and that the pain is random. Our explanation is that when someone is slightly below the threshold, what a non-event is for a normal person is often stressful enough to throw a #2 over the threshold and into symptoms.

At position #3 is the individual who has mild but persistent symptoms that wax and wane. This is the person who is 'surfing' the threshold. Symptoms associated with #3, while seeming to be almost always present, occasionally drop below threshold only to come back inexplicably. The person at position #3 usually experiences chronic but more or less tolerable pain and dysfunction.

At position #4 is the individual who has chronic and intractable pelvic pain and/or dysfunction. He or she doesn't drop below the symptom threshold. When asked to describe the frequency and severity of symptoms, this person will report that the symptoms are always present, 24 hours a day, seven days a week, and that the symptoms strongly impact his or her life. Our treatment aims to lower baseline pelvic pain, tension/neuromuscular irritability of individuals in positions #2, #3, and #4 to that of the position #1.

Anxiety increases symptoms

Most of the patients we see with chronic pelvic pain syndromes have what we have referred to earlier in this chapter as trigger points in their pelvis and related muscles. To reiterate, a trigger point is a taut band within a muscle that is painful either spontaneously or when touched, and which creates pain at the site palpated or refers pain to a site remote from it. Trigger points are exquisitely sensitive and it is not uncommon for the patient to jump when the trigger point is pressed. We determine the presence of a trigger point through a digital/rectal or digital/vaginal examination for internal trigger points. The doctor inserts a finger inside the rectum or vagina and presses on the muscles to assess the tissue and to find trigger points. External trigger points are evaluated using the methodology described by Travell and Simons in *Myofascial Pain and Dysfunction: The Trigger Point Manual.*

A 1994 study sheds much light on the relationship between trigger points and stress. McNulty, Gevertz, Hubbard, and Berkoff inserted a needle electrode directly into a trigger point and monitored its electrical activity with a machine called an electromyograph. It appears that the higher the electrical activity in a trigger point, the higher the level of pain.

Patients were given the stressful task of doing mental arithmetic. The scientists wanted to determine what the effects of stress were on the trigger points being monitored and the differences, if any, between the responses of the trigger points and the responses of the adjacent non-sensitive tissue without trigger points. Results indicated that the electrical activity of the trigger points increased during this stressful activity while the adjacent, non-trigger point tissue remained essentially electrically unresponsive.

This kind of experiment has been replicated hundreds of times. These findings are remarkable. They suggest that in some way the nervous system that is connected to the stress of emotional activity and arousal is selectively connected to trigger points and not to non-trigger point tissue. Understanding this, it becomes clear why patients with pelvic pain and dysfunction routinely report that their symptoms are aggravated by stress.

Anxiety, anger, fear and sorrow, which are expressions of nervous system arousal, can cause increased pain in areas that have trigger points. Furthermore, your fearful attitude toward your body and symptoms can stress you. If you are aware of pain every day during urination or sexual activity, and you feel anxious each time you are aware of your pain, it is helpful, in our experience, to shift your thoughts and attitude about your symptoms.

Plato taught that we need to be kind to each other because each of us is engaged in a mighty, yet unseen, struggle in our lives. Compassion for the most difficult of people comes from understanding their struggle. Like letting go of anger and fear toward difficult people, letting go of fear and anxiety toward a painful rectum and genitals is simply an expression of your understanding and compassion for your own struggle. Discovering compassion toward oneself and one's body is part of our protocol. As patients understand the language of the pelvic floor and their struggle with their habit of chronically tightening it, their attitude can change from fear to compassion and understanding.

What is the role of inflammation?

As one views the maladies and aberrations that occur in the human body to create suffering, the evidence for inflammatory conditions underlying a great preponderance of these disorders is plentiful. These conditions include coronary artery disease, arthritis, inflammatory bowel disease, multiple neurologic disorders, diabetes, infectious diseases, etc., and the list goes on and on. We have no reason to think that chronic pelvic pain disorders may not also be an inflammatory condition.

A few things are known and others strongly believed. There is a large body of literature that shows that inflammation produces anxiety. But there is also significant evidence that the reverse is true. Anxiety may worsen inflammatory conditions and may even worsen cancer deterioration. Whether it is surgery, infection, arthritis, cancer, coronary disease or bowel disease, stress and distress can worsen inflammation. Stress is well known to delay wound healing. For example, if you are among those who score in the top one-third of anxiety behavior, you will take four times as long to heal a duodenal ulcer. In discussing inflammation, we want to be clear that the symptoms associated with what is typically called "prostatitis" seem to have little relationship to inflammation. That said, the association between anxiety and inflammation, in our view, particularly in relationship to interstitial cystitis and what was formerly known as urethral syndrome, is another reason that makes it imperative to bring ongoing anxiety under control.

Some inflammatory conditions of the body are obviously harmful to us. Parts of our body become inflamed and often suffer from the internal war our body wages when anything that remotely threatens our survival becomes involved. Certain kinds of defense cells found in the inflammatory response secrete noxious and toxic biochemicals that cause pain. Inflammation almost always overshoots the mark and then we have to suffer from it. The scientific evidence would suggest that reduction of anxiety can promote healing and reduce the inflammatory response. With regard to pelvic pain, inflammatory reduction may be particularly helpful in interstitial cystitis and urethral syndrome.

The tension-anxiety-pain cycle: the heart of the problem

Chronic pelvic pain has been resistant to effective treatment because of what we call the *tension-anxiety-pain cycle*. This is a cycle in which chronic tension has shortened the muscles in the pelvic floor and created an environment in which the pelvic floor can be said to be functioning like a clenched fist. The pain is a kind of alarm to which the body responds with protective bracing and a heightened state of arousal or anxiety. Anxiety always produces increased tension, which then produces more pain, which then produces more anxiety.

The Tension-Anxiety-Pain Cycle

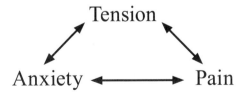

We propose that the tension-anxiety-pain cycle is the heart of the problem of most chronic pelvic pain syndromes we treat. Once the pelvis becomes sore, painful and the normal functions are disturbed in some way, the sore and painful pelvis becomes hyper-sensitive to anxiety. Anxiety results in the tightening of the muscles in preparation for fight, flight or freeze. This tightening of the pelvic floor and surrounding musculature tends to be reflexive and usually happens out of a person's awareness. Some level of anxiety is what almost all patients with chronic pelvic pain syndromes live with day in and day out. Anxiety can regularly exacerbate the condition fed by the patient's catastrophic thinking, the isolation of sharing one's feelings with very few, and a medical establishment that can't help.

In the presence of anxiety and reflexive protective guarding, the sore contracted pelvis can't fully relax. This relaxation is necessary for the healing of the sore pelvic tissue. Added to an individual's anxiety is the puzzlement of the doctors whom the individual sees for this problem. As we have discussed, the doctor is often frustrated about his inability to help the problem and is not infrequently worried that perhaps he has missed something. Doctors are problem solvers. As we have discussed, certain doctors do not respond well to their helplessness to solve the problem of pelvic pain. Any anxiety, uncertainty or helplessness of the doctor is almost always communicated to the patient – a communication whose impact, as we have discussed, is profound.

Pelvic pain is hugely affected and perpetuated by anxiety. This is why the placebo effect reduces the anxiety that helps fuel the condition. This is also why many people have a reduction in symptoms after they read this book. Finally something makes sense about what is going on and offers some intuitively viable solution.

We often see patients in pain who are very emotionally upset about their pain. Their hands are often cold and clammy; they are agitated and can't seem to sit still. These patients are caught in the active grip of the *tension-anxiety-pain cycle.* The difficulty of intervening effectively on behalf of these patients is illustrated in the children's jump rope game called "Double Dutch." In this game, two children facing each other, turn two ropes, one clockwise, and the other counter-clockwise, as one child jumps both ropes simultaneously.

The difficulty in Double Dutch is found in entering through both swinging ropes into the jumping space. Children who successfully "jump Double Dutch" are able to watch the two ropes as they follow closely one after another and are able to determine the split second when there is a space through which they can enter. Even for an athletic and bright child, Double Dutch is a challenge. Similarly, the events that occur in the *tension-anxiety-pain cycle* follow so closely one after the other, that we could call this "Triple Dutch." Entering into these events to stop the cycle is not a small challenge.

Pelvic pain triggered by the biological mammalian response of pulling the tail between the legs in states of fear

In 2009, after the printing of the 5th edition of our book an insight occurred to us about pelvic pain. This insight helps clarify the pervasiveness of muscle-related pelvic pain and a biological basis for it.

It is common knowledge that a dog will pull his tail between his legs when he is fearful. Other emotions have been attributed to this tail-pulled-between-the-legs behavior, including shame, submission, dread, defeat or shyness. For the present discussion we propose here that the common denominator running through the various emotions associated with the tail-pulled-between-the-legs behavior is fear.

In the typology of Walter Cannon, the great Harvard physiologist of the early 20th century who introduced the phrase *fight, flight, freeze* to describe the varieties of survival behavior in mammals, a tail-pulled-between-the-legs is an expression of the survival behavior that he termed, *freeze.* This *freeze* behavior expresses the organism's attempt to self-protectively hold fast, while waiting for danger to pass. The behavior of a waving tail has been associated among animal watchers with the emotions of excitement or aggression, contrasting sharply to the tail-pulled-between-the-legs behavior. Most cat and dog owners, for example, intuitively read their animals' emotional states, in large part, by what the tail is doing.

In humans, the tailbone is commonly understood to be what remains of the tail inherited from our humanoid ancestors. This tailbone (coccyx) is sometimes called the vestigial tail. In humans, the coccygeal, iliococcygeal and pubococcygeal muscles of the pelvic basin are attached to the coccyx or tailbone and are responsible for its movement, in conjunction with other pelvic floor muscles.

The phrase, "a tail between the legs" exists in the vernacular of many languages to describe behaviors of fear, shame, submission, cowardice or defeat. For example, in French, the term, *la queue entre les jambes* is commonly used and is identical in meaning to "pulling his tail between his legs." In modern Greek, the transliterated phrase "Autos einai san to skylo pou vazi tin oura mes ta skelia tou" translates as "he is like the dog who puts his tail deep down below." Greeks use this phrase all the time to describe someone who is fearful, anxious, nervous, ashamed, or beaten down by life. Interestingly as well, he said that the phrase is often used to describe someone who can't make a decision, who is "frozen" by choices before him, who obsesses over which decision to make.

The phenomenon of pulling the tail between the legs requires that specific pelvic floor muscles, particularly involving the coccygeal muscles, participate in this muscular event. In this act of muscle contraction, this set of pelvic muscles contracts, causing the tail (tailbone) to pull in. We offer the insight here that in terms of evolution, the tail-pulled-between-the-legs is an active behavior associated with the experience of fear, and whose aim is likely to protect the anorectal area and genitals of the organism. This behavior also signals to a predator or competitor that the animal offers no threat.

Sitting pain and the reflex of pulling the tail between the legs

To our knowledge, in the scientific discussion of pelvic pain, there has been no discussion of what we believe to be the intimate relationship between tail-pulled-between-the-legs behavior, anxiety and pelvic pain. Here we introduce this idea and the therapeutic implications of this surprisingly clinically important relationship.

From the beginning of our research, we have known that pelvic pain was related to chronic self protective muscle tension that formed a self-feeding cycle of tension-anxiety-pain and protective guarding. In the original publication of our book, A Headache in the Pelvis, we summarized our understanding as follows:

We have identified a group of chronic pelvic pain syndromes that we believe is caused by the overuse of the human instinct to protect the genitals, rectum, and contents of the pelvis from injury or pain by contracting the pelvic muscles. This tendency becomes exaggerated in predisposed individuals and over time results in chronic pelvic pain and dysfunction. The state of chronic constriction creates pain-referring trigger points, reduced blood flow, and an inhospitable environment for the nerves, blood vessels, and structures throughout the pelvic basin. This results in a cycle of tension, anxiety, and pain, which has previously been unrecognized and untreated.

Understanding this tension-anxiety-pain cycle has allowed us to create an effective treatment. Our program breaks the cycle by rehabilitating the shortened pelvic muscles and connective tissue supporting the pelvic organs while simultaneously using a specific methodology to modify the tendency to tighten the muscles of the pelvic floor under stress.

We have been impressed by the pervasiveness of pelvic pain internationally. Every month our website is visited by individuals from over 90 countries. The biological instinct for animals to pull the tail between the legs exemplifies why pelvic pain, to one degree or another, exists in human beings regardless of race, gender or country of origin.

Muscle related pelvic pain comes from a universal, biologically based behavior that appears hardwired in vertebrates

The insight that pelvic pain is related to tail-pulled-between-the-legs behavior has both theoretical as well as practical applications. The practical application more clearly identifies what we believe is the therapeutic strategy necessary to treat posterior symptoms like sitting pain, coccygeal pain and post-bowel movement pain in particular, along with associated pelvic pain and dysfunction in general.

The tail-pulled-between-the-legs muscles are the muscles most associated with pelvic pain

Upon examination, the muscles involved in the tail-pulled-between-the-legs behavior are among the most common with trigger-pointed, shortened and painful muscles in patients with pelvic pain. In the data we have collected from patients who have visited us for treatment of their pelvic pain, we have very often been able to recreate pain associated with sitting, coccygeal pain and post bowel movement pain by palpating the ileococcygeus, pubococcygeus, sphincter ani, and piriformis muscles.

It is also important to say, that physical trauma or injury to the pelvis can also trigger this protective tail-pulled-between-the-legs behavior. In other words, the tail-pulled-between-the-legs behavior can occur outside of states of chronic anxiety or fear.

The tail-pulled-between-the-legs phenomenon is essentially invisible to our fellow humans because we do not have a visible tail to inform each other of our states of fear and anxiety. Because muscle related pelvic pain likely has its origins in this biological instinct, it makes sense that this disorder consists of various spastic or chronically contracted muscles that tighten the entire pelvic floor, and are fed by tension, anxiety, pain and protective guarding. Once set in motion, this syndrome takes on a life of its own and forms a self-feeding cycle, even when the fearful event or trauma has passed. Additionally, the act of sitting on sore muscles reinforces a protective contraction that perpetuates sitting pain and makes it difficult to treat.

Pulling the tail between the legs is a muscular event primarily involving contraction of the puborectalis, pubococcygeus, ileococcygeus, sphincter ani, gluteus maximus and related muscles. From the data of patients that we have treated over the last several years in our *Wise-Anderson Protocol* clinics, we found in a large number of cases of patients with sitting pain that palpating trigger points in the muscles listed above recreated sitting pain symptoms. The rehabilitation of these muscles and the modification of the tendency to chronically pull the tail in under stress are essential to the amelioration of sitting pain.

Beyond the necessity of softening taut, chronically tensed muscles that come from a biological impulse to pull the tail between the legs in states of fear, is the necessity to lower the default level of nervous system arousal that keeps the tail chronically pulled in.

Lowering the default level of nervous system arousal requires ongoing practice in reversing the thinking process representing the world as a dangerous place in which we must remain protectively guarded. Paradoxical Relaxation provides a regular time during the day, when you can release your protective guarding, free yourself from fear and inwardly rest. In the moments of being free from anxiety, the biological reflex to keep the tail pulled in is interrupted and the pelvic floor can get accustomed to being relaxed.

**Fear, anxiety, dread, resentment, and anger
are the breeding grounds of pelvic pain:
the necessity of modifying the tendency
toward dysfunctional emotional states**

It is easy to get lost in the narrow focus of pelvic pain and its related symptoms. Some professionals who work with pelvic pain say that they specialize in conditions 'between the belly button and the knees.' The narrow focus just on fixing the area from the belly button to the knees or briefly reducing the pain, has generally failed to offer any real resolution. Indeed, the tendency to tighten the pelvic floor is no accident. It is one of the central ways most individuals with pelvic pain, usually unconsciously, deal with the stresses of life. And yet especially when it arises, *pelvic pain is perpetuated in an internal atmosphere of fear, anxiety, dread, resentment, and anger.* These feelings are usually subterranean. These states exist below the surface and are usually invisible to others or even to one's self.

We know that when you have pelvic pain, you usually live with some level of anxiety and/or depression. Our recent study at Stanford shows a greater early morning rise in salivary cortisol in pelvic pain patients as opposed to normal, non-symptomatic control subjects; findings which suggest heightened anxiety in individuals who suffer from pelvic pain syndromes. We have discussed the increased level of psychological distress in those with Interstitial Cystitis, as well as how dealing with pelvic pain syndromes is equivalent to dealing with the same kind of stress people deal with who have heart disease or Crohn's disease. Absent are studies of levels of dread, resentment and anger in those who deal with pelvic pain, though it is our anecdotal experience that such emotions often punctuate the lives of many of our patients.

Most people with pelvic pain are only rarely aware of the impact of these underlying emotions on their symptoms. The reason for this is that if you live, for instance, in a marriage where there is ongoing resentment, a work situation in which you deal with frustration and disappointment regularly, or live with a sense of dread because of a general psychological tendency to jump to catastrophic conclusions, you get used to these emotional currents and think they are just a part of life. You may not connect the dots in seeing their relationship to your symptoms. When you live in water, you don't notice that you're wet.

I'm determined to see things differently; the intention to rehabilitate a tendency toward dysfunctional thinking and mood

In *A Course in Miracles,* a self-help primer that focuses on teaching the reader about how to be happy, the student of the *Course* is taught to take a different perspective on normally troublesome events. The major premise of this self-help text corresponds to the general assumptions of cognitive therapy – that suffering comes from your viewpoint and not from the things about which you have a viewpoint. The *Course in Miracles*, in part, consists of 365 lessons aimed at helping someone rehabilitate their habitual way of thinking which keeps them in fear, anxiety, dread, resentment and anger. The *Course's* purpose is to both help readers become aware of how their thinking creates their dysfunctional emotional states, and also to dissolve them.

Early on, one of the 365 lessons in *A Course in Miracles* is entitled 'I am determined to see things differently.' Its placement in the lessons follows a discussion of how our thinking creates our unhappiness. This lesson emphasizes that once you see that the cause of your suffering is your point of view, there is no other alternative, if you want to be happy, but to change your viewpoint to one that does not upset you. This viewpoint, reiterated over and over again, invites the reader to see things differently: to see things in a way that permits forgiveness for all of your grievances.

The *Course* goes in the right direction. When you see how releasing yourself from thoughts that promote fear, anxiety, resentment and anger profoundly affects your symptoms, you most likely will find the real motivation to do something about these problematic emotions.

This is a huge enterprise. One of the gifts of pelvic pain is that it can provide the motivation to begin this process – a motivation usually lacking when life goes on relatively untroubled.

In other words, pelvic pain can provide the impetus to decide to see things differently, because seeing things differently can reduce your symptoms. It is part of our language to distinguish between optimistic and pessimistic viewpoints by using the analogy of 'seeing the glass half full or half empty.' It is not a lie to say the glass is half full or half empty; they are both equally true. But for someone who usually sees glasses as half empty, and suffers from such a viewpoint, it takes a decision and effort to choose the 'half full' perspective, because the half empty perspective is so strongly ingrained.

One of the major obstacles to finding a way to live free from the disturbing emotions described here, is that most people dealing with pelvic pain are not aware that such emotions go on inside them or are significant in their condition. When you are able to relax and let go of a level of anxiety you normally live with, and you witness a dramatic improvement in your symptoms, you usually find the wherewithal to earnestly do something about your normal level of anxiety. It's all about seeing the relationship between cause and effect.

Unfortunately, at this time, contemporary medicine has not been interested in the profound relationship between pelvic pain and ongoing dysfunctional emotional states. This is the reason why, in our view, conventional treatments have failed. *The rehabilitation of attitudes that promote chronic states of anxiety, fear, dread, resentment or anger is essential for anyone who is serious about stopping their pelvic pain.*

The new paradigm implied in the treatment protocol for muscle related pelvic pain developed at Stanford University

If we look at the slang related to the anal sphincter, we typically will hear someone on the street referring to someone as a "tight-ass" or being "anal." Using this term to refer to someone tends to mean that they are perfectionistic, withholding, cheap, or obsessed with detail. It relates the tightness of the anal canal to such psychological and characterological traits. The "tight-ass" is just a certain kind of person. These terms imply that your character (and the state of your pelvis) is like the color of your eyes or the enduring characteristics of a personality. It is remarkable to notice how these terms have become part of the vernacular, when they first originated in obscure psychoanalytic theory. What Freud referred to as "anal" was derived from a psychological fixation associated with the anal phase of development.

It is a new paradigm to think you can voluntarily relax your habitually tight core which includes the anorectal area. When you call someone a "tight ass," the implication is that such a person is characteristically in a chronic state—someone who is "tight-assed" or "anal" is considered a kind of person whose habitual tendency is to be perfectionistic, compulsive or picayune and cannot be reformed. Our protocol is based on the understanding that concerted voluntary efforts to behaviorally change the default tone of the anal sphincter and other muscles of the pelvic floor, can change one that is tight and chronically contracted to one that is relaxed and at ease. This new understanding asserts that "tight asses" can become "relaxed asses."

Like the insights of the new paradigm of neuroscience regarding the plasticity of the brain, we propose that the chronically tensed core of us, including the intestines and pelvic floor muscles, can be trained to be relaxed. We propose that the tendency to chronically brace the viscera under stress can be modified without surgery or drugs. It can be modified with training in calming down a chronically vigilant nervous system. In other words, the visceral reaction of chronic tension associated with nervous system arousal can be, with a certain level of training, brought under our voluntary control.

Changing this habitual inner posture is not brought about by drugs or surgery, but can be brought under the control of the patients' disciplined consciousness. For those patients who come to our clinic, the suffering with pelvic pain is what we believe provides the motivation for someone with a tight gut and pelvic floor to learn to control catastrophic thinking, an upset nervous system, and the pelvic pain related to them. *We are proposing that ultimately resolving chronically tight insides can't be done by anyone else except by the person who is suffering.* Over a lifetime, we believe that teaching people to calm down their insides under their own volition is the most cost effective method of dealing with pelvic pain that exists, despite the fact that initially training people to do this has its costs. In our view, the psychophysical treatment of the *Wise-Anderson Protocol* represents the best framework within which someone can modify a chronically contracted core.

Unfortunately, behavioral treatment for anal fissures to reduce the high muscle tone of the anal sphincter is not generally a focus of colorectal surgeons who are consulted for this problem. If you seek treatment from a colorectal surgeon, you will often end up with surgery. This approach does not take into consideration the fact that someone with a tight anal sphincter can learn to voluntarily loosen it with proper physical therapy and behavior instruction, as our protocol has been shown to demonstrate. The idea that the anal sphincter can be worked with and one can learn to relax the anal canal is not within the framework of conventional medicine. The tight anal sphincter is considered to be a chronic state, somehow essentially unreachable by voluntary means.

If you go to an orthopedic surgeon and complain of tight neck or back tension, they would never consider cutting the trapezius muscle or the muscles of your back. Nor would an oral surgeon consider cutting the masseter muscle in a patient suffering from jaw pain. In fact, patients would be horrified at such suggestions. Why would one consider cutting the muscles of the anus to relax it? The idea that one can learn to voluntarily relax the anorectal area is novel and outside the conventional medical model.

The willingness of a doctor to cut a tight anal sphincter and not even consider cutting a tight shoulder or jaw, in a certain peculiar way, may be reflective of the general disownment and rejection of the anorectal area in the culture. The genitals and anorectal area are considered dark, mysterious, often unclean, sinful, and dirty. The idea of patiently working with this area in yourself to rehabilitate its chronic tightness is a peculiar activity in a society where there is a generally fearful and rejecting attitude toward the anus. We believe that this new paradigm requires a re-owning of the genitals and anorectal area; an acceptance, appreciation and respect of them. And considering them with acceptance, as Steven Levine has said, involves bringing this area into the sphere of your heart and caring. When you care about this area you would be loathe to cut it before you did everything in your power to learn to relax it.

Changing the habit of contracting your inner core is not won easily. A sufficient amount of pain experienced over time provides the incentive for many of our patients with a tight gut and pelvic floor to learn to relax it. We propose that changing the posture of tight insides to relaxed insides is by far most effectively done by the person who is suffering.

A gentle approach to break the tension-anxiety-pain cycle

The *Wise-Anderson Protocol* intervenes in all aspects of the tension-anxiety-pain cycle. *Paradoxical Relaxation* lowers pelvic tension and anxiety by lowering autonomic nervous system arousal in general, and habitual pelvic tension in particular. *Trigger Point Release* and certain myofascial release methods, including what we describe as *skin rolling* and *pelvic floor yoga,* deactivates trigger point pain, lengthens chronically contracted muscles, and makes the pelvic muscles more capable of relaxation. We have found that an effective way of beginning therapy when someone is caught in the grips of the *tension-anxiety-pain* cycle, is to start *Trigger Point Release* gradually. If the patient cannot tolerate any pressure inside the rectum or vagina, we begin the physical part of our treatment by simply inserting a finger with no pressure anywhere. If they cannot tolerate the insertion of the finger, we hold the finger gently, touching the opening of the rectum or vagina without moving at all. In backing up and reducing the intensity of the treatment to a tolerable level, we find a baseline from which to begin.

John J., a patient from Minneapolis, could not tolerate any pressure inside his pelvic floor. When we instructed his wife in the *Trigger Point Release*, we told her to simply insert her finger inside his rectum and not press anywhere. She did this on a daily basis for a week, and with our instruction, she began slightly pressing on a trigger point. Gradually, as her husband could tolerate more, she increased the pressure. After a few months, he was able to tolerate the pressure that we are usually able to exert at the beginning of treatment with most other patients. Similarly, John J. was not able to lie down and do the first lesson in the relaxation training for more than three minutes. We instructed him to do *Paradoxical Relaxation* for two minutes each day, which he did for a week or so. Following this, we asked him to increase the relaxation time gradually until he reported actually relaxing for over a period of half an hour.

The aim of the Wise-Anderson Protocol is to rehabilitate the chronically tensed and shortened muscles related to pelvic pain and dysfunction, restore their original length and flexibility, substantially reduce nervous system arousal and change the habit of continually squeezing them and the nerves, blood vessels and structures they contain. In focusing on this, we have been able to help many patients help themselves in substantially reducing or completely abating their symptoms.

Our understanding is a significant departure from the conventional view of prostatitis and chronic pelvic pain syndromes. We see pelvic pain as a physical expression of the way a person copes with life. We propose that *pelvic pain is the result of a neuromuscular state perpetuated by anxiety and chronic bracing in both men and women and not the result of a foreign organism in the prostate gland in the case of prostatitis, an autoimmune disorder, or other contemporary explanations of pelvic pain in men and women.*

When certain predisposed individuals focus tension in the pelvic muscles, this chronic tension, over time, creates an inhospitable environment in the pelvic floor that gives rise to a cycle of tension, anxiety, and pain. *Once the cycle of tension, anxiety, and pain is set into motion, it takes on a life of its own. Our treatment aims to restore the capacity of the pelvic tissue to relax, to perform its normal functions, and to return to a pain-free and dysfunction-free state.* This rehabilitative protocol consists of the simultaneous use of *Paradoxical Relaxation* and *Trigger Point Release.*

Pros and Cons of Our Treatment

The cons

Ours is the slow fix, not the quick fix

On the negative side, *ours is the slow fix, not the quick fix.* Our intention is to provide your sore and irritated pelvic muscles and structures with an opportunity to heal. Our method for doing this is 'low tech' and not 'high tech.' We ask you to do a good hour and a half of self-treatment daily, usually divided up into 45 minutes in the morning and 45 minutes or more in the evening. This typically goes on for many months and sometimes a few years. We tell our patients that our program is like getting a pilot's license; you have to put in the hours. Furthermore, you are instructed to practice relaxing the habitual tension in your pelvic floor many times a day by doing *Moment-to-Moment Paradoxical Relaxation.* This is not a small matter.

Trigger Point Release can be painful at first

Trigger Point Release is not something you would do unless you felt it was necessary. It is not uncommon, especially during the first number of sessions of *Trigger Point Release* inside the pelvic floor, for there to be a flare-up of symptoms, often lasting between a few hours to several days or longer.

Our treatment is inconvenient

Our treatment is inconvenient in that the clinic we hold is six days in length and with travel usually requires setting aside seven to eight days. As we said above, home practice can often take 1½ hours or more per day until symptoms quiet down. In short, receiving and practicing elements of our protocol is time-consuming and inconvenient.

Insurance often covers only a small part of the cost of treatment

Health insurance usually covers some but often does not reimburse all components of our treatments. To date, medical insurance usually covers diagnostic and routine office visits but is spotty or low in its reimbursement of relaxation training and physical therapy for pelvic pain.

Our treatment does not help everybody

While we believe that our treatment is by far the best method to resolve chronic pelvic pain syndromes in general, our treatment does not help everybody.

The only way to know the effectiveness of treatment is to do it

The full effectiveness of our protocol for an individual cannot be known until after it is actually done and the effects are evaluated. We always evaluate the appropriateness of our treatment according to a patient's symptoms and recommend it after a urologic evaluation when it is clear that there is no gross pathology and according to our experience, the patient is likely to benefit. In other words even if you fit our criteria as an appropriate candidate and we believe you are likely to significantly benefit from our protocol, there is no way of determining the exact level of effectiveness of our treatment for you until you do it earnestly and observe the results.

The pros

Our treatment does not use medication, surgery, or invasive procedures

Our approach does not use drugs or surgery or invasive procedures. In fact our goal is to help patients off of all drugs. Every patient is examined with a traditional urologic work up, and disorders of infection, obstruction, or neurological abnormality are treated appropriately.

No known significant side effects

To our knowledge, no one we have seen has suffered any sustained side effects from our treatment. Patients often experience pain, especially at the beginning of the physical therapy part of treatment. This pain, however, tends to diminish as therapy proceeds.

The purpose of our clinics is to make you independent of doctors and health professionals – the majority of treatment is done at home

We teach you how to help yourself. Both in the relaxation training and the physical therapy, we act as consultants, and you are the one responsible for doing the treatment. While a partner is not necessary for the success of our protocol, whenever possible we enlist the help of a partner. Typically, if a partner is willing, he or she will come in at the beginning sessions of *Trigger Point Release* and will be instructed in how to administer the *Trigger Point Release* at home. This helps reduce cost and the inconvenience of having to come to the doctor's or therapist's office as frequently. When someone does not have a partner and there are trigger points that they cannot deactivate themselves, we encourage patients to enlist the services of a physical therapist or doctor from time to time for the specific purpose of deactivating those trigger points and releasing those areas of restriction.

Our protocol can help a select group of patients significantly reduce their symptoms or become symptom-free

The most important benefit is that our protocol has the real possibility of helping selected individuals with muscle related pelvic pain significantly reduce their symptoms or essentially become symptom-free. Because pelvic pain tends to reoccur under periods of stress, our protocol gives the patients the tools that empower them to help resolve their own symptoms. This is of great value. Furthermore, as symptoms reduce, a continued improvement in symptoms tends to be ongoing with many patients if they sincerely comply with the protocol and competently manage their response to stress.

Our values and assumptions in the treatment of pelvic pain

1. Above all, do no harm
2. Help our patients by putting them beyond the need for our help
3. Wisdom is recognizing that change is easier than suffering
4. Eagerness and earnestness make the possibility of our protocol helping you most likely
5. Action is the proof of earnestness
6. Faith and belief is not necessary in doing our protocol—daily practice of our protocol is essential
7. It is what you do that counts. The only way to know the extent to which our protocol can help you is by doing it and seeing the results
8. Pelvic pain didn't start overnight and it doesn't go away overnight
9. Resolving muscle related pelvic pain ultimately is an *inside* job
10. The aspiration to become friendly with fear, discomfort and tension makes our protocol most likely to work.

CHAPTER 4

THE WISE-ANDERSON PROTOCOL: PARADOXICAL RELAXATION AND TRIGGER POINT RELEASE

The protocol in this book was originally called the *Wise-Anderson Protocol* in the first edition of this book published in 2003. It became popularly known on the internet as the *Stanford Protocol* because it was developed in the department of Urology at Stanford University. In this book, the *Wise-Anderson Protocol* and the term *Stanford Protocol,* when it is used, refer to the identical treatment for pelvic pain.

It is not uncommon for people inquiring as to whether the *Wise-Anderson Protocol* can help them with their pain and dysfunction, to be unclear about the exact nature of their diagnosis. People will often complain of seeing numerous doctors who give them different and conflicting diagnoses. We typically see individuals diagnosed with prostatitis, interstitial cystitis, pelvic floor dysfunction, chronic pelvic pain syndrome, levator ani syndrome, urethral syndrome, pelvic floor myalgia, dyspareunia, among others.

The symptoms that the *Wise-Anderson Protocol* may be able to help are listed below. Few people (although some) have all of the following symptoms. Typically, the number of symptoms someone has that the *Wise-Anderson Protocol* can help varies from a few to many of the following:

- Discomfort/aching/pain in the rectum (often described as a "golf ball" in the rectum)
- Sitting that triggers or exacerbates discomfort/pain/symptoms
- Discomfort or flare-up during or hours or a day after orgasm
- Reduced libido (reduced interest in sex)
- Urinary frequency (need to urinate often, usually more than once every two hours)
- Urinary urgency (hard to hold urination once urge occurs)
- Discomfort or pain in the genitals
- Ache/pain/sensitivity of testicles
- Suprapubic discomfort or pain (discomfort/ pain above the pubic bone)
- Perineal discomfort or pain
- Coccygeal discomfort or pain (discomfort/ pain in and around the tailbone)
- Low back discomfort or pain (on one side or both)
- Groin discomfort or pain (on one side or both)
- Dysuria (discomfort or burning during urination)
- Nocturia (frequent urination at night)
- Reduced urinary stream
- Sense of incomplete urination
- Hesitancy before or during urination
- Anxiety about having sex
- Discomfort or relief after a bowel movement

Reading the list above, it is no wonder that patients and physicians arc bewildered and confused as to the nature or treatment required to effectively treat these symptoms.

Introduction to the methodology

- *Paradoxical Relaxation* trains patients how to relax the muscles of the pelvis, how to modify the habit of focusing tension in the pelvic floor under stress, and how to regularly reduce their level of anxiety and nervous system arousal that potentiates the cycle of pain and dysfunction. The skill is developed by repetitive practice of the proper technique.

- Pelvic floor related *Trigger Point Release* is a manual technique of deactivating pain referring trigger points, and stretching, loosening, and lengthening the contracted tissue inside and outside the pelvic floor, thereby enabling it to relax. The technique focuses on trigger points and areas of spasm and constriction related to pelvic pain. Patients are taught to self administer Trigger Point Release inside and outside the pelvic floor.

Once a patient has been diagnosed and considered appropriate for our treatment, he or she begins training in the self-treatment of *Paradoxical Relaxation,* intrapelvic and extrapelvic *Trigger Point Release,* and related myofascial methods.

The practice of *Paradoxical Relaxation* aims to release the grip of pelvic tension and heal the consequences of its chronic state of hypertonicity and irritability. *Paradoxical Relaxation* is often done after *Trigger Point Release* as a way of helping to reacquaint the pelvic floor with extended periods of being in a pain-free and relaxed state. Our goal is to help a patient become skilled in a lifelong practice that allows deep relaxation of the pelvic muscles.

Trigger Point Release aims to help our patients free the muscles in and around their pelvis of active trigger points, and to restore the muscles of the pelvic floor to a flexible, lengthened, soft and supple state. This is done by teaching patients a specialized type of internal and external therapy that deactivates painful trigger points and rehabilitates the soft tissue of the pelvic floor. In this aspect of treatment, a patient is in direct digital contact with the physical sites of the pain and constriction. The purpose of this intervention is to slowly stretch the constricted pelvic tissue to a normal length and level of flexibility. We teach patients to do *Trigger Point Release* on themselves. When there are trigger points or areas of restriction that a patient cannot reach him or her self, a partner or therapist is enlisted for those areas of the body. Our strong emphasis however, is for patients to do as much of the treatment themselves as they can.

It is our view that *when either Paradoxical Relaxation or Trigger Point Release is done without the other, the potential reduction or elimination of most pelvic pain symptoms is substantially reduced.*

Who is appropriate for the methodology?

We determine that someone is an appropriate candidate for our treatment after a thorough diagnostic evaluation. This evaluation is necessary to rule out organic conditions that might be mimicking the symptoms of the conditions we treat. It is essential that we know what we are treating.

One of the goals of the *Wise-Anderson Protocol* is to get patients off of all drugs. This often is not possible at the beginning of treatment. Many patients have been given antibiotics, alpha blockers, muscle relaxants and pain killers. Not infrequently, patients have grown reliant on pain-reducing analgesics in order to cope with their symptoms. *While it is sometimes possible for patients to wean off of these medications before treatment, this is in no way essential.* We now suggest patients remain on their medications and slowly wean off of them, under physician supervision, once their self-treatment begins to reduce their pain.

We have had our best results when we have been able to find trigger points internally and/or externally, or stretch contracted or spastic muscles that tend to recreate some aspect of a patient's symptoms. Determining this is a skill in which few physicians or physical therapists have experience. Determining whether or not someone has trigger points usually requires our evaluation or the evaluation of someone very experienced in *Trigger Point Release* and physical therapy for pelvic pain. In our chapter on *Trigger Point Release*, we describe and show illustrations of the most common trigger points related to pelvic pain.

Some individuals have written us to ask if an unremarkable biofeedback reading rules them out for our protocol. In another section of this book, we have indicated *that a pelvic floor biofeedback reading is an unreliable criterion for determining the appropriateness of our protocol. In other words, a rectal or vaginal biofeedback sensor that indicates a normal amount of tension on any particular machine is not a reason to rule out the appropriateness of our protocol. Pelvic floor electromyographic evaluation of the anal sphincter or the opening of the vagina is one of those medical tests in which a positive finding may be significant and point toward the proper therapy, whereas a negative result does not prove anything.*

In general, we do not believe in the use of narcotic pain medicines because they tend to lower a person's pain threshold and often lead to habituation or addiction. We of course recognize that some individuals' pelvic pain is so great and debilitating that narcotic medication has been the only relief, or partial relief, that they have had. There are patients we have helped who began treatment while taking narcotic medications and have been able to wean themselves off of these medications during the course of their self-treatment.

A strong motivation to do our rigorous protocol is essential to the success of our treatment. If someone is not adequately motivated, it is unlikely that the person will be a good candidate for our work.

Assessing the Symptoms of Our Patients

Below are the forms we use to evaluate people's symptoms before treatment begins. When we are able to follow up with patients using the same forms, these scores allow us to compare the scores over time and to assess a patient's progress. The form is divided into sections on pelvic pain, urinary dysfunction, and sexual difficulties. The *Pelvic Pain Symptom Score* questionnaire used with our *Wise-Anderson Protocol* is a modification of a survey developed by Dr. J. Krieger, and incorporates survey questions from the American Urological Association.

Pelvic Pain Symptom Score Form (Male)

Name _____ Date _____

Over the past month or so, including today, how much were you bothered by:

	Not at all		*Moderate*		*Extreme*
Pain in the lower back	0	1	2	3	4
Pain in the lower abdomen	0	1	2	3	4
Pain during urination	0	1	2	3	4
Pain with bowel movements	0	1	2	3	4
Pain in rectum	0	1	2	3	4
Pain in the prostate gland	0	1	2	3	4
Pain in the testicles	0	1	2	3	4
Pain in the penis	0	1	2	3	4

Number of days experienced pain in the last month _____ days

How bad is the pain on average now?   0 _____ 10

                                   no pain   *worst pain*

Total Pain Score _____

Difficulty postponing urination, hard to hold it (urgency)	0	1	2	3	4
Need to urinate again less than 2 hours after urinating (frequency)	0	1	2	3	4
Number of times urinating at night	0	1	2	3	4
Bladder does not feel completely empty after urinating	0	1	2	3	4
Stopping and starting several times while urinating (intermittency)	0	1	2	3	4
Weak urinary stream	0	1	2	3	4
Having to push or strain to begin urination	0	1	2	3	4

Total Urinary Score _____

Lack of interest in sexual activity	0	1	2	3	4
Difficulty getting an erection	0	1	2	3	4
Difficulty maintaining an erection	0	1	2	3	4
Difficulty reaching an ejaculation	0	1	2	3	4
Pain with ejaculation	0	1	2	3	4
Pain or discomfort after ejaculation	0	1	2	3	4

Total Sexual Score _____

In addition, men also fill out the National Institutes of Health-Chronic Prostatitis Symptom Index as a comparison tool.

Pelvic Pain Symptom Score Form (Female)

Name_____ Date _____

Over the past month or so, including today, how much were you bothered by:

	Not at all		*Moderate*		*Extreme*
Pain in the lower back	0	1	2	3	4
Pain in the lower abdomen	0	1	2	3	4
Pain during urination	0	1	2	3	4
Pain with bowel movements	0	1	2	3	4
Pain in rectum	0	1	2	3	4
Pain in the urethra	0	1	2	3	4
Pain in the vagina	0	1	2	3	4
Pain with menstrual period	0	1	2	3	4
Pain with intercourse	0	1	2	3	4

Number of days experienced pain in the last month _____days

How bad is the pain on average now?　　0 _____ 10

　　　　　　　　　　　　　　　　　　no pain　　　　　*worst pain*

Total Pain Score _____

Urinary urgency/frequency	0	1	2	3	4
Number of times urinating at night	0	1	2	3	4
Difficulty emptying the bladder	0	1	2	3	4

Total Urinary Score _____

An overview of what happens in treatment: the six-day intensive clinic for the *Wise-Anderson Protocol*

We currently offer treatment in the *Wise-Anderson Protocol* through a monthly six-day intensive immersion clinic that is designed for both local and out of town patients. This venue for treating pelvic pain is by far the most effective we have used. In an intensive period of time, its aim is to teach patients the elements of the protocol in order for them to be able to go home and do it on a daily basis.

Originally we treated patients with *Paradoxical Relaxation* and the *Wise-Anderson Protocol Trigger Point Release* in conventional office visits. After initial instruction, patients were given an audiocassette course in *Paradoxical Relaxation* to be used daily at home. Follow-up was provided by regular consultations at Stanford or followed up by telephone or Internet consultations for those who lived at a distance.

The intrapelvic *Trigger Point Release* was originally performed over a number of months in a series of office visits. The typical course of treatment involved ten to forty individual sessions, each lasting between thirty to sixty minutes. Our protocol usually began with two or three physical therapy sessions per week, tapering down as the rehabilitation of the pelvic floor occurred. This form of treatment has all been superseded by training our patients to do all of their own myofacial and trigger point release themselves.

The intensive treatment offered in our six-day program has had side benefits we did not anticipate. Most patients with pelvic pain have never met anyone else with their symptoms or who could relate to their situation. When patients meet others who have been through the same experience with pelvic pain, they often feel relief. Furthermore, the support and interaction between patients at the clinic appears to aid their learning of the protocol. It is a format that may have application for other medical treatments.

Taking ownership of your pelvic pain: like Home Depot we say that 'you can do it and we can help'- The *Wise-Anderson Protocol* is ultimately a do-it-yourself protocol

Home Depot is a home improvement store that has become an institution on the basis of providing the materials and support for people who wish to renovate their home themselves. Whether you want to build bookshelves, tile a bathroom counter top, or frame up a new room on your house, Home Depot sells the tools that enable you to do this. You can buy tile, tile cutters, cement board, grout, bathroom sinks, counter tops, plywood, framing saws, nail guns and air compressors. All of these materials are aimed at giving you the tools to *do-it-yourself.*

There is another way to do home renovation. You go into the yellow pages and look under contractors and find one who will build your bookshelf, tile your counter top, or frame up a new room. You can find a general contractor whom you can hire to do anything you wish to do in your house. All you have to do is agree on what to do and a price and off you go. You don't have to touch a hammer, carry a 2x4, or clean up a speck of saw dust. It is all done for you. This is often the paradigm of *I-don't-know-how-to-do-it-myself* or *I-don't-want-to-do-it-myself.* For various reasons, the *do-it-yourself* paradigm has taken the country by storm. Not only is there the self esteem that comes from the independence of doing it yourself, but the economic savings are considerable in this route toward home improvement

The *Wise-Anderson Protocol* is a *do-it-yourself* protocol. This is in contrast to the conventional kind of medical treatment in which the doctor is the expert and you submit to the doctor's treatment that is done to you or done with you as a relatively passive recipient of it. This is our conditioning. Something is wrong with our body or we are worried that something is, we go to the doctor and say "is there anything wrong?" If there is, we are used to having the doctor give us medicine or do a procedure or surgery to fix it. This is simply what we have grown up with and almost everyone with pelvic pain has gone down this route in an attempt to resolve their symptoms.

Almost without exception, those who come to see us for treatment have taken multiple drugs. The less fortunate have undergone surgical procedures. For almost all who have come to see us, the drugs and surgeries have failed. Active participation of the patient in his or her treatment is essential to our protocol. The ownership of the problem must be assumed by the patient. Can the dental hygienist keep your teeth clean? She can do a cleaning and show you how to keep your teeth clean, but she can't follow you around in your life to keep your teeth clean. You have to be the one to take that responsibility.

Similarly, in our view, the practitioner you see for pelvic pain, be it a doctor or psychologist or physical therapist, cannot fix the pelvic pain. Like your teeth, you must be responsible for keeping your teeth, clean unless you hire your dental hygienist to follow you around and clean your teeth once or twice a day. Beyond this absurd idea, it's up to you. Dealing with a pelvic floor that habitually tightens is similar. You must learn to quiet down your nervous system regularly and stop tightening up the pelvis. We have found that the repetitive daily self-treatment of pelvic floor relaxation and internal and external *Trigger Point Release*, and the use of myofascial release methods done by the patient on him or herself, is by far the most effect way to rehabilitate the pelvic floor.

Most people who attend our clinic who do well with our protocol, undergo a shift away from the idea that the doctor or psychologist or physical therapist is the person who is the source of their salvation from pelvic pain. Our message is very clear. For the most part, you the patient are the best practitioner to help yourself with your pelvic pain. You must take ownership of the problem and the solution. You must do it. And we show you how.

We have discovered that the best way to do our protocol is in the form of a six-day intensive clinic which we do monthly. In our 6-day intensive clinics, patients immerse themselves in the protocol. Patients learn the relaxation protocol more easily and more thoroughly, having many hours to experience the method, deal with the difficulties that normally arise and have their questions cleared up. Absence from their regular life and routine often provides an opportunity for the nervous system to significantly quiet down although this initial quieting is only the beginning.

The physical therapist in our clinic has an opportunity to see the patient daily, to follow up on what transpired in the session the day earlier, and to go into a depth of exploration of the pelvic floor that is often not possible in a single weekly office visit. *Most important, we have the luxury of time to teach the internal and external self-treatment protocol and make sure patients are practiced and competent in it.*

In the past, when someone has had a willing partner, we taught the partner how to perform the *Trigger Point Release*. With patients learning their own physical therapy self treatment, a partner is not essential for our treatment to be successful.

Our Purpose is to Make a Pain-Free State the Normal State

Tissue memory: nerves, muscles, and blood vessels adapt to their situation

Researchers in the area of pain have tried to understand why pain becomes chronic even in the absence of any objective physical findings. The explanation that is emerging revolves around the idea that the tissues themselves have memory and can 'remember' and recreate the pain even when the original source of it has gone away.

We see the evidence of tissue memory in our work with pelvic pain and dysfunction. Earlier we discussed some patients with pain and dysfunction from interstitial cystitis who opted for surgery to have their bladders removed. Choosing such a radical approach was based on the idea that if the source of the pain was removed, which presumably was the bladder, the pain would be gone. Unfortunately, after surgery, the pain remained unabated in these patients.

From the point of view of tissue memory, we might say that the bladder originally may have been one of the sources (along with the pelvic floor) of the pain. The nerves, muscles, and blood vessels that connected to the bladder may have "remembered" the pain circuits even when the bladder was removed. The removal of the bladder did not address the tissue memory that participated in and enabled the pain in the first place, nor did it in any way address pelvic floor pain.

Adapting to chronic pain

No one with pelvic pain and dysfunction says that their symptoms feel comfortable or normal. However, it may be that your body has adapted to your pain and dysfunction as a normal state. In other words, your pelvic pain and dysfunction at a certain level may become 'home' and a place that feels stable.

Repetition is the mother of retention

It is often the case that patients will experience significant relief from symptoms after both *Paradoxical Relaxation* and *Trigger Point Release*. This relief is often brief, with symptoms re-emerging after hours or days. In our view, the 'normal' setting was shifted from one of pain to one of less or no pain. This setting needs to be reestablished as 'normal' by repeating treatment over and over again. *One purpose of Paradoxical Relaxation and Trigger Point Release is to retrain the nerves, muscles, and blood vessels so that freedom from pain and dysfunction feels like home.*

An example: getting used to not stuttering

In 1971 Dr. Martin Schwartz, professor of speech science, department of surgery at New York University, noted spasms of the vocal cords in a patient who stuttered during blocked efforts at speaking. When she was able to speak again, her vocal cords slightly relaxed, enough for air to pass through and vibrate them. This insight led him to a new treatment for stuttering that allowed most stutterers using his method to stop stuttering within a few minutes. Success was achieved by learning a simple respiratory maneuver that prevented the vocal cords from locking immediately prior to speaking.

The biggest challenge to stopping stuttering, Schwartz reported, was changing the stutterer's unconscious resistance to not stuttering. For stutterers, stuttering is known territory. Though uncomfortable and dysfunctional, stuttering and everything associated with it is familiar and known. As one stutterer reported to Dr. Schwartz, "I don't stutter now, but my problem is not knowing how to talk to people."

A dysfunctional state can become home. Fluent speech, to the unconscious mind and highly practiced conditioning of the stutterer, can feel destabilizing and threatening.

Schwarz states "Give them effective techniques, have them practice the techniques regularly so they become semi-automatic, and then take them through a hierarchy of situations graded with respect to stress, moving from initially low stress to increasingly greater degrees of stress." The Schwartz method enables stutterers to overcome their anticipatory fear that drove their stuttering. It is a method that enables many stutterers to make fluency feel like "home."

Paradoxical Relaxation and the Profound Relaxation of the Pelvic Floor

The aim of *Paradoxical Relaxation*

People with chronic pelvic pain have a tendency to focus tension in the pelvic floor under stress. Over time this focus of tension shortens the pelvic muscles and makes an inhospitable environment for the muscles, nerves, tissues, and structures involved in the pelvic floor. This inhospitable environment contributes to the symptoms we normally associate with chronic pelvic pain.

The shortened state of the muscles inside the pelvic floor does not allow for normal relaxation, flexibility and function of the tissue. *Trigger Point Release* is necessary to unknot the pelvis and deactivate the pain-referring trigger points and to loosen the constricted muscles, making it possible for them to relax.

One aim of *Paradoxical Relaxation,* therefore, is to change the habit of automatically tensing the pelvic floor. The relaxation of the pelvic muscles helps to create the essential healing necessary for the irritated nerves, tissues, and structures of the pelvic floor. The repetitive relaxation of the pelvic floor allows for the regeneration of tissue, proper oxygenation, nutrition, and waste management of the tissues. Regularly quieting the autonomic nervous system helps the pelvic muscles get used to no pain or dysfunction as the normal state, and to reduce trigger point sensitivity.

It is not obvious how to begin to teach individuals to relax when they are in pain. Without any training, people in pain clearly have difficulty relaxing. They remain tense as the body tries to guard itself against the pain. This is understandable, even natural, but in the long run, it is not helpful. *In the Wise-Anderson Protocol, Trigger Point Release helps to restore the length and suppleness of the contracted pelvic tissue so that it has the capacity to remain relaxed using Paradoxical Relaxation described here.*

Soft tissue of the pelvic floor must remain soft in one's life to be out of pain

The pain and dysfunction in the conditions we are describing in this book derive from the contracted state of *soft tissue*. Temporarily releasing this *soft tissue* while not changing the habit of inappropriately tightening it, tends not to be effective in the long term. *Paradoxical Relaxation* is the practice of regularly restoring the pelvic floor to a pain free state. *Soft tissue* of the pelvic floor must remain soft in one's life to be out of pain.

When you are relaxing while you are in pain, a realistic goal is to subtract tension and discomfort rather than aiming to entirely eliminate it. Having realistic goals is important in undergoing the *Wise-Anderson Protocol*. In this section, we will discuss the origins of *Paradoxical Relaxation* and the details of its technique.

Origins of *Paradoxical Relaxation*: the work of Edmund Jacobson

The foundation of *Paradoxical Relaxation* began about 100 years ago with the work of Dr. Edmund Jacobson. Jacobson is considered the father of relaxation therapy in the United States and his method of *Progressive Relaxation* has been used in one form or another throughout most of the twentieth century. Over the years, many research studies have been done on the effect of *Progressive Relaxation* on conditions varying from constipation to ringing in the ears. Despite much misunderstanding about *Progressive Relaxation*, even by professionals who use it, Jacobson's method has stood the test of time.

Jacobson was born in 1888 to a middle class family in Chicago. A brilliant student, he graduated from Northwestern University in two years. At the age of 18 he attended Harvard University where he was the youngest at that time to receive a Ph.D. in psychology. He taught physiology at the University of Chicago and later went to Rush Medical College where he received a degree as a Doctor of Medicine.

Jacobson related that when he was eight years old, a fire broke out at an apartment house owned by his parents in turn of the century Chicago. Tragically, a close friend of his parents was killed in the blaze and his parents became distraught and hysterical over this shocking loss.

The level of his parents' upset deeply disturbed the young Jacobson. He reported later in his life that at the time of the fire, he vowed never to get upset the way his parents had gotten upset. This desire to remain calm and relaxed stayed with him through adolescence.

Later, when dealing with his insomnia as an undergraduate at Harvard, he began to experiment with his own methods of relaxation. As he developed a technique that allowed him to go to sleep, he chose to write his Ph.D. dissertation on an experiment showing that tense subjects responded acutely to a stressor (two metal bars clanging), while subjects trained in relaxation hardly reacted at all.

Jacobson was the master of his method. A newspaper reporter who interviewed Jacobson toward the end of his life wrote that she acutely felt the level of her own nervousness through the mirror of being around such a profoundly calm man. It was his ability to relax deeply and reduce his metabolic requirements for oxygen that allowed him to stay underwater for several minutes.

When he demonstrated his relaxation method in front of students, he was able to relax so deeply in a minute or two that he looked like a corpse because the only muscles that had any appreciable tension were the muscles required for the functioning of his heart and for respiration. Perhaps the greatest demonstration of his mastery of relaxation was his long life of 95 years, especially in light of the fact that both his parents had died at relatively young ages.

Jacobson's life was devoted to applying the principles he developed to the treatment of many psychosomatic disorders. In 1924, he treated women with *globus hystericus*, a condition in which the patient feels that there is something stuck in the throat. Jacobson documented the narrowing of the esophagus in this condition by capturing images of the esophagus with a fluoroscope. He then trained these patients in *Progressive Relaxation* and fluoroscoped the esophagus after the relaxation training. Not only were the subjective symptoms resolved, but the fluoroscopic images verified a widening of the constricted portions of the esophagus.

For the next 60 years, the conditions Jacobson successfully treated included hypertension, spastic esophagus, spastic colon, headache, functional cardiac disorders like heart palpitation and arrhythmia, as well as the gamut of psychological disorders including anxiety disorders, depression, and mania. He documented the success of his treatment in the many studies he published. What is perhaps more remarkable is that Jacobson proposed the link between stress and illness many decades before it became fashionable. It is also remarkable that he actually treated patients and conducted scientific research on the subject at a time where there was very little interest and awareness on the relationship between body and mind.

In the mid-1940s, Jacobson wanted to develop a machine that would be able to independently verify the efficacy of his method. There were no reliable independent findings that could indicate whether someone was relaxed or whether there was any change in their level of relaxation as the result of Jacobson's intervention.

In conjunction with Bell Telephone Laboratories, he developed the first *electromyograph*, an instrument able to detect electrical activity in muscles with a sensitivity of up to one millionth of a volt. With this machine, the formerly undetectable physiologic effects could be easily and scientifically demonstrated. The *electromyograph* could *objectively verify* whether someone was tense or relaxed and the extent to which *Progressive Relaxation* had an effect.

Although the *electromyograph* formed the basis of the first biofeedback machine, Jacobson was never interested in incorporating the technological wonder he created as a tool in the clinical setting. He took a position that one could not learn to relax while looking at a meter or listening to a tone. He felt that the very act of looking or listening was tension producing and interfered with dropping into the profound states of relaxation for which he was aiming.

Progressive Relaxation is not about contracting and relaxing muscles

Progressive Relaxation is best known for its instruction to contract and relax muscles at the beginning of relaxation. In fact, many practitioners who have not understood *Progressive Relaxation* have thought that it simply involves voluntarily tightening and then relaxing muscles as a way of promoting relaxation in the muscles. This is a fundamental misunderstanding.

Jacobson was clear that his instruction to tense and then relax a muscle was intended to only highlight tension so that the patient could consciously recognize how it felt. *The ability to recognize subtle degrees of tension is a master skill in Progressive Relaxation.* The most difficult patients to treat are those who report that they feel very little or no tension, even though they have obvious tension by objective measures.

The contract/relax instruction in large part was meant to help patients who were out of touch with their bodies to become re-acquainted with sensations of tension. *The intention of contraction and relaxation was never to fatigue the muscle or to do anything to it to make it relax. Instead, its purpose was to help recreate tension in order to become aware of subtle tension that remains after one voluntarily relaxes.* This tension, which Jacobson called *residual tension*, was the most important tension to release. Releasing residual tension ultimately produces the most profound relaxation.

Jacobson's main work was described in his book *Progressive Relaxation*, first published in 1929, and then revised in 1939. Throughout his lifetime he wrote books and published many articles. He was quick to point out that *Progressive Relaxation* was fundamentally different from hypnosis or psychoanalysis which were popular during his time. He had little respect for either of them. *Progressive Relaxation*, Jacobson contended, did not operate in an altered state or because of transference or suggestion but in a conscious, *unaltered* state and where transference was not a factor in its effect.

One of the main points he made throughout his life was that 'the mind' was not simply found in the brain but in the peripheral muscles and nerves as well. This was the point he made in his last book, *The Human Mind*. One of the ways he demonstrated this point was by hooking subjects up to an electromyograph and asking them to imagine riding a bicycle. He found that when the subject imagined riding a bicycle, simultaneously the parts of the body involved in riding a bicycle including the hands, arms, feet and legs, subtly contracted as if the subject were actually riding. Understanding that the mind was also in the muscles of the body enabled him to control the mind by relaxing the muscles.

He introduced the then radical idea, which he demonstrated and validated objectively in his work with the relaxation of the gastrointestinal tract, that the arousal of the autonomic nervous system, long thought to be out of one's control, could be controlled voluntarily. This was a startling insight at the time.

The key to profound relaxation: the relaxation of the eyes and speech muscles

Perhaps Jacobson's greatest insight came from his discovery that visualization, as well as conceptual and abstract thinking, are always accompanied by small muscle movements of the eyes and apparatus of speech. He found that when you picture an apple in your mind, your eyes actually move and focus as if they were looking at an apple in real life. Similarly, the speech muscles, including the lips, tongue, jaw, and throat move slightly when you think in words and sentences.

The significance of this insight may escape you unless you realize that *it was Jacobson's goal to learn how to relax the muscles of the eyes and the speech apparatus as a way of stopping thought.* This quiet state of mind allows for the body to relax very deeply. The idea that you can quiet the mind by relaxing the muscles of vision and speech has been almost entirely overlooked by medicine and psychology.

As an example of the clinical usefulness of his insight, Jacobson had a patient who obsessively thought about killing her child. This obsession profoundly disturbed the woman who went to different doctors in search of help. Jacobson worked with her by helping her examine what position her eyes were in when she had this obsessive thought. He then taught her to relax her eyes and let go of inwardly looking at this image. Over time she was able to stop this obsessive thought by simply relaxing her eyes when her mind went to it. This ability to control her mind resulted in the restoration of her good mood as well as a rise in self-esteem, confidence, and long term relief from the anxiety and obsession. This *positive feedback loop* is what benefits many people who become competent in *Progressive Relaxation*.

Quieting the eyes to stop visualization and quieting the speech muscles to stop 'inner talk'

Jacobson's discovery that relaxing the eyes and speech muscles could stop thinking is a master skill. Over the centuries, the world's major wisdom traditions have understood that the noisy and discursive mind blocks the experience of one's own unconditioned nature and sense of cosmic union. Certain ancient Yogic, Taoist and other esoteric meditation traditions have focused on the relaxation of the eyes and the speech muscles as a necessary preparation for accessing the deepest meditational states.

Jacobson's discovery is as simple as it is profound. One aspect of visualization is muscle activity in which the eyes focus as if they were looking at an object even though the eyes are closed. Visualization, therefore, is not only a 'mental' activity somehow separated from the body, but involves corresponding physical responses. Similarly, Jacobson found that during the process of thinking there are slight movements of the speech muscles, which could be called thinking-associated subvocalization. Thus, thinking is a form of talking involving subtle movements of the lips, tongue, throat, and vocal cords.

When you relax the eyes and speech muscles, you relax profoundly

The human organism is designed to adapt and respond to constantly changing circumstances in order to survive. All of these responses involve some degree of muscle tension. When we learn to still the mind and body and quiet the impulse to respond, we can profoundly relax and rest deeply.

We see the evidence of this in the deep rest that occurs with non-REM (non rapid eye movement) sleep (or dreamless sleep). Rapid eye movement sleep is an important aspect of the sleep cycle and indicates that the person sleeping is dreaming or having visual images while sleeping. Non-REM sleep, however, is the most restful and restorative. The most profound, restful kind of sleep occurs when there are no visual images or dreams as indicated in the absence of rapid eye movement. Absence of thought in *either* the sleeping or waking state is indicative of a state of the deepest rest.

If we have no thoughts going on in awareness, except in moments of immediate threat, there is no triggering the body's 'emergency responses' to brace and protect itself. *A profoundly quiet mind means that there is no issue about survival in that moment.*

Peace of mind means no thinking

We normally think about peace of mind as a lofty and ongoing state of the old and the wise. Jacobson made the understanding of 'peace of mind' comprehensible, practical and attainable. Peace of mind means a quiet mind with no thoughts. Peace of mind allows you to relax and allows your emergency center to put the "all clear" message out. Peace of mind stops the rise of adrenalin and other stress response hormones in your blood stream allowing the body to be at peace.

The relaxation of the eyes and speech muscles is the advanced practice of Progressive Relaxation

Before you can discern the activities of your eyes and of your muscles of speech, you must learn to relax the body as a whole. Once you have established a certain level of bodily quiet, it is easier to pay attention to the subtle, easily missed stream of pictures and thoughts that cross through your mind. As you become able to witness these pictures and thoughts, you can begin the subtle practice of 'letting go of inner looking and inner talking.'

Most patients can relax the body sufficiently to reduce or stop pelvic pain and dysfunction without training in the relaxation of the eyes and speech muscles. There are some, however, who cannot become sufficiently quiet without learning this advanced skill.

Paradoxical Relaxation developed from Jacobson's work

Relaxation of muscles and quieting of the nervous system is an effect of feeling safe. In the practice of *Paradoxical Relaxation,* this state of safety is achieved by learning to direct your attention towards accepting tension, relaxing the muscles, and stilling thoughts that trigger survival responses.

All methods of relaxation direct your attention. Some methods direct your attention to pleasing scenes. Others ask you to relax or warm your body. Jacobson asked patients to lie down and instructed them to 'discontinue effort' or 'go negative' as a way of telling them what to do with their attention in order to relax. It was the mastery of his own method that gave him such charisma and influence in the field of relaxation and autonomic self-regulation. However, his language was from the nineteenth century, and it is not the most useful language to communicate what we know in the twenty-first.

Jacobson tended to be brusque and patriarchal, telling his patients what to do without offering any reassurance or softness in style. In fact the very title of his book, the only one currently in print, *You Must Relax*, demonstrates the limitations of his language in communicating his insights about relaxation. Furthermore, as we have mentioned, Jacobson wanted to make sure that no one confused the success of his method with hypnosis, transference or the giving of reassurance, or because of a placebo effect. When he taught *Progressive Relaxation* to professionals, he was adamant that it was wrong for the teacher of *Progressive Relaxation* to offer any reassurance to the patient. He felt the results of relaxation should be their own reassurance. While his own view represented his high level of integrity and faith in the effectiveness of his method, instructions in relaxation associated with these considerations can be off-putting.

Finally, because Jacobson was very concerned that his method might be regarded as some offshoot of yoga, meditation, or spiritualism, his language tended to be mechanistic and rigorously conforming to the scientific and objective language of his peers. This language was sometimes not helpful, instructive or accessible to those reading his work.

During Jacobson's time, the prevailing religion was science, and any hint that a method was spiritual or mystical made the method suspect among the illuminati of the time. Jacobson shunned any hint that his method bore any relationship to so called spiritual practices. In truth, the method of *Progressive Relaxation* is in the finest tradition of the world's wisdom practices.

There was little understanding during Jacobson's time of the healing potential of acupuncture, chi gung, yoga, and meditation. This is in contrast to the present when the efficacy of these and other similar methods is even documented in the scientific literature.

We have modified the technique of *Progressive Relaxation* to make it more accessible to the modern era. We use a different language to communicate its insights and methodologies to relax the muscles of the pelvic floor. Importantly, we have specifically modified the method to help someone relax in the presence of pain. *This modification of Progressive Relaxation is what we call Paradoxical Relaxation.* Just as the modern car stands on the shoulders of the Model T, so *Paradoxical Relaxation* stands on the shoulders of *Progressive Relaxation*.

Medical monitoring in the practice of *Paradoxical Relaxation*

Occasionally patients may have a condition requiring medical monitoring. If you have high blood pressure, asthma, or epilepsy, you should inform the doctor who is teaching you *Paradoxical Relaxation*, as medications may need to be adjusted as you become more relaxed. For example, if someone has high blood pressure and continues the regular dose of antihypertensive medicine while more and more deeply relaxing, the medication may prove to be too strong for the improved state of relaxation and will need to be reduced.

What is paradoxical about *Paradoxical Relaxation*?

A paradox is a statement that seems to contradict itself, but nevertheless is true. Examples of paradoxes tend to be found in philosophical writings. For example, the premise of Alcoholics Anonymous is that you can only gain control over the addiction to alcohol by admitting you are powerless over it. In *A Course in Miracles* it says, *to have, give all to all* which means that if you want something for yourself, give everything you have away. In Zen, Suzuki Roshi, a renowned Zen master wrote that *if you want a horse to be close to you, give it a big pasture.*

The paradox of *Paradoxical Relaxation* is as follows: accepting tension, relaxes it. As Jacobson correctly understood, relaxation has to do with letting go of effort. *Letting go of effort* means letting go of 'doing' anything. Muscle tension generally is involved, at some level, in 'doing something.' This 'doing something' involves all actions we do in our life from riding a bicycle to cutting carrots. This 'doing something' may involve issues of survival, like bracing to prepare for a blow, tensing in preparation for flight, or contraction of the muscles in preparing to attack. 'Doing something' is intimately a part of muscle tension, even when you're lying down. You can call this 'doing something' when you're lying down, "micro-efforting." The relaxation of these micro-efforts is the focus of *Paradoxical Relaxation*. We discuss this in detail in the next chapter.

If we tell you to relax, your mind will probably interpret this instruction being asked to 'do' something or make some effort, when in fact, relaxation means discontinuing effort. Relaxation means the a*bsence of* doing. What a peculiar idea the 'absence of doing' is. What does it mean to 'not do?'

The state of relaxation that occurs when the pelvic floor is relaxed is a state of *being*. It contains no action or volition. Notice how it feels if someone tells you to, 'be.' You may find such an instruction disconcerting because generally speaking you can't do anything to 'be.'

Relaxation and being are not states that you can make happen. *The closest one can get to telling someone how to relax, we have discovered, is to ask them to be present with their current and immediate state without trying to change it. Our relaxation curriculum involves pointing the way to being effortless in relationship to tension and pain. Hence we discover that when we step back and feel and accept our tension with no intention to do anything about it, after awhile, relaxation occurs.* Notice that we say *relaxation occurs* instead of saying *you relax yourself.* Relaxation *occurs* as a natural consequence of letting go of doing. *You can't make yourself relax.*

When you accept something, you no longer exert effort in relationship to it. You let it be. When you accept your tension, you stop all conscious effort in relationship to it. This is another way of saying you relax it. This identity between the acceptance of tension, and the cessation of effort in relationship to tension, is the seminal insight of *Paradoxical Relaxation.* In other words, the way to relax tension is to accept it.

Hariwansh Lal Poonja once said that what is *not* the state of being has been eloquently described, but *what is* the state of being has never been described. So it is with words aimed at directing someone to relax a painful pelvis. You can say that relaxation is the cessation of doing anything, or trying, but there are few ways to explain exactly what it is. *Paradoxical Relaxation* borrows from this perennial wisdom that you let go of effort by fully accepting it the way it is.

Understanding the method of *Paradoxical Relaxation*

The aim of Paradoxical Relaxation is to be able to allow your body to rest deeply and allow tissue restoration and rebuilding. Its aim is to help allow your pelvis to heal from the chronic irritation of its tensed and shortened muscles and the effect of these muscles on the structures, nerves, and tissues within the pelvis. Paradoxical Relaxation is most effectively used in conjunction with the intrapelvic Trigger Point

Release in the same way that Trigger Point Release is most effective when used together with Paradoxical Relaxation.

There are pitfalls that students of *Paradoxical Relaxation* can encounter, of which they are often unaware. Similarly, the interior of the pelvis is not an area that someone untrained in its anatomy and physiology should enter into without the close supervision of an experienced professional. The information we share here is educational. Our protocol is not intended to be a how-to method that one can use by reading this book in the absence of competent instruction.

A fifty-five year old surgeon came to us for treatment after suffering with chronic pelvic pain syndrome for over thirty years. He was a strong and determined man who was used to doing something concrete and seeing the immediate results of his efforts.

When we first began our instruction in *Paradoxical Relaxation,* he asked us how the seemingly innocuous instructions, aimed at helping him relax his pelvic muscles, could possibly make a dent in a condition that he felt had been ruining his life. His incredulity about the effects of relaxation on his condition had to be addressed so that he could practice it wholeheartedly.

Modern medical treatment will use needles, pills, creams, or scalpels against offending parts as a way of making them normal again. The idea that practicing a shift in attention onto a part of the body that is tense, and then accepting that tension, is a radical departure from the conventional medical methods.

Chronic tension eventually feels normal

When you learn *Paradoxical Relaxation,* you focus on detecting subtle sensations of effort in your body. These sensations are unremarkable, and if someone did not tell you to pay attention to them you probably wouldn't give them any notice. Learning to relax means paying attention to the small and unremarkable efforts to which we normally pay no attention. In fact, these tensions usually feel normal.

A patient told us a story which illustrated the process of how tension can become what one feels to be normal. As a teenager, he went to summer camp with an odd fellow who found a pair of thick black glasses that contained no lenses. At the beginning of camp, our patient recalled, this odd fellow wore these glasses despite the disparaging and perplexed comments of other children. People told this fellow that he looked strange and asked him why he chose to wear glasses without lenses. The fellow shrugged and did not respond to the comments of others. Instead, he wore them day and night throughout the course of the summer. Eventually, people got used to him and his glasses. We can get used to almost anything.

Toward the end of the summer this fellow lost the glasses. Our patient remarked how strange it was that the very people, who disparaged these glasses at the beginning of the summer, asked this fellow what had become of his glasses toward the end of the summer. These glasses had become part of the identity of this odd fellow, and as strange as it was to others when he began wearing them, it was equally strange when he stopped.

Relearning to let go of effort

We have described how the body gets used to chronic tension in the pelvic floor. Like the glasses of this fellow, *you can get used to your chronic tension and effort*. Learning to relax requires that you be aware of your chronic states of tension. If you are not aware of this tension, it will tend to remain with you. The first step of *Paradoxical Relaxation* involves paying attention to subtle degrees of tension that normally you would give no mind to. Learning to feel and rest with this subtle tension usually makes it is possible to relax the pelvic floor profoundly.

When you fail to be able to relax, you usually miss the essential point that letting go of effort means accepting your unconscious refusal to let go. Letting go of effort means ceasing the attempt to change tension that doesn't easily let go.

Relearning to come back into your body

Imagine you are given a luxurious two-hour massage in an elegant European spa. The room in which the massage takes place is soft, comfortably warm, and beautifully appointed. The masseuse is sensitive and knows what muscles allow for the easing of your tension. There are no distractions or discomforts. However, in order to fully enjoy this experience, your attention must be on the massage, not elsewhere. Your attention must be in your body or you miss the experience.

If there are areas of discomfort in the body, we tend to avoid them. This is true for pelvic pain. Your attention tends to want to focus anywhere but on the discomfort. We are programmed to pursue pleasure and avoid pain. The practice of *Paradoxical Relaxation* requires that you direct your attention back into your body even if it is initially uncomfortable to do so.

Paradoxical Relaxation and insomnia

Added to the distress of chronic pain and dysfunction, people who suffer from chronic pelvic pain commonly struggle with insomnia. Whether it is anxiety, continual pain, or nocturnal urinary frequency and urgency, many of our patients describe the havoc of being awakened several times during the night, not being able to fall back to sleep, and not getting a good night's rest.

Edmund Jacobson remarked that the quality of relaxation during the day tends to determine the quality of sleep at night. In our experience, the same is true for chronic pelvic pain. *Paradoxical Relaxation* helps with both the difficulty of falling asleep as well as with the difficulty of going back to sleep after one has awakened. Until all symptoms are *substantially* reduced, however, a good night's sleep can remain problematic.

Falling asleep tends to be easier to solve than going back to sleep, but we can help our patients with both difficulties. The help that

Paradoxical Relaxation can offer in falling asleep is simple. If you have any facility in *Paradoxical Relaxation*, there is usually a high likelihood that doing this relaxation will enable you to fall asleep.

Going back to sleep after waking up in the middle of the night

Going to sleep with pain often makes going to sleep difficult. Waking up in the middle of the night in pain is always difficult. Not infrequently, in the midst of trying to get back to sleep, there is additional anxiety about having awakened early and becoming sleep-deprived. It is a period of time that can be quite distressing. In this section we will discuss a strategy for going back to sleep after you have woken up anxious and in pain

Using your early morning cortisol rush as your muse

The word 'muse' was originally used in 1374 to mean protectors of the arts, from the Greek mousa meaning muse, music, and song. Muse is generally thought of as that which inspires inspiration. We offer here the unlikely idea that if you wake up anxious in the morning, you can use that as your muse for getting things done, especially in matters involving creativity. This time of anxious early morning awakening can also be used to do the physical therapy portion of our protocol. Following the constructive use of this early morning state, using Paradoxical Relaxation can be most effective to go back to sleep.

Cortisol is a neurochemical and hormone essential to the proper function of the body. Cortisol is produced by the adrenal glands and is often referred to as the "stress hormone" as it is secreted in times of stress and anxiety. It functions to increase blood sugar and stores of sugar in the liver as glycogen. In doing so, it temporarily puts the immune function on hold. While there is normally an increase in cortisol in the morning, in a study we did at Stanford we found that men with pelvic pain had much higher levels of morning cortisol compared to men without pain.

Think of your early morning cortisol rush as a gift of 1½ hours of strong energy

The early morning cortisol peaking time can be intensely energetic. It can enable sustained and energetic focus. Some people do their best work during this time, when the most of the world is still asleep and they are undisturbed.

While waking up anxious is no fun, as with everything in life, it is the viewpoint you have about cortisol-driven wakefulness that is more important than the wakefulness itself. If you wake up anxious in the morning, we suggest that you consider looking at this 1½ hour period (this is usually how long the cortisol rush lasts) as a gift of strong energy. It can be used proactively and productively in your life. Also, using this energy can dissipate it constructively and clear the way for the nervous system to be able to go back to sleep more easily.

If you find yourself typically waking up anxious early in the morning, we suggest you consider accepting it and factoring it into your day. You may wish to go to bed a little earlier to make up for this time. In doing this, the early morning time can be a time that is appreciated rather than dreaded.

In other words, one of the best and most productive strategies we suggest for dealing with early morning anxiety and unwanted wakefulness is to 'spend' this energy on work or self treatment in the midst of the cortisol flurry. You can work on a report, paint a picture, write a story or involve yourself in some other project or creative enterprise. You can do stretching, trigger point release and other aspects of our home physical therapy self treatment. You can also clean the house.

Journaling in the early morning

Some of our patients 'journal' when they bring themselves to wakefulness in the midst of the early morning cortisol rush. Journaling is a modern term for keeping a diary. When you journal, you keep a file in your computer or have a special book dedicated to writing down whatever you feel like writing. When people keep journals, they usually write down what they are thinking or feeling about what is most pressing in their minds.

In a journal, you usually practice introspection, that is to say you bring your attention inside and in a certain sense share with yourself what is most intimate and often troubling. You can think of keeping a journal as an ongoing letter to the most trusted of friends, sharing what is going on in your life and your heart. In a journal you share your thoughts and feelings about conflicts, concerns, worries, hopes, projects, and relationships in your life —whatever you would want to share with your most trusted confidante. It is often possible to process and resolve what is troubling your heart and mind when you write in a journal.

Journaling is a way of transferring thoughts and feelings that can go around and around inside of you to paper or pages on a computer monitor. In transferring these thoughts and feelings, difficulties can be evaluated and considered in a way that is not possible unless they are externalized and considered in a safe and unhurried environment. Aside from exploring feelings and thoughts, journaling can simply be a practice in writing down your stream of consciousness—whatever comes into your head. Journaling is an excellent activity during the early morning cortisol rush.

After an hour and a half or so of whatever kinds of activity work best for you, the cortisol driven early morning anxiety state tends to abate and you can use Paradoxical Relaxation to fall back into the most delicious and relaxed sleep.

CHAPTER 5

PARADOXICAL RELAXATION

Moment-to-Moment and *Intensive Paradoxical Relaxation*

The word relax comes from the old French word *relaxer* which means "to make less compact or dense, to loosen, or open" and from the Latin word *laxus* which means "to be wide, loose, open, slack or languid." Indeed tension is a state of denseness, tightness, constriction, and contraction. *Paradoxical Relaxation*'s intention is to restore someone's ability to reverse a dense, tight, constricted, contracted state of the body. In the case of pelvic pain, it reverses a dense, tight, constricted, and contracted pelvic floor basin.

In our treatment protocol, we use *Paradoxical Relaxation* in two different but complementary ways. *Moment-to-Moment Paradoxical Relaxation* is used throughout your normal day to regularly interrupt the habit of tensing the pelvic muscles. Doing *Moment-to-Moment Paradoxical Relaxation* can involve many brief relaxations during the day. As you become more skilled, this practice takes less time and is done almost automatically. The intention here is for you to abort the old, dysfunctional chronic habit tensing. *Intensive Paradoxical Relaxation* requires setting aside time that is devoted to the practice of the technique, without the distractions that occur during your normal everyday life. This is best practiced two to three times a day with each practice period lasting approximately 30 to 45 minutes.

Moment-to-Moment Paradoxical Relaxation does not offer the depth of relaxation achieved by *Intensive Paradoxical Relaxation* and by itself can have clear but limited effects. The intensive practice represents the laboratory in which the skill of the method is developed. It represents the heart of the practice and produces the most benefit. The skill of feeling, accepting, and resting with tension that can make it possible for pain to reduce or disappear, is honed in the *Intensive Paradoxical Relaxation* practice.

Moment-to-Moment Paradoxical Relaxation

Patients are often surprised at the number of times each day that they tense their pelvic muscles or find them in a continual state of contraction. Changing this habit is not a small matter.

Under normal circumstances most people would never be willing to devote the time and attention to change this habit. The energy required to change it comes from the strength of the desire to stop the pain and dysfunction. Most patients will devote the time and effort required to change this habit when they feel doing so reduces their symptoms. This motivation is the gift of this condition, even though it rarely feels like a gift when the symptoms exist unabated.

How to relax your pelvic muscles throughout the day

Our instruction to our patients regarding *Moment-to-Moment Paradoxical Relaxation* goes something like this, *"It is necessary that you become aware of your habit of tensing your pelvic muscles on a moment-to-moment basis and change this habit. Throughout the day check for tension in your pelvic muscles so you can apply the technique of relaxing it. You may want to tie a string around your finger, or paste a colored piece of paper to your bathroom mirror, or paste a tiny iridescent dot on the face of your watch. Anything that you can do to remind yourself to feel your pelvic tension and relax it can help. Do this many times, as long as these mini relaxations don't interfere with your functioning during the day." Moment-to-moment relaxation is not a Kegel exercise of tightening and then relaxing.* Kegel exercises were originally done to strengthen weak pelvic muscles.

It is sometimes useful to use a small and inexpensive device called *The MotivAider*. Recently, certain vibration watches have come on the market that can be set to vibrate for certain set periods of time. These devices vibrate silently and repeatedly like someone tapping you on the shoulder at times you designate, to remind you to let go of any tension you might be unnecessarily holding in your pelvis. You can set one of these devices to vibrate every ten minutes, or every hour, as a private reminder to relax the pelvic muscles.

Sensing pelvic tension

Most people can feel tension in their pelvis and let go of this tension to some degree or another when they are aware of it. Others cannot. If you are one of those who cannot discern pelvic tension or how to relax pelvic tension you can become sensitive to it in the following way. While you are sitting on a toilet, notice how your sphincter, rectum and genitals slightly drop and relax when you begin to urinate. The sensation is very subtle and will occur out of awareness if you're not paying careful attention. These muscles naturally relax when you begin urination. These are the muscles that you want to learn to relax throughout the day for these muscles are part of the guarding response that keeps the pelvic floor tight and tense.

Up tight and stuck up

Someone with chronic pelvic pain tends to have pelvic muscles that are held 'up' and 'tight.' The relaxed, dropped state of the pelvic muscles tends to be absent with pelvic pain. Another way to conceive of what goes on in the pelvic floor is to understand that the tight and contracted pelvic muscles are stuck in a contraction and held up in such a contraction. Hence we can describe the pelvic floor in most pelvic pain patients as 'up tight' or 'stuck up.'

It is necessary to rehabilitate this pelvic floor posture so that the default mode of the pelvic muscles is 'down' and 'relaxed.' If you have difficulty feeling and relaxing your pelvic muscles, you can practice doing this in the following exercise. Sit on the toilet and feel the slight relaxation of the muscles in your pelvic floor as if you are about to urinate, except do not urinate. This maneuver is simple and easy and requires fine motor control in that you relax the tightened muscles, to whatever extent you can, without actually beginning urination. The flow of urine should not begin during this pelvic letting go. You shouldn't even get near it.

These instructions might make this relaxation sound much more complicated than it is. Most likely, you will feel a slight dropping of the muscles around the rectum as you prepare to urinate. The muscles you relax in this exercise are the same muscles you should be relaxing with *Moment-to-Moment Paradoxical Relaxation.* In fact, it's quite simple and most people easily get the hang of it.

Moment-to-Moment Paradoxical Relaxation in a nutshell

Moment-to-Moment Paradoxical Relaxation is the practice of allowing the pelvic muscles to drop and relax all day. Whether you remind yourself spontaneously or are reminded by a vibrating timer like *The Motiv-Aider* or by some other means. Don't look for immediate results. Don't strain in any way. It should just take a moment to notice and do and should hardly take any attention away from what you're involved in. Remember that your voluntary relaxation of these muscles at first will rarely cause much of a sense of relaxation in them. It is best to expect that your voluntary relaxation will only help a little to relax the pelvic muscles. Even if this method is effective for you, you may only experience slight relief of symptoms for days or weeks. Nevertheless, it is important to do this relaxation on an ongoing basis until this relaxation becomes a habit that replaces the tendency of chronically tightening the pelvic floor.

Hints on the application of the
Moment-to-Moment Paradoxical Relaxation

1. It takes time to learn

It takes time to learn how to do *Moment-to-Moment Paradoxical Relaxation* so that it does not interrupt your day. Doing it should take only a moment or two.

2. Make sure that you do not exert effort

Make sure you do not exert any effort to relax. Just as you don't exert effort to initiate urination, don't exert effort to do this momentary relaxation. Don't push down as in the Valsalva maneuver to accomplish relaxation. Instead let go of any tension that you can easily let go of.

3. Continue to practice even if no results seem to occur

The *Moment-to-Moment Paradoxical Relaxation* practice is aimed at subtracting tension from the pelvic muscles throughout the day. It is like using a thimble to empty water in a row boat. Occasionally the effect on symptoms is dramatic; often it is not. *We tell our patients to continue to do it whether you have results or not.* Practicing this conscientiously for weeks has helped some patients reduce their symptoms. Some experience no benefit from doing this. Although quite unusual, when we published the first edition of our book, one man said doing this for several months reduced his symptoms by 90%.

Intensive Paradoxical Relaxation preparation

The preparation for doing *Intensive Paradoxical Relaxation* (or simply called *Paradoxical Relaxation*) is essential for its effectiveness. We encourage our patients not to be disturbed for the period of time that they are doing the relaxation. This might mean asking their spouse to make sure that their children don't come into the room in which they are relaxing. If possible, we suggest disconnecting the telephone and turning off the television or stereo. Relaxation needs to be done with out distractions.

When possible, we tell our patients to do their relaxation practice at a time when they do not have an important appointment immediately afterwards that requires them to be alert and tense. We suggest our patients are alone in the room, undisturbed by pets or other distractions.

Bath or shower and stretches

A warm bath or shower can be very helpful in easing pelvic discomfort. Furthermore, the warm water is a good preparation for *Paradoxical Relaxation.*

Under ideal circumstances, we suggest that our patients do some form of aerobic exercise, take a comfortable warm bath or shower, do their home physical therapy program, including appropriate skin rolling, *Trigger Point Release,* and stretching, and then do *Paradoxical Relaxation. While taking a bath and doing stretching prior to relaxation is advisable, it is not always possible and is not essential for the success of the relaxation.*

Timer

We have found that it is best to set a timer that will ring at the end of the relaxation session. When someone falls asleep during the relaxation period, the timer will indicate that the period is over. Because the relaxation is done first lying down, we advise the use of a pillow or two under the knees as a way of reducing stress on the lower back.

If patients have many things to do during the day, it is a good idea to write them down on a piece of paper so that they will have less of a tendency to carry them in their head during relaxation. Also, we have found it is good to have a paper and pencil nearby while doing the relaxation. If a pressing thought arises, it can be jotted down and relaxation can be continued.

Relaxation, eating, drinking, and the bathroom

It is best not to eat any substantial amount of food prior to relaxation as it tends to make one fall asleep. While falling asleep is not bad, it is better to remain awake throughout the entire relaxation session. Furthermore, we advise patients to avoid caffeine, sugar or other stimulants prior to relaxation.

In order to remain as comfortable as possible, we advise people to urinate before a period of relaxation, especially if they feel uncomfortable holding in the urine. It is also usually better, if possible, to avoid drinking fluids prior to relaxation, especially if there is urinary frequency and urgency. Finally, most patients are more comfortable when they loosen their tie, belt, or anything constricting.

Setting up the room

We advise patients to partially darken the room in which they are going to relax and to use an eye pillow. An eye pillow is a small sack, often made of velvet or cotton and filled with flax seed or rice that can be bought at a health food store. It has the advantage of darkening the field of vision even in a room with a great deal of light. The eye pillow also tends to be soothing to the eyes and is usually helpful for relaxation.

Paradoxical Relaxation can be done lying down or in a chair. At the beginning of training it is advised that it be done lying down with the knees bent but not resting on each other, especially if there is increased pain while sitting. A bed, a couch, a futon, or a carpeted floor will work. Sometimes patients are more comfortable lying on their side with a pillow between their knees, though this may tend to promote falling asleep. Because the key is comfort, it is acceptable to use as many pillows as necessary.

While it is good to have a comfortable regular place for relaxation, the practice can be done almost anywhere. It is possible to do *Paradoxical*

Relaxation in a hotel room, on a bus, in a plane, in an office chair, in a park on the grass, or on a towel in the sand.

What about falling asleep?

It is not uncommon to fall asleep during *Paradoxical Relaxation*. Falling asleep is more likely if you are tired and if you do the relaxation during a part of the day when you tend to become fatigued, such as the afternoon or evening.

Paradoxical Relaxation is not taking a nap. Often, however, one can fall asleep especially if one is sleep deprived. Falling asleep is of little concern, especially in the beginning of relaxation training. It is preferable to doze rather than to tense for the purpose of staying awake. The experience of sleep during *Paradoxical Relaxation* tends to be different and usually more beneficial than simply falling asleep at night. When patients seem unable to remain awake during relaxation, we suggest that, if possible, they sit up and make sure the room is not overly warm. When someone is in treatment and have committed themselves to two periods of relaxation a day, we suggest that relaxing before sleep not be counted as one of the two periods of practice. An additional session would need to be done to comply with our protocol.

The best time to do *Paradoxical Relaxation*

The best time to do Paradoxical Relaxation is when you have the most energy. Most people find that they have this kind of energy in the morning. However, this is not universally true. Some people have more energy and ability to pay attention in the afternoon.

Paradoxical Relaxation requires energy because this practice is attempting to modify a habit of inner tension that has been practiced countless times. Establishing a new habit in the face of such a practiced habit is very ambitious. It is for this reason that each practice period must 'really count' by virtue of the earnestness and level of attention with which it is done.

It is best to get into a routine doing *Paradoxical Relaxation* so the body gets used to a regular time of quiet. A routine also helps avoid missing relaxation sessions. While we normally advise people to do *Paradoxical Relaxation* at least once a day, when possible it is preferable to do it twice a day. The best times tend to be in the morning and afternoon or evening, but before a major meal.

Beginning *Paradoxical Relaxation*

After the Respiratory Sinus Arrhythmia (RSA) breathing, which we will soon discuss, the cassette recordings of *Paradoxical Relaxation* instruction that are given as part of our monthly clinics have made the practice relatively simple. All of the instructions for the practice are provided in the forty-four lessons in the taped series. A small cassette player with a headset that goes over the ears is usually used. Noise-canceling headphones, like ones from PlaneQuiet or Bose are sometimes useful when the relaxation method is used on a plane or in a noisy place.

Daily checklist

Patients are asked to keep a record of their experience during the relaxation. Over a period of time the answers to the checklist provide an understanding of the effect of the relaxation upon symptoms.

Daily Checklist for *Paradoxical Relaxation* Training

Do item 1 before the relaxation session and the rest of the questions after your session

Name_____ Date _____ Session # _____

Number of tape you are listening to _____

1. Global symptom level before relaxation

    0   1   2   3   4   5   6   7   8   9   10
    (No discomfort)   *(Worst discomfort)*

2. Global symptom level after relaxation
0	1	2	3	4	5	6	7	8	9	10

    (No discomfort)   *(Worst discomfort)*

3. At what time did you do the relaxation? _____

4. Did you fall asleep during relaxation?   Yes   No
    If yes, approximately what percentage of the relaxation period were you asleep? ___ %

5. Were you alone and undisturbed by outside factors?   Yes   No
    If no, describe disturbance _____

6. Did you understand the instructions on the tape?   Yes   No
    If no, explain _____

7. What did you do well during relaxation?_____
    With what did you have difficulty? _____

8. Is the concept of accepting tension / resting with tension clear to you?
    Yes No If no, explain _____

9. What level of success have you had in accepting or resting with tension?
0	1	2	3	4	5	6	7	8	9	10

    (No discomfort)   *(Worst discomfort)*

10. Did you listen to the entire tape?   Yes   No

11. How intrusive was the pain/discomfort in your pelvis when you were doing the relaxation?
    Very intrusive   Somewhat intrusive   Slightly intrusive   Not intrusive

12. How closely are you listening to the instructions on during the relaxation?
    Very closely   Somewhat closely   Not closely

13. Questions/comments

Accepting tension to relax can seem counter-intuitive

All of the instructions of Paradoxical Relaxation are aimed at assisting our patients to let go of effort. Most of us can remember times in our lives when we felt peaceful and happy. In those times, there tended to be no trace of strain, tension, or effort. Those times felt easy. The experience most patients have is not one of effortlessness or ease, and yet it is what patients most deeply yearn for.

Relaxation = feeling and accepting tension without trying to relax

You will discover how relaxation results from feeling and accepting tension by giving yourself this instruction and seeing how it affects you. We have found that using the instructions 'feel and accept tension' or 'feel the tension without trying to do anything about it' are a few of the useful phrases in our repertoire of instruction to teach someone to cease straining. To *try* comes from 15th century Anglo-French *trier* which means "to subject to some strain" (of patience, endurance). As the etymology of the word implies, trying involves straining and is the opposite of relaxation. This is why you can't *try* to relax.

It is important to note that the method of *Paradoxical Relaxation* asks the patient to make a distinction between pain and tension. While pain needs to be acknowledged and not resisted, the focus of our methodology is on tension and not on pain. In other words, in doing *Paradoxical Relaxation*, the foreground that one chooses to focus on is the sensation of tension. Pain, then, is not directly focused on but is allowed to remain in the background. An experienced teacher can help the student of *Paradoxical Relaxation* understand this essential distinction.

It is in practicing how to accept tension that you learn how to do it

Accepting tension is like learning to ride a bicycle. Let's imagine you have never ridden a bicycle and we present you with a simple balloon-tire, old-style, one-speed bicycle. We can say, "Put your leg over the bicycle and sit on the seat and push off with one leg while the other leg is in the stirrup of the other pedal and when you start falling to the left, lean to the right, and when you start falling to the right, lean to the left."

For those of us who can ride a bicycle, it is clear that these instructions will not go very far in teaching you how to ride a bicycle. In the end, the only way to learn how to ride a bicycle is to get on it and ride. Knowing this, parents will often teach their children how to ride a bicycle by letting them get on the bicycle while the parent runs along side of it and holds it upright. Training wheels are sometimes used as a replacement for the parent running alongside the child.

The example of riding a bicycle makes it obvious that the only way you learn is by doing. Instructions may be helpful, but do not substitute for actually being on the seat of the bicycle and having to contend with the forces that are pulling you off-balance at every moment. While it is helpful to have a coach who is practiced in the skill you wish to master, all such skills are ultimately learned through direct experience. So it is with *Paradoxical Relaxation*.

Respiratory Sinus Arrhythmia breathing (RSA breathing) in preparation for *Paradoxical Relaxation* and *Trigger Point Release*

RSA breathing, as we describe it here, is sometimes used as part of *Paradoxical Relaxation* in the *Wise-Anderson Protocol*. We have recently incorporated it as part of the *Trigger Point Release* methodology that we use. Using RSA breathing in conjunction with *Trigger Point Release*, as we will describe, is a way of making the *Trigger Point Release* more effective by breaking sympathetic arousal at the time of the *Trigger Point Release*.

RSA breathing is a description of the relationship between heart rate and breathing and refers to the heart rate varying in response to respiration. RSA is a phenomenon that occurs in all vertebrates. You can experience the phenomenon of RSA by taking your pulse and noting that when you breathe in, the heart rate increases slightly and when you breathe out the heart rate decreases slightly. There is considerable research that indicates that when there is balance and health, the heart rate and the breath move robustly together. In a normal healthy individual, as inhalation occurs, heart rate increases, and as exhalation occurs, heart rate drops.

Under circumstances of mental or physical disease, the relationship between breathing and heart rate is interrupted. When individuals suffer panic attacks for instance, RSA is disturbed. When they recover from panic disorders their RSA breathing becomes more coordinated, stronger, more balanced, and robust. The higher, stronger and more coordinated the heart rate is with respiration, the more balanced and healthy the individual. For example, healthy children generally have very robust RSA breathing in which the heart rate can sometimes vary 40 beats or more between inhalation and exhalation.

Disturbed RSA is thought to be an indicator of an adverse prognosis for people with heart disease. Generally, disturbed RSA is indicative of early problems in the healthy functioning of the autonomic nervous system as it relates to a number of diseases. It has been suggested that one measure of the therapeutic effect or safety of a drug is whether it positively or negatively affects RSA.

It is usually possible with our RSA method to voluntarily strengthen RSA and bring it into balance when it is unbalanced. Restoring RSA can facilitate autonomic quieting and a reduction of anxiety by consciously coordinating the heart rate with respiration. We use this practice as part of *Paradoxical Relaxation.*

RSA focused breathing should be done under the supervision of a professional. Occasionally, RSA can trigger benign ectopic or missed heart beats. Lightheadedness or a sense of not getting enough air can occur when the correct technique is not used. If there are any problems that occur such as lightheadedness or not getting enough air during the RSA breathing, we ask our patients to immediately let us know so we can help them adjust their use of this method. RSA can be a useful method to quickly quiet sympathetic nervous system arousal, reduce anxiety, and allow one to be at a deeper level of relaxation at the beginning of *Paradoxical Relaxation.*

Practicing RSA breathing

It is generally agreed that slow, abdominal breathing in which the abdomen rises during inhalation and falls back during exhalation can be important in relaxation of the body and in the reduction of autonomic arousal. Slow abdominal breathing maximizes the possibility of breathing and heart rate coming into synchronicity with each other. While there is no absolute formula rigidly defining how many respirations per minute should occur to permit deep relaxation, 6 deep abdominal breaths per minute is more or less considered an optimal respiration rate. Again 6 breaths per minute is ideal and breathing rates that accomplish preliminary quieting of the body can vary from 2 to 9 breaths per minute depending on idiosyncrasies, experience, and metabolic requirements of the particular patient.

More important than having an idea of what the ideal number of breaths per minute should be is the understanding that one's level of comfort in breathing is the most important criteria in fine tuning one's respiration rate during RSA breathing. When our patients slow their breathing to approximately 6 breaths per minute, as we will describe below, we ask them to adjust this slower respiration rate up or down to fit individual levels of comfort.

Computing the number of heartbeats per breath in RSA breathing

In *Paradoxical Relaxation*, RSA breathing is done for approximately 5 minutes immediately prior to following the instruction on the taped audio course our patients receive at the end of our clinic. Below are the instructions about doing RSA breathing. In order to determine how many heartbeats should be devoted to inhalation and how many heartbeats should be devoted to exhalation, we use the following computations (these computations may appear to make the technique more complicated than it is).

In conjunction with instruction from someone experienced in RSA breathing, patients are asked to take their pulse to determine their heart rate. Generally speaking, the heart rate is taken and monitored using the thumb of one hand to feel the pulse in the wrist of the other. Counting how many heartbeats occur in a 15 second time frame, and then multiplying that number by 4, is an easy way to determine the pulse rate per minute.

We ask patients to divide their heart rate by 6. If for instance someone has a heart rate of around 60 beats per minute the computation would be:

$$\frac{60}{6} = 10 \text{ (Represents the number of beats allocated for a full in and out breath in order to breath 6 times per minute)}$$

We then would divide 10 by 2 to get the number 5. If someone has a heart rate of around 72 beats per minute, 72 divided by 6 = 12, and 12 divided by 2 = 6. The number 6 in this case or the number 5 before, represents the number of heartbeats allocated for a single inhalation or exhalation.

Patients lie down in preparation to do *Paradoxical Relaxation*. We ask them to be in a comfortable position while feeling their pulse. Sometimes pillows are placed under the elbows to reduce the tension in the arms and hands while feeling the heart rate. This makes it easier to feel the pulse on an ongoing basis.

Once relaxed and feeling the pulse comfortably, patients with a heart rate of between 55-64 are instructed to inhale over a count of 5 heartbeats and exhale over a count of 5 heartbeats. Similarly, if the heart rate is between 65-74, 6 heartbeats are counted during inhalation and 6 heartbeats are counted during exhalation. If one's heart rate is between 75-84, 7 heartbeats are counted during inhalation and 7 heartbeats are counted during exhalation.

The amount of air taken in can vary. If patients feel that they are not getting enough air, they take in more air. If they feel uncomfortable getting too much air, they reduce the intake of air. Breathing in or out more can be done more quickly at the beginning, middle or end of the appropriate heart beat count depending on what feels comfortable.

Breathing must be *comfortable*. Comfort level is the most important fact in considering whether to breathe in or out more or less, or whether to breathe more quickly or slowly at any given part of the breathing cycle. As in *Paradoxical Relaxation,* attention is returned over and over again back to the sensation of the breath, away from attending to visual or conceptual thinking. Usually after about 5 minutes, *Paradoxical Relaxation* is begun without regulating or paying attention to the breath at all.

RSA breathing and quieting down urinary frequency and urgency

Some patients have reported that the practice of the RSA breathing has quieted down the urge to urinate. One of our patients, who felt the urge to urinate, was stuck on an airplane runway, and had to remain seated for an hour. He did the RSA breathing and reported that he was nearly able to stop his sense of urinary urgency. We have had others who have reported that they have been able to use skin rolling (discussed later) to accomplish this as well.

RSA breathing during *Trigger Point Release*

As we mentioned earlier, we have incorporated the practice of RSA breathing with patients for a few minutes prior to and during, both self-*Trigger Point Release* and *Trigger Point Release* with our physical therapist. There is some evidence that RSA breathing reduces sympathetic nervous system tone during the actual *Trigger Point Release* session, and makes the effects more effective and longer lasting.

Finding tension

If most people are asked to locate some area of tension or tightness in their bodies, they usually can. Sometimes, some of our patients cannot seem to find any tension whatsoever, except in their pelvis. This is usually because the pelvic tension and discomfort is so great that it masks any other sensations of tension, or because the individual has been tense for so long that the tension feels completely normal and is not identified as such.

A preliminary exercise in beginning *Paradoxical Relaxation* directs patients to do an inventory of tension throughout the major muscle groups of the body. Forehead, face, jaw, neck, shoulders, arms, upper back and chest, lower back and stomach, pelvis, legs and feet are carefully examined and any tension in these areas is identified. Practice begins in finding a part of the body, other than the pelvis, that feels any degree of tension. It does not have to be any great or unbearable tension, just a simple sensation of tension. Tension in the shoulders or neck, however unremarkable, is a suitable area to focus on for the purpose of this exercise.

A word about what constitutes tension in *Paradoxical Relaxation* instruction. The slightest, tiniest bit of tension is considered significant even though most people would never notice it or regard it in any way as significant. As we have discussed, the relaxation of the tiny or what is also called 'residual' tension, is the key to reducing nervous system arousal and to permitting profound pelvic floor relaxation. The understanding that a tiny bit of tension is essential to identify and work with is emphasized in early stages of instruction.

At first, it is preferable to *not* focus on the pelvic muscles since they are uncomfortable and there is usually a great desire to feel relief from this discomfort. This strong desire, especially for the beginner, makes the practice of accepting tension more difficult. It is for this reason that in the first few months of relaxation training, the pelvis is not the primary object of attention.

Inwardly locating the tension

The outside world is familiar to us when we open our eyes and look across the room or across the street. If we are asked where the street corner is, we will easily locate it. Similarly, if we were to look at our left knee, we would not have any trouble in finding it. If we were to look at our right hand, again, we would not have any difficulty in locating it.

The inner world of sensation, thought, and emotion is not so clear. For example, when we close our eyes and direct our attention to the sensation of our neck, while its location may generally be clear, the sensation of our neck usually does not have the discreet boundaries and precise location that appear when we see our neck with our eyes open. In learning *Paradoxical Relaxation*, we practice locating sensations inside the body. Tensing and relaxing a part of the body is designed to teach us to locate the tensions in the body while the eyes are closed.

In the beginning of relaxation training, attention is directed inside the body in order to locate tension that does not relax. Patients are asked to feel the tension without trying to modify it or reduce it. The purpose of this initial focus on tension is to acquaint the patient with the practice of feeling, accepting, and resting with tension.

There is a quality of attention that can help more clearly locate and relax tension in the body. When patients are first learning *Paradoxical Relaxation,* they are asked to be more receptive than active in perceiving it. They are asked to allow the sensation to come toward them, so to speak, rather than actively reaching out toward it.

To best achieve this receptive attitude, it is important to practice being steady with one's attention. Patients are asked to feel the tension in the body without trying to define its borders or its exact location within. Sometimes we use the analogy of a self-focusing camera. The camera is simply pointed in the direction of the object to be photographed. This triggers an automatic focusing of the camera's lens. The photographer simply has to turn this point-and-shoot camera in the direction of the object and everything else occurs automatically.

Attention works like a point-and-shoot camera. Point attention at inner tension, sustain it there, give attention a chance to settle down and the sensation of the tension usually comes into focus without effort. We ask patients to tolerate that the sensation they are focusing on may be subtle, vague, and not clearly differentiated. We ask them to take that sensation exactly as it shows up in their awareness. Again, we ask patients to not be concerned about gaining a sense of the precise boundaries of the tension. The sensations of the tension usually come on their own terms, like the smell of jasmine wafting into awareness on a warm summer night. The scent of jasmine need not be grabbed. As the aroma finds its way into the nostrils, so the sensation of tension finds its way into awareness with the very simple act of focusing and resting attention upon it.

Relaxation occurs when attention rests in sensation and not in thought

We all understand what it means to think what can be called a picture thought, a verbal thought, or an abstract thought. If you imagine an apple, what you're seeing in your mind's eye can be called a picture thought. When you think about what you said to a friend yesterday, your focus is on what can be called a verbal thought. When you add 420 to 816, your focus is on what can be called an abstract thought. Thoughts are symbolic representations in the mind.

Sensation can be felt directly without the need for thought. When you feel a cold wind on your face, your attention is directed to sensation directly. No thought is necessary.

A central premise of Paradoxical Relaxation is that relaxation occurs when attention rests in sensation and not in thought. In fact, relaxation is most profound when no thought is present in awareness. Learning *Paradoxical Relaxation* requires that you can make the distinction between a thought and a sensation and that you can rest attention in sensation.

Directing attention to sensation and not to thought or mental pictures

It is essential to become practiced in focusing attention on sensation and not on a picture or thought of it. When you slip into a warm fragrant bath, you feel the warmth and support of the water and smell the fragrance in it. The bath experience is a sensory one and not an intellectual one.

It is important to understand that correctly focusing on sensation in no way means that thoughts should not come into your awareness. Very often one can be absorbed in sensation while peripherally noticing thoughts coming in and out of awareness. This is absolutely fine. Becoming an adept in *Paradoxical Relaxation* means that you can stay focused on sensation as thoughts float in and out of awareness and not have your attention be pulled away by these thoughts.

Getting good at 'coming back'

Morihei Ueshiba, known as the father of the modern martial art of Aikido, was reputedly asked by one of his students how he remained so present and apparently unperturbed in the midst of a fight. Whether apocryphal or not, he is reputed to have said that he did not consider himself particularly good at being continuously present in a fight but what he was really good at was 'coming back' from being distracted.

When people first begin *Paradoxical Relaxation* training, almost universally they report that their major difficulty is staying focused. Their distress about being distracted is usually allayed when they understand that the practice of *Paradoxical Relaxation* involves, like the skill of the Aikido master, getting good at 'coming back' from distraction. One learns to be tireless, remorseless, and unperturbed by the tendency of one's mind to wander away from the object of focus.

Neophytes often feel various degrees of frustration, irritation and remorse when they find that their attention has wandered off into what they're having for lunch or some distressing thought about their symptoms. As one progresses in this relaxation practice, one learns to return attention to the chosen sensation they are focusing on without any emotion or internal comment about being distracted. Coming right back from distraction without emotion or internal comment is what it takes to get good at 'coming back.' There is no quick way to achieve this—practice, practice and more practice is the often unwelcome secret.

Subtleties in the practice of *Paradoxical Relaxation*

Engaging in the activity of quieting down your nervous system and relaxing your pelvic muscles is a peculiar activity, unlike any other. The skill involved in doing this involves the subtle control of your attention. It involves the micromanagement of your emotions and attitude in the moment of practicing *Paradoxical Relaxation*. Absent the development of these skills, *Paradoxical Relaxation* fails. In this section we will discuss these subtleties.

How can you tell the difference between paying attention to sensation and thinking?

When you rest attention in neutral sensation, your mind and body tend to quiet down. When you pay attention to sensation, you have to be in the present, neither going back to the past nor considering the future. Thoughts may flit in and out, but your attention rests on the sensations you are feeling. When attention shifts to thinking, some increase in tension and discomfort usually occurs.

During *Paradoxical Relaxation*, when you pay attention to slight amounts of tension in a part of your body, you typically notice fleeting thoughts. It is best to continue your focus on this slight amount of tension, resolutely returning when you are distracted by these thoughts.

The following metaphor can be useful in understanding how to keep attention focused on sensation rather than on thought. When walking down a crowded city sidewalk, many faces come toward you as they continue in the opposite direction. If you are clear about where you are going, you continue in your direction. While you may see many of the faces through the periphery of your vision, you don't stop to have conversations with these people. You simply go in your direction.

We suggest that patients do the same thing with the thoughts that cross their awareness as they focus on feeling the sensations of tension. It is fine to be aware of them as they pass, but keeping your attention focused on the sensation, without stopping and getting involved or carried away with these thoughts, is a central practice of this method.

Accepting tension includes accepting your resistance to accepting tension

As you continue to rest your attention on the sensation of tension, you may notice an aversion or resistance to doing this. If this resistance or aversion could talk it might say, "Hey, this is no fun. This does not feel good. I don't like it. I want to move. I want to feel better. I want to do something. Yuck! I want to get out of here!"

This resistance is normal. The human organism is not programmed to focus on discomfort or tension. It is programmed to move toward pleasure and away from pain.

Unless you include this resistance in your sphere of acceptance, it will stalemate you. Resistance is usually experienced as stubborn tension. The unacknowledged resistance stays put as long as it is unacknowledged and unaccepted. Acknowledging and accepting the resistance, in practical terms means, feeling this sensation of stubborn tightness and permitting it to be present without having to do anything about it. In acknowledging and accepting the resistance, you open the door for it to leave.

The freedom to not have to change anything

Most people feel a peculiar sense of freedom and ease when choosing to permit everything in their experience to be in the moment. Paradoxically, with nothing to change, nowhere to go, nothing to do, nothing to make different, and feeling everything, including your tendency to resist feeling discomfort, you are most likely to go beyond what is uncomfortable and into the experience of ease and comfort.

Making the distinction between pain and tension, and focusing on the tension

As one's ability to focus improves, relaxing the pelvic floor directly becomes easier (in general, it is not the best idea to try to relax the painful or tense pelvic floor muscles in the beginning of the relaxation training). It is important when relaxing the pelvic floor or any other part of the body in which one feels discomfort, to distinguish between the sensation of tension and the sensation of pain or discomfort. The tension usually feels tight, closed, gripping, squeezed or contracted. The pain or discomfort can feel burning, torn, raw, ripped, hot or achy. While focusing on a painful area, we suggest allowing the painful sensations to exist in your awareness without blocking them out or defending against them.

In relaxing a tense and painful pelvic floor, it is as if you are having a conversation with one person while the person's partner is jumping up and down right beside you. Acknowledge and allow the jumping up and down of this person, while continuing your dialogue with the person to whom you are talking. Feel and accept the sensation of tension while allowing, but not focusing on or trying to influence the sensation of pain or discomfort. If the pain or discomfort reduces while you are relaxing, that is fine. If it does not relax, that is also fine.

It is as if you are saying to your tension and pain, "I feel you, tension, and I feel you, pain. I am focusing my attention on the tension now. You are not remarkable, tension. However, I am feeling you now. I feel you, pain, as well. I wish you weren't here. I want you to stop. However, I am going to include you in my experience and allow you to be here along with my desire to get rid of you. I am doing my best not to tense up against you or push you away. I am allowing you to be here now, but I am paying attention to feeling and accepting the tension."

Nowhere to go, nothing to do, no goal to achieve

As you feel the tension now, remember that there is nothing to achieve. *Our instructions here are simple; feel the sensations of tension and all the resistances that arise in doing this without fixing on a goal of relaxation.* Notice that when you find yourself just *hanging out* with your tension, your conditioning and natural inclination may be to "do something" about it.

It is important to remain aware of the inclination to do something about the tension you are feeling. In the beginning of *Paradoxical Relaxation* people sometimes report feeling restless which may incline them to want to wiggle or move to relieve their sense of uneasiness in the tension. In the first few minutes of relaxation, we usually suggest that the patient allow this wiggling or movement. As the relaxation proceeds, this inclination to wiggle tends to diminish and with practice, the nervous system and the muscles tend to quiet down.

Continuing to feel the bodily sensation in the area upon which you have chosen to focus

You may notice that the tension subsides as you continue to feel and accept it. You may feel this as a kind of easing. If tension in your shoulders is your focus, you may notice the shoulders drop slightly.

This experience of relaxation (or the easing of the tension) tends to regularly occur when you accept whatever sensation remains after you have relaxed whatever easily relaxes. You may find that as tension eases, a new and lower level of tension appears. It is like opening one door and walking down a hallway to discover another closed door.

This second closed door is the natural reaction of the body to resist sudden precipitous change.

Understood in this way, the new lower level of tension is simply a way station along the way to complete relaxation. It is the body saying, "Okay, I can let go, but I can't let go all the way right now—so I'll let down a little."

The tension or other sensation you are accepting is dynamic and changes and shifts regularly

When you hold a baby, you will often be aware of the baby's squirming and movement in your arms. The experienced and loving parent knows to hold the baby loosely but firmly, allowing the squirming when it occurs, but keeping a solid hold on the baby.

Accepting tension is like holding a baby. The tension will usually move and shift over and over again. Doing *Paradoxical Relaxation* involves holding or allowing the shifting and squirming of the tension or other sensation as you attend to it and accept it. Remember the tension is your own unconscious holding. You are focusing on and accepting your own holding. This holding at first doesn't know what to do with such attention, as it is used to your resistance to it. Allow sensation to simply be there, and allow it to move and shift, release and tighten, relax and squirm. Be present with any tension and accept it like you would hold and accept the squirming of your beloved infant.

Grasping for more

What often happens when one door opens only to find another is that the desire for complete relief is ignited. We could call this desire a grasping for pleasure and relief, which results in increased tension. You move from an inner attitude of openness and allowing to an attitude that is not in harmony with the inner closed door. Any grasping involves increased tension.

When you are able to feel the relaxation of tension without becoming attached to more, you can relax very deeply, very quickly. There is no secret to doing this. Follow the instruction of accepting whatever tension arises at whatever level. This is a practice of postponing gratification. Paradoxically, the result is an increase in gratification in the form of deeper and deeper relaxation.

You give it up to get it

Our purpose for doing *Paradoxical Relaxation* is to achieve profound relaxation of the pelvic muscles and a significant reduction of nervous system activity. *Understanding this principle of giving up attachment to relaxation while feeling and accepting whatever sensation remains after you have relaxed your tension as much as you can, will allow you a level of relaxation not available otherwise.*

Pay attention to the moments when you are trying to manipulate yourself to relax by accepting tension

The key to accepting tension involves *sincerely* accepting tension. Notice when you have not sincerely committed yourself to accepting your tension. Most of us are reluctant to give up our grasping for relief and pleasure. Most people go through a stage of trying to manipulate themselves to be in a state of acceptance of tension, while not truly inhabiting that intention. You can't experience the fruits of a sincere acceptance of tension by pretending to accept tension.

When there is a part of you that refuses to sincerely accept the tension, that refusal can be felt as additional tension and discomfort. This refusal exists in most of us, and again, it is a problem only if it is unrecognized and the tension of it unaccepted. In other words, feel the tension that is part of the refusal to sincerely accept your tension. What we are talking about here may make little sense to you without doing *Paradoxical Relaxation*.

The effort error

Dr. Edmund Jacobson described failure to understand the principle of 'giving it up to get it' as the 'effort error.' Jacobson described relaxation as the practice of 'letting go of effort.' *Any attempt 'to relax,' which you can understand to mean doing anything, is trying to use effort to discontinue effort. Efforting to stop effort does not work.*

Accepting tension or other sensation is letting go of effort

When you focus on sensation which may include tension, with the goal to simply feel it and accept it, you are practicing the essence of Paradoxical Relaxation. When we instruct you to feel the tension we mean to let the tension be there without adding to or subtracting anything from it. When we say *rest with the tension,* we are instructing you to feel the tension and do your best to quiet yourself down while experiencing it. You are not trying to change the tension and there is no effort involved. This effortlessness allows for relaxation.

Imagine that you are lying directly on a wood floor without any pillows or blankets and you have not had any sleep in two days. You are completely exhausted and can hardly keep your eyes open. Now imagine that you are right on the edge of falling asleep. At that moment your muscles relax even though you are aware of the hardness of the wood.

You can consider your tension in the same way you consider the wood floor. You are intimately connected with the tension as you are intimately in contact with the wood floor. In accepting tension, you are allowing yourself to rest deeply on the wood floor of your tension. *The difference between resting on the wood floor and resting with tension is that in resting with the tension, the tension itself will tend to relax as well, whereas the wood floor will not.* Your residual tension responds to your accepting attitude toward it.

Accepting 'what is'

When you accept tension or discomfort you are neither adding anything to, nor subtracting anything from, the discomfort. You are 'laying alongside' the tension. You are not doing anything to it except being present and feeling it.

The Japanese form of poetry known as Haiku demonstrates the pure intention to accept 'what is.' Here are some examples:

> *The crisp autumn leaves*
> *Rustle softly in the breeze*
> *And then blow away*

> *A red hawk soars high*
> *With no effort and no sound*
> *near a soft white cloud*

> *Warm and fragrant air*
> *Gently fills the valley floor*
> *While the blue bird chirps*

In these poems, the poet simply reports his experience of what is in front of him. There is no embellishment, no judgment, no interpretation to what is perceived, no 'spin.' The poet reports what is directly.

Be patient with yourself. It takes practice to be present with discomfort, tension, and whatever other sensation you focus on. The more you are able to accept what may not be comfortable without judging it, interpreting it, or trying to change it in any way, the better. In fact, the more likely it will be that what you're focusing on will change. *Whatever arises in your awareness as you feel your tension and discomfort, or other remaining sensation, continue to apply the basic instruction of feeling and then accepting what arises. This allows for the deepest relaxation.*

Applying the basic instruction to whatever arises

In the practice of *Paradoxical Relaxation,* we offer you a strategy for dealing with the fear and aversion that can arise when you are relaxing with your discomfort. Instead of being focused on and distracted by the fear or aversion, we suggest you simply allow these feelings to be present in your experience. Coexist with them. Hang out with them. Allow them to present without having to do anything about them.

Your tension responds to your unconditional acceptance in the same way that you respond to someone else's unconditional acceptance

Imagine you spend time with somebody who accepts you unconditionally. Imagine they communicate to you their commitment in the following way:

"I want to be present with you exactly as you are. I am not asking you to change in any way. While I may have preferences about how I might want you to be, I am committed to letting go of those preferences in favor of letting you be exactly the way you are. You may change from one moment to the next, and I am committed to being fully present with you on a moment-to-moment basis and to feel and accept you however much you change. No matter what happens in this moment, I am determined to let you be as you are with an open and sincere heart."

Most people would be very grateful to have a friend like this. When someone is present with us like this, we can relax. There is no danger of attack or judgment. The organism's emergency systems can rest, for there is no need to defend or to ensure survival. No need for vigilance. The attitude of such a friend is true support.

The tissues of your body respond to this unconditional attitude as you do. Your tissues are imbued with your intelligence. The tissue has the same consciousness as you do. It recognizes the presence of such an accepting attitude.

Most people are looking for relationships in which they are regarded in this unconditional way. In *Paradoxical Relaxation,* you are asked to be this kind of friend to yourself.

Paradoxical Relaxation necessarily requires attention training

When you first begin *Paradoxical Relaxation,* you will inevitably struggle with keeping your attention focused. While this can be disconcerting, it is everyone's experience. *The ability to stay focused, like any ability, comes with practice. When the mind wanders from its focus, it must be returned to the object of focus, again and again.* It can take an hour or two of daily practice, for several months to gain a modicum of competence in managing this wavering of your mind where you can hold your attention relatively still for periods of 30 to 60 seconds. Holding attention still for three or four minutes at a time can take much devoted practice.

Attention is the joystick of the nervous system

At the beginning of the 20th century when airplanes first came on the scene, the lever that controlled their movement and direction was named the *joystick.* Over the decades, the term *joystick* has been used to describe any lever-like switch for controlling, manipulating, guiding, or the like. As the age of computers matures and video games become more a part of the culture, the *joystick* is used to control all of the video game action on the screen. The *joystick* is the control center.

Attention is the *joystick* of the nervous system. *If you are able to control your attention, generally speaking, you will be able to exercise significant control over your nervous system.* For example, if you direct your attention toward something upsetting, your nervous system will immediately respond with arousal and disturbance. If you direct your attention toward what is peaceful and uneventful, your nervous system will remain quiet. All things being equal, when you can control your attention, you most likely control whether your nervous system is quiet or not.

If you want to "pull someone's chain," as the modern vernacular goes, you will say something that directs their attention to what arouses them. If you want to make someone feel good you will direct their attention to something that is soothing to their nervous system. The optimist directs their own attention to what is hopeful and not disturbing. In a classic movie, Pollyanna is taught by her father to play the 'Glad game' in which you deliberately look for what you are glad about in any situation. When Pollyanna is sent to live with her misanthropic and miserable aunt and must confront a harsh reality, her stubborn 'Glad game' transforms her experience and everyone else around her. The 'Glad game' is simply an intention to direct attention in a certain way.

The pessimist directs his attention to what is hopeless and disturbing. The cheerful person regularly pays attention to what is cheerful. The anxious person regularly pays attention to what is fearful. In the 'glass half-full' analogy, the way you view the glass is all about what you do with your attention in relationship to it. As we see with Pollyanna, the only difference between seeing the glass half-full and half-empty is related to what aspect of reality you direct your attention.

You can think of the human organism as a 'response machine,' adjusting and responding to the different circumstances in the environment in order to survive. A central function of the nervous system is to respond with arousal to danger, to fight/flight/freeze. When attention is not directed to anything fearful or disturbing, the parasympathetic branch of the autonomic nervous system is activated and restorative activities of tissue rejuvenation, healing and rest would dominate your experience. On the other hand, if you only paid attention to what was threatening, scary, ugly, and disturbing, the sympathetic branch of your nervous system is aroused and activated. You can think of an aroused system like a car engine that is racing and a quiet nervous system as an engine that is quietly and smoothly idling.

The point in Paradoxical Relaxation is to rest attention in sensation and to turn attention away from the thoughts and interpretations that pass through awareness. In *Paradoxical Relaxation* we practice simply receiving sensation directly, bypassing any filter through which the sensation usually passes. Absent any attention to thought, the nervous system remains quiet, electrical activity in the trigger points of the pelvic pain patient becomes unremarkable as demonstrated by the many experiments of Gevirtz and Hubbard and the likelihood of pelvic pain and discomfort reducing in that moment is very high. Controlling attention without strain is the key to the success of *Paradoxical Relaxation*.

Brain activity and attention training

When you look at the hands of a carpenter used to holding heavy hammers, and saw lumber, you will notice that his hands invariably will be large and muscular. Similarly, when you examine the legs of ballet dancers who daily practices leaping and dancing en pointe, their legs are strong and muscular. Your body and mind develop to support any activity that you do repetitively. As your body and mind develop by doing something repetitively, what you are doing, you do more easily and skillfully. Generally, you get better at whatever you practice.

While it is unremarkable to see the development of a carpenter's hand enabling him to more skillfully use a hammer, the scientific field of *neuroscience* has recently documented dramatic changes in the brain associated with repetitive activities. For instance, the part of the brain that is associated with the muscular activity of the fingers of the left hand of violinists shows dramatically more blood flow than the part of the brain associated with the activity of the fingers of the right hand, which simply hold the bow and aren't involved in the gymnastics of the fingers of the left hand. The same increased brain activity exists for the part of the brain associated with the fingers involved in piano playing.

There is a story of a prisoner of the Korean War, captive for a number of years, who practiced golf in his mind while confined to a cage-like jail cell. Every day he would imagine the tiniest aspects of playing golf, from morning to evening, during his captivity. This included gripping the golf club, planting his feet, all the way through the swing for a long drive, to the short putts on a putting green. Remarkably, when he was freed and came home, his reputed scoring was under 100 in his very first golf game after having not physically touched a golf club for years.

This story is consistent with the recent discoveries about *neuroplasticity* in modern neuroscience, which has documented the development of the brain in simply mentally rehearsing some activity. Indeed, it appears you can practice the piano without even touching it and you will be supporting the brain activity associated with playing the piano.

What is remarkable in the fledgling research emerging from neuroscience about attention is that paying attention is a peculiar kind of brain state, involving blood flow in parts of the brain that typically do not operate at the same time. Furthermore, those who have practiced paying attention for thousands of hours demonstrate the development of brain activity associated with paying attention that is unseen in the brains of those who have practiced no attention training.

The point here is that just like a carpenter who has to have strong hands to be holding a hammer all day (and has to have developed increased brain activity to support accurate hammering), so the brain develops to support the activity of sustained continuous attention. It has been estimated that to develop mastery in a musical instrument, one must have invested 5,000 to 10,000 lifetime hours of practice. Similarly, the development of competence in focusing attention requires many hours of practice to develop the brain activity associated with it.

Now, now, now and more now

Be present now. Feel the tension now. Rest with the tension now. Take your mind back from wandering now. Feel the tension without interfering with it now. Accept the tension now. These and other instructions in *Paradoxical Relaxation* are intimately tied to the present. *Paradoxical Relaxation* only works as your attention is here and now. Voluntary relaxation of the pelvic muscles almost always occurs when attention is focused on the present moment.

The commitment to keeping your attention in the present moment often flies against the ingrained habits of thought, that carry you back and forth from the past to the future. Being in this present moment often requires that you experience the discomfort and dysfunction that are hallmarks of pelvic pain. *It is the commitment to keeping your attention in the present moment that can allow the voluntary undoing of the discomfort and dysfunction.* While doing relaxation, thoughts about past and future must be ignored in favor of the currently felt sensation. Disregarding thoughts of the future and being present now are requirements of effective practice. All of the instructions in *Paradoxical Relaxation* are done *now*.

Practicing non-resistance

In Paradoxical Relaxation we practice non-resistance. We practice resisting nothing and permitting everything. When we practice not resisting our resistance, it is most likely for our resistance to soften or disappear. We practice not trying to stop anything but instead allowing everything in our experience in the moment.

Paradoxical Relaxation is not taking a nap

When you take a nap, you let go of controlling your attention, you relax and let your attention go wherever it likes. And you usually fall asleep. In *Paradoxical Relaxation,* you are intentionally focusing your attention on the sensation of a particular part of your body. While you may drift in and out of sleep, you aspire to stay relaxed and focused.

The attention of the novice at *Paradoxical Relaxation* is usually undisciplined. Focusing this attention is not easy and the beginner quickly notices how easily his or her attention is distracted. Losing your focus usually occurs hundreds of times at the beginning of relaxation training and beginners have to redirect attention away from thinking and daydreaming, back to the effortless attention on the sensation which is the object of their focus.

Paradoxical Relaxation, in large part, is a special kind of attention training. Ramana Maharshi described meditation as a *royal battle* in which one fights to keep one's attention on the object of one's focus. As you get used to keeping attention focused, there is less struggle and eventually, as you get to taste the fruits of controlled attention, the battle ends and the attention willingly and easily rests where you want it to rest. When you have relaxed tension as much as it will easily relax, accept whatever sensation remains; accepting *tension often makes it go away*. In *Paradoxical Relaxation* we instruct patients to rest with the remaining sensation on an ongoing basis without looking for an outcome, and to continue to focus continuously on the remaining sensation, doing their best to let go of evaluating or looking for benefit.

Presence of mind and *Paradoxical Relaxation*

Presence of mind means that your attention is here and focused in this moment. It implies having good judgment because your attention is fully here, attending to what needs attending to and not somewhere else, remote from the issue needing to be addressed. Unless you are here with whatever the problem is that you are confronting, your ability to address it is impaired. People get into accidents using cell phones because their attention is distracted from being here in this moment, fully paying attention to driving.

Presence of mind means that in this moment your attention is not distracted. It means that in considering what you are paying attention to, you are all there. It is a highly positive state, universally valued. To have presence of mind means that you can see clearly what you are focusing on and being in this state implies that, being in full possession of your faculties and the facts of the situation, you know best what to do.

This 'clear seeing' is why developing your ability to pay attention with regard to quieting down your nervous system and relaxing a chronically tight pelvis is so important. When you can focus, when your mind (or attention) is fully present with your tightness and nervous arousal, you can feel *that it is you doing the tensing*, and relaxation of what has been chronically tense becomes easy. It is easy because you have the presence of mind (i.e., the ability to focus your attention) to be able to feel the tension that formerly you have been simply tightening automatically and out of your awareness. Again, presence of mind brings into your conscious awareness the experience of your agency regarding the tension, *that it is you doing the tensing that formerly you felt was just happening to you.* Most importantly it permits you to let this tension go. Patients have reported that when they have been able to focus their attention competently, the primitiveness of the tension – how their tension has been protectively guarding out of fear, became clear to them.

When you have presence of mind focused on your own tension and lack of relaxation, you see all of this in a flash. It is not theoretical or intellectual, and you experience it directly. It becomes clear whereas before the noise of your anxiety and continually held tension (which is another word for chronic tension) is something you have gotten used to and has come to feel normal (although never comfortable).

Often, people intuitively feel a sense of vulnerability in letting down. The letting down of the chronic tension however almost always feels like a huge relief, a kind of 'oh my God I can't believe how good this feels.' This great pleasure and relief comes from releasing an inner burden that has sometimes been carried for years. And when you have pelvic pain, this relief almost always involves a reduction of pain or the absence of pain in that moment. This experience is always profound, especially the first time it happens.

Typically, the symptoms of pelvic pain patients wax and wane. Not uncommonly, patients have reported that on vacation or when stress in their life is significantly reduced (by the way, vacations are not always stress free and sometimes patients have increased stress and symptoms on vacation), their symptoms significantly drop or disappear, only to return upon re-entering their normal life.

The ability to voluntarily reduce or relieve symptoms is a large event in someone's life and brings with it a level of satisfaction, self confidence and gratitude that usually does not come with the unbidden, uncontrolled reduction of symptoms. Symptoms of pelvic pain syndromes usually depress people and leave them feeling helpless. Being able to focus on the inner holding and apply the principles of *Paradoxical Relaxation* that result in, even a temporary reduction or disappearance of symptoms, is the best anti-depressant for pelvic pain.

The relationship between attention training and the profound relaxation of the pelvic floor

There is much to say about attention training and relaxation. Below we present various points on the subject.

- Sustained, focused attention is essential to reliable, profound relaxation in general and the reliable, profound relaxation of the pelvic floor in particular.

- The naïve and unskilled practitioner of relaxation often assumes that relaxation means letting go of control over one's attention. The misunderstanding of those who try to relax but are not able to, is that they think relaxation is rather like taking a nap, where you let go of focusing your attention and let your mind go wherever it wishes.

- If you are not able to sustain long periods of focused attention, your ability to profoundly relax the pelvic floor and lower the activity of the autonomic nervous system will have little chance of becoming reliable or deep.

- The tendency of a person's attention to flit from one mental object to another is generally part of the fight/flight/freeze mechanism not unlike the flitting of a bird's attention to scan for danger. Normally, one's attention necessarily moves around and is involved in scanning the environment for danger. Focusing attention takes control over this scanning tendency that keeps the body vigilant.

- Learning to reliably sustain attention takes you beyond the default programming of your body to scan the environment.

- REM (rapid eye movement) sleep is the sleep involved in dreaming where attention moves around. Non REM sleep is the deepest, most restorative level of sleep and involves the profound reduction of wandering attention.

- When attention cannot be sustained long enough to permit you to become aware of the unconscious holding and guarding you are doing, this guarding tends to remain in place.

- One of the cornerstones of *Paradoxical Relaxation* is the practice of maintaining seamless continual attention on a part of the body, while at the same time resting and using as little effort as possible to remain focused. In other words, the task is to remain focused and simultaneously relinquish any unnecessary effort in doing so.

Identification vs. being the witness

Identification vs. being the witness is easy to understand if you are not put off by these peculiar and rarely used terms. When you are identified with your anxiety and fearful thoughts, you see no difference between these thoughts and feelings and yourself. You are merged in them. You see no difference between your fearful thoughts and reality, they are one and the same and they control you. In our view, being identified in your fearful thoughts and feelings about your pelvic pain is the greatest suffering of the condition.

When you become a witness to your fearful thoughts and feelings there are two things present: you, who is witnessing and the fearful thoughts and feelings. In becoming a witness you step back from identifying with your fearful thoughts and feelings. In becoming a witness, you 'disidentify' from your fearful thoughts and feelings. You perceive them as your thoughts and feelings and not necessarily what is real and not making up all of you. Disidentifying from your scary thoughts and feelings is the first step to dissolving them. Both the relaxation and the attitude shift of the cognitive therapy we describe later, by themselves can help reduce pelvic discomfort and symptoms. We'd like to note that disidentification from scary thoughts and feelings is of huge value, well beyond the subject of pelvic pain and its treatment.

The map is not the territory

The words that communicate what to do in order to relax can be called the 'map' of the territory of voluntary relaxation of the pelvic floor. They are not the 'territory.' The territory of relaxation, which could be called its skillful practice, can only be found in the depths of many hours of practice.

It is often scary to lie down with the discomfort/pain and anxiety usually connected to suffering from pelvic pain. Most people with pelvic pain are afraid of what the pain means, that it will never go away, that it is something bad, that accepting it means that you are giving up. Being still and voluntarily focusing on these sensations is not a small accomplishment. The scary thoughts and feelings that arise when people open themselves up to focusing on their tension can be impediments if they are heeded. We suggest that when these thoughts and feelings arise during relaxation, they be treated like any other thought and attention be turned away from them back to the object of focus.

The words and concepts that describe the practice of what is necessary for the possibility of relaxing a painfully tensed pelvis and quieting an agitated nervous system can be summarized in the following way. These points relate to what our patients must learn to do with attention during relaxation practice.

- Understand the difference between resting in sensation and being involved in thinking.

- Practice disidentifying with the fearful thoughts and feelings that come into your awareness, in favor of being a witness to them and returning attention to the place upon which you've been focusing.

- Focus *continuously* on whatever part of your body you have chosen to focus on.

- Accept tension which means you must be willing and able to feel tension/constriction/bracing/guarding in your body, rest with it and do nothing about it.

- Cease to regard as dangerous or bad, the discomfort or pain in the area you are focusing on or in the periphery of your awareness.

- Distinguish tiny amounts of tension that normally you would not pay attention to and rest your attention there.

- Rest wherever you can in the body while simultaneously focusing continuously on the area upon which you've chosen to focus on.

- Be willing to have and accept your experience in the moment in favor of trying to have some other experience. In other words, in the moment, practice giving up what you prefer in favor of what you have.

- Earnestly be committed to returning your attention to the chosen site you are focusing on without disappointment, frustration, or remorse for having lost focus.

- Give up trying to relax.

- Give up trying to achieve anything during relaxation sessions.

- Give up measuring your progress in the
  moment of doing relaxation.

- Give up trying to figure out what is going on
  in the moment of doing relaxation.

- Become conscious of and permit your discomfort, pain,
  anxiety, and restlessness in the moment of relaxation practice,
  rather than struggling against these sensations/emotions.

These are some of the concepts that describe what you have to do if you wish to relax profoundly. But these concepts occur in the *map* of the *territory*, the *map* of conceptual understanding. While this *map* is important, the intellectual concept is, to use another metaphor, like a finger pointing to the moon. It is not the moon. In order to see the moon you have to be looking at it. Seeing the moon is different from seeing the finger that points to it.

The *territory* that you must enter repetitively is the territory of lying down and practicing these instructions. Many of these instructions can at first feel complex and overwhelming to understand and practice. This sense of complexity is only found in trying to decipher the *map* of relaxation training. In the *territory* of relaxation practice, when you are focused inside yourself, these instructions are ultimately simple and clear. However, the catch is that most people feel some fundamental resistance to keeping the mind focused. One must come back to this resistance over and over again, permitting the resistance to paying attention.

Again here is the paradox. When you do not get frustrated at the tendency for your mind to wander, it gets easier to focus. It does not work to fight the resistance to staying one pointed. However much your attention seems to fight your control of it, with great patience and resolve, you must continue to focus. In doing this, you must let go of frustration, the desire to feel better, the feeling that you don't want to do this – all of the ways that your conditioning has to stop you from focusing continuously and thereby training your attention. There must be no force, frustration, or impatience. Desire for quicker results must be abandoned. The best attitude is 'I am here forever with what I am focusing on and no matter what happens, I continue to return my attention when I find my mind wandering.' This means postponing gratification. At first it requires having faith that you will reduce or stop your pain even though you are being asked to give up wanting that in the moment.

When you are able to practice this skill, you too will probably have difficulty explaining the practice in words, as we stumble here with the words. But the words are not the *territory*. They are the *map* of the *territory*.

Kriyas, fasciculation, fluttering, jerking, feeling of falling, body heaviness, limb tingling, and floating

As one gets into deeper states of relaxation, particularly states that go past the normal range of nervous system quiet that one is familiar with, several unusual kinds of sensations and phenomena can occur. One can experience a kind of jerking and temporary tightening and relaxation of certain muscle groups at certain stages of Paradoxical Relaxation. These are due to a kind of psychophysical ambivalence of letting go of vigilance beyond a certain point. It is as if the body and mind are saying: 'I am letting go now but as I let go I am not comfortable letting go to the extent I find myself letting go... so I tighten back up to guard against letting go too much, then I let go and go past the point of comfortable letting go and so I tighten up again..." Sometimes episodic jerking is accompanied with a feeling of falling. The jerking is a defensive response to the sense of falling. At other times deeper levels of relaxation are accompanied by feelings of heaviness of the limbs and a tingling in the arms, hands and feet. Sometimes, momentarily, someone has the feeling that they cannot move (although they always can). Again these are all characteristic of deeper states of relaxation

In yoga, these movements are thought of as involuntary movements, the release of physical, mental or emotional tension as the life force of *kundalini* moves through areas of tightness. Kriyas are thought to be cleansing and indicative of moving toward a more developed state of consciousness.

It is common, as a very tight pelvic floor begins to relax, for one to feel a kind of fluttering or fasciculation in the muscles of the pelvis. It is usually pleasant and is usually accompanied by a reduction or stopping of pelvic discomfort or pain. Again this feeling represents a kind of pelvic ambivalence of letting go as if the muscles of the pelvic floor can't decide whether to relax or tighten.

When one becomes very quiet during Paradoxical Relaxation, one often experiences a feeling of floating and weightlessness. This is enormously pleasurable and the term bliss is not too strong to describe it. Floating almost always is accompanied by a significant reduction in or absence of pelvic pain. Floating is effortless and there are instructions for what to do during the experience of floating that involve letting go of focusing attention until thinking occurs again.

Some people have followed the relaxation protocol as described in this book and have had some of these experiences and became alarmed by them. In fact, all of these experiences are good news and are signposts on the road to training the body to come out of its habitual contraction of vigilance and learning to relax a painful pelvis.

Faith and patience

Practicing *Paradoxical Relaxation* is practicing patience. The trio Crosby, Stills, and Nash sang a famous lyric, "If you can't be with the one you love, love the one you are with." In *Paradoxical Relaxation* "the one we love" is ease and comfort. "The one we are with" is often tension and discomfort. Being present with "the one we are with" and letting go of grasping for "the one we love" cannot be done without patience. We tell our patients that our treatment is the "slow fix" not the "quick fix." This slow fix requires the postponement of gratification.

There are inevitably many ups and downs. Flare-ups are simply part of the process. We advise our patients not to celebrate when they feel better, nor to despair when they feel worse.

Resolving pelvic pain means that you learn to live with a relaxed 'insides'

Most people with pelvic pain have symptoms that profoundly and fundamentally interfere with their ability to be happy. When we have pelvic pain, our life, our loves, our joys, sorrows and stresses all have to pass through the filter of pelvic pain and constriction and the fearful thoughts about those symptoms. When we suffer from pelvic pain, at some level or another, pelvic pain colors all of our experience.

Conventional medicine tends to focus on the narrowest of pictures when it looks at and treats our pelvic pain. The pelvic pain alone is seen as the problem. The doctor tends to direct his efforts toward the pelvis or a specific organ or structure within the pelvis. But this is looking at the problem of pelvic pain through a keyhole rather than looking at it by opening up the door. The resolution of pelvic pain, in our experience is not simply found by focusing on the pelvis.

Our purpose in writing this book is to present a bigger picture of pelvic pain. The kind of pelvic pain we treat and describe in this book is the result of someone's innards, being in an ongoing kind of knot. *Pelvic pain means your guts, your insides, are tight and constricted.* This tightening usually happens simultaneously with the tightening of other parts of the body. This tightening often affects one's breathing, digestion, bowel function and other parts of the body that are seemingly unrelated. *You live in a body whose core tends to be chronically knotted up when you have pelvic pain.*

As we have described earlier, this chronic knotting up inside, under certain circumstances, can simply let go and one can feel normal again. It is not uncommon for someone with chronic pelvic pain to be on holiday, fall in love, or be released from some major ongoing stress and, in the matter of a few hours, feel almost normal and without pain. Many patients have reported this. Usually, however, the normal circumstances in one's life resume and the old pain and attendant inner contraction reasserts itself.

If you remember peak moments in your life, moments of deep satisfaction and happiness, you may recall that your chest, belly, and pelvis felt good. With the deep relaxation of your body come feelings of hope and love and peace and seeing the goodness in others and in life. A chronically knotted up pelvis, and sometimes attendant knotting up of the innards of the abdomen, do not allow one to feel peaceful.

Resolving pelvic pain means that we have changed this inner knotting up. It means that our stomach can relax, that we can feel the joy of a complete bowel movement, the relaxation that comes with urination, the deep rest and joy that comes after orgasm. It means that our insides are capable of letting go and being relaxed.

Generally speaking, the state of your pelvic muscles reflects the level of the state of your anxiety and emotional disturbance. Chronic fear and anxiety knot up our insides, and tighten our stomach and pelvic muscles. People with pelvic pain who have chronically knotted up insides tend to get used to inner constriction. This is often because they have experienced it for so long. This inner knotting up feels uncomfortable but normal. Different compensations enter into one's life, trying to calm down one's insides. Overwork, psychoactive and pain medications, substance abuse, over eating, and distractions of various kinds are the common compensatory behaviors in many people with pelvic pain.

Resolving pelvic pain means changing what you do with your insides. It means living your life with substantial periods of time when you are not anxious. It means learning to relax your gut and live your life in some large way with a relaxed gut and pelvis. Usually this means living life with patience, understanding, compassion for yourself and others, and making the quality of your own life and relationships more important than money, career or ego. Having a relaxed pelvis means somehow skillfully managing life in the crazy modern world.

On the methodology of *Paradoxical Relaxation*

We are slaves to what we do not know;
of what we know we are masters.
Whatever vice or weakness in ourselves
we discover and understand its causes
and its workings, we overcome it by the very knowing;
the unconscious dissolves when brought into
the conscious.
The dissolution of the unconscious releases energy;
the mind feels adequate and becomes quiet.

Nisargadatta

In this section, we will discuss the often over-looked issue of unconscious psychological resistance to profound relaxation. Conventional relaxation training is usually done without paying attention to the resistance to letting go of defenses. In our view, however, the management of this resistance is central to being able to profoundly relax.

Identifying the thought: "If I am not tense, I am not safe"

The chronically tight pelvis tends to be part of the habit of conditioned vigilance—this vigilance which says, "Beyond a certain point it's not safe for me to relax and take my attention off of the external world." The chronically tight pelvis often is an expression of an early conditioning that says: "If I am not on my guard, I am in danger."

So almost universally, individuals with pelvic pain who tend toward anxiety bump up against a stubborn barrier to quieting down, to relaxing their muscle tension and allowing their level of arousal and guardedness to release. It is common for individuals with pelvic pain to feel that if they take their attention off the pelvic pain, they are somehow unsafe. This stubborn barrier to relaxation is not arbitrary. We believe when it is present, it is most likely to have been conditioned early in life. It is often a scary experience to relax this barrier.

If you name the inner refusal to fully let go 'resistance'—resistance that is defending against relaxation, let us be clear that there is no way to cheat this defense. In our view, it is unlikely that hypnotizing someone and waving the magic wand of therapeutic suggestion for example, or giving medication or doing surgery, or using other interventions that work from the outside to the inside, will bypass or short-circuit this conditioned resistance.

The road less traveled

Paradoxical Relaxation is the road less traveled. This is a territory not known to most. And it is usually only of interest to those who have to deal with pain and have run out of options or those who understand the fruits of this practice.

In *Paradoxical Relaxation,* you make friends with your own chronic holding rather than hating it. You abide with it. You practice releasing your attachment to immediate relief in favor of accepting, relaxing with, opening up, and remaining continually present with what is not the most pleasant of experiences. It is in this training to give up one's preference, in favor of resting with what is, that what is, is most likely to change and become what one originally preferred. The experience of this is found in the trenches of the ongoing and devoted practice of this understanding.

Why we don't sell stand-alone relaxation tapes

(Part of David Wise's reply to the webmaster of the ChronicProstatitis.org chat group responding to the question of selling the recorded *Paradoxical Relaxation* course on a stand alone basis.)

"I do not sell the audio *Paradoxical Relaxation* course on a stand-alone basis. There are numerous relaxation tapes that can be bought from many different sources and people are free to buy them. I could sell the recorded relaxation course I use on a stand-alone basis. I have certainly had enough requests, but choosing not to do this is neither a casual nor a self-serving decision on my part. I have a short answer and a long answer to explain why.

Here is the short answer. I have little confidence that someone can learn to relax a painful pelvic floor from a relaxation tape without both instruction from someone who is competent in the method himself or herself and without pelvic *Trigger Point Release.* There are patients who have gotten a hold of earlier tapes in the recorded relaxation training course and have attempted to learn the protocol by listening to the tapes without competent instruction. Sometimes a physical therapist who has copies of these earlier lessons gives a copy of these tapes to a patient and says, "Here are some tapes to try." The patient goes home and listens to these tapes for a while, comes up against some difficulty and usually abandons their use. The tapes wind up on the shelf and the patient is convinced that relaxation of the pelvic floor isn't possible. This is a great shame in my opinion. It closes off what I believe is a critical component in recovering from pelvic pain. I speak from my own experience and many patients that I have treated.

Like learning the piano or learning carpentry, I believe you need a real teacher who is a true pianist or carpenter. Taped recordings of relaxation instruction without the communication of the skilled teacher to the earnest student usually fail in my experience. Furthermore, you can only teach someone to go as far as you yourself can go with any skill particularly with the profound relaxation of the pelvic floor. I don't support anyone teaching *Paradoxical Relaxation* who is not skilled in it and who does not do it regularly him or herself.

I had the best teachers in relaxation, including having the privilege of working with Edmund Jacobson for a number of years, and even with such support and access to unequalled instruction, learning relaxation was hugely difficult and took me years to learn. There is no quick way here. I know this personally. I do not want to associate myself with making available a half-measure that appears to offer something substantial but does not.

When I was symptomatic, I tried many remedies that all seemed reasonable but ultimately failed to help me. They left me hopeful at first, then disappointed, and disheartened. A stand-alone relaxation tape, in my opinion, is a half-measure. Half-measures give little chance of offering real recovery from chronic pelvic pain syndromes. I have decided that if I am to err, I will err in the direction of not offering anything instead of offering a half-measure in which I have no confidence."

In summary, *Paradoxical Relaxation* is a psychotherapeutic method aimed at lowering pain-exacerbating anxiety, dysfunctional thinking and habitual pelvic floor hypertonicity

The group therapy sessions in *Paradoxical Relaxation* combine guided relaxation training, behavior modification and psychotherapy. As thoughts and feelings arise during relaxation, patients often experience support and relief in hearing others share the experiences common to most patients with pelvic pain. Unkind physicians, the loneliness of having no one to speak to, ongoing and catastrophic thoughts, sexual dysfunction and pain, stress on interpersonal relationships, problems in parenting, difficulties in courting for the unmarried, helplessness in controlling the pain and dysfunction, dealing with the impulse to socially withdraw, guilt and shame, social isolation, questions about being able to function at work, changing careers, insomnia, and general hopelessness about any symptom resolution are all common themes that arise as patients practice the methodology and interact during treatment. *Paradoxical Relaxation* supports developing a new relationship with the pelvis and introduces the concept that the pelvis is not the enemy and is best treated with kindness and understanding. Gestalt therapy methods are sometimes used as part of *Paradoxical Relaxation* in order to help patients be able to communicate with and relax a painful, hypertonic pelvic basin. Cognitive behavioral therapy with regard to thoughts arising during relaxation is also part of the *Paradoxical Relaxation* methodology.

CHAPTER 6

TRIGGER POINT RELEASE AND MYOFASCIAL RELEASE INSIDE AND OUTSIDE THE PELVIC FLOOR

Defining *Trigger Point Release* and *Myofascial Release*

There is often confusion on the part of patients that we see as to what *Trigger Point Release* and *Myofascial Release are.* The typical reference to *Myofascial/Trigger Point Release* makes it appear that they are one method when actually they are two different methods. While we use *Myofascial Release* methods, *we believe that they are not by themselves an effective treatment for pelvic pain.* We wish to be clear that in the *Wise-Anderson Protocol*, the strong emphasis is on *Trigger Point Release*, though we do use some *Myofascial Release* methods as well. Absent the effective release of trigger points related to pelvic pain, we do not think that most pelvic pain syndromes have the possibility to resolve.

We will briefly describe these terms here as we describe them in more detail later. *Trigger Point Release* is a method of identifying and releasing knots or taut bands in muscles that refer pain, either at the site of the trigger point or to a site remote from the actual trigger point. *Myofascial Release* is a name given to stretching the fascia or connective tissue around muscles that over time has tightened up and restricted the muscles that it surrounds.

Teaching patients to use *Trigger Point Release* and *Myofascial Release* on themselves

Some of the greatest suffering of pelvic pain has to do with not knowing whether your symptoms are going to get better, get worse, or never go away. When patients come to our clinic, they are both excited about the possibility of getting real help and simultaneously (depending on someone's tendency to catastrophize) worried about whether their hopes will be fulfilled.

In the pursuit of calming down the suffering, people with pelvic pain will often compulsively search the Internet for answers and reassurance. Typically the Internet scares people instead of reassuring them and leaves them more anxious. The Internet is a blessing and a curse because it democratizes access to information, but at the same time exposes us to the spectrum of ideas about pelvic pain that are variously weird, crackpotted, without scientific merit, scary or disempowering.

> Give people fish and they eat for a day. Teach
> people to fish and they eat for a lifetime.

What reassures patients the most is the experience of their symptoms dramatically improving or going away. Reassurance by professionals or other patients is often helpful as well. The management of doubt and fear, however, is one of the most important things to handle when you are dealing with pelvic pain. We tell our patients that they don't have to believe anything during the clinic. They don't even have to get rid of their anxiety or tendency to catastrophize. The most important thing is that they sincerely and earnestly do the protocol and watch the results. Ultimately the results will speak for themselves and we will help those we help and won't help those our protocol will not help. We have found in our clinic that we are most likely to help patients when we train them in self treatment that enables them to reduce or stop their symptoms themselves.

> "The only help worth giving is helping someone to become free from further help."
> Nisargadatta

Our treatment has evolved over the past twelve years and our experience has taught us that patients do best with our protocol when they learn to use it on themselves. Therefore our treatment involves teaching patients how to interrupt the self-feeding cycle of tension, anxiety and pain, which is the heart of the pelvic pain syndromes we treat, and how to keep the muscles in the pelvis loose and unrestricted. The resolution of pelvic pain is an inside job.

From this understanding, we became aware of the limitations of our more conventional office visits for pelvic pain. Just like taking on the responsibility of brushing one's teeth or showering, we have come to see the necessity of patients' taking on the full responsibility of effectively dealing with the tendency to tighten, and the consequences of having tightened their pelvic muscles. Our 6-day intensive clinic format has proven to be more effective in teaching patients the essentials of self-treatment.

As our treatment has shifted into an intensive 6-day clinic, the focus of our physical therapy now is to identify and map trigger point locations and areas of restriction related to our patients' pelvic pain. We then teach our patients to locate and deactivate their own trigger points inside and outside the pelvic floor and to teach certain *Myofascial Release* methods for them to use in self-treatment as well.

As we have discussed elsewhere, we teach willing partners to do internal *Trigger Point Release* that a patient cannot reach him or herself. While sometimes it is necessary for someone to see a physical therapist for internal *Trigger Point Release* for trigger points that they may not be able to reach themselves, *our goal is to limit patient dependency on professionals in favor of patients knowing how to take care of themselves.*

Deactivating trigger points and rehabilitating the chronically knotted up pelvic floor

We teach patients how to do this for themselves using *Trigger Point Release*, stretching, self-massage, and other methods that communicate to the pelvic floor muscles that it is okay to be relaxed and out of pain. *Trigger Point Release* has the aim of rehabilitating the tissues in and around the pelvic floor. We want to deactivate symptom-referring trigger points, restore the capacity of the pelvic floor muscles to relax, restore the competence of the blood vessels that serve this area, to soften the muscles around the nerves and to re-introduce the experience of a quiet pelvic floor.

Why one's finger is superior to any instrument used for internal self-treatment

It may seem like a challenge for most people to reach inside the pelvic floor with a gloved, lubricated finger, rectally or vaginally, in order to release pelvic pain related trigger points, spasm, and areas of restriction. In fact, it is relatively easy to do once one's initial reticence and awkwardness is overcome. Indeed, while doing internal *Trigger Point Release* may sound strange, people do far more invasive kinds of self-treatment, like routinely injecting themselves with insulin, or catheterizing themselves in order to urinate, along with other similar routine kinds of self-treatment for certain conditions. *Trigger Point Release* especially at the beginning of therapy, in the scheme of things, is relatively unremarkable.

We have heard from many people with pelvic pain who have bought some kind of sex toy which they inserted internally for the purpose of doing *Trigger Point Release*. Generally speaking, we have been unimpressed with the effectiveness of this kind of instrument. The sex toys available are designed more for sexual stimulation than any kind of therapeutic purpose.

We believe that the impulse to use an instrument inside the rectum or vagina may be the expression of a person's shame and aversion to the area of the pelvic floor. People who are embarrassed about their genitals or anal/rectal area often want to use an instrument because they don't want to get too near this area. They feel afraid or squeamish about this part of their body and want to keep it at bay.

There are doctors who use needles inside the pelvic floor to do *Trigger Point Release*. We generally do not think this is a good idea for a number of reasons. First of all, it is difficult to identify a trigger point and then accurately insert a needle into it inside the pelvic floor. Secondly, the area cannot be made sterile and for reasons related to hygiene and infection there is some risk involved. We have had patients who have had severe reactions to needles being inserted inside the pelvic floor, from the inadvertent piercing of a blood vessel that filled the abdomen with blood, to painful flare-ups that lasted months after a nerve was probably nicked. Furthermore, the use of needles promotes the idea that the pelvic floor cannot be helped by oneself but only by a professional. This is an idea we do not want to support.

In general, we think that a self-treatment tool inserted inside the pelvic floor is useful only where one cannot reach with one's own finger. Toward this end, we have been developing an experimental trigger point wand to deactivate internal trigger points that are difficult for a patient to deactivate manually.

We think that the finger is superior to any instrument because when you use your finger, you are the therapist and the patient at the same time and your feedback to yourself is immediate. In other words, you can feel the area that you are working on, as well as feel and adjust the level of pressure you are exerting.

With some practice in stretching and loosening of muscles in the arms and torso, it is possible for most people to effectively work on the large majority of their external and internal trigger points. Finally, with regard to teaching patients to do internal *Trigger Point Release*, we believe that a professional should be able to do internal self-treatment on him or herself before teaching a patient to do so.

A word about lubrication for internal *Trigger Point Release*. We use and recommend a sterile, water-based lubricant like K-Y® Jelly. Novelty lubricants, lubricants that warm the tissue, spermicidal lubricants or petroleum based lubricants are not recommended.

The necessity of repetitive treatment

Trigger Point Release needs to be done repetitively so that offending trigger points become quiet and that the pelvic muscles remain relaxed when there is no need for them to be tense.

The actual number of self-treatment sessions varies. We encourage patients to use *Trigger Point Release* and *Myofascial Release* when needed as life's stresses trigger pelvic-related contraction and trigger point activity. These methods have to be used repetitively in order to override the tendency of the pelvic floor to remain shortened and contracted when it has been so for a prolonged period of time.

In doing *Trigger Point Release*, we are saying to the tissue: *"We know you are distressed, we know you are hurting, we know you are tense and contracted. We are going to press on painful trigger points in you to release them. We are going to stretch you to give you room to breathe, to be nourished and to rest. At first it will probably hurt because you are used to being tense and contracted, so any stretching that we do to you will probably feel uncomfortable and unknown. You are used to being uncomfortable and so any sense of comfort, while feeling good, may not feel like 'home' to you. With a finger, we remind you over and over again that it is okay to lengthen and soften and relax. We are going to stretch you regularly so that the lengthened state becomes normal for you. As we do this, the stretching most likely will be both painful and paradoxically may also feel good. It may feel like sometimes the discomfort of what is being done to you during a session 'hurts so good.' We do this as your friend and want the best for you. We know that when you learn that it is okay to be out of pain, you will want to stay out of pain. We want you to feel safe. Let's work together."*

What to expect during an initial *Trigger Point Release* session

When you first come for *Trigger Point Release*, first our physical therapist will examine you externally, look at your posture and feel and evaluate all of the muscles that relate to your pelvic floor. Then we will determine the strength of these muscles and whether there are trigger points or constriction in them. We will press on trigger points to see if they refer pain into the areas where you are symptomatic.

The external examination first assesses muscles of the trunk and lower abdomen, looking for acute trigger points that may refer symptoms to the pelvic region. The internal examination is done through the rectum in men, and either through the vagina or the rectum or both in women. Before we do an internal examination, we will review the anatomy of your pelvic muscles with you. We review with you how our finger will enter inside and what we will be doing inside as we feel for trigger points and areas of soft tissue restriction.

We will be clear that in order to evaluate how your muscles are related to your pain and dysfunction, we will have to press on areas that likely will be painful. We will tell you that if the pain becomes too intense, that you are in control of the session and all you need to do is tell us to stop if you want us to stop, or slow down and lighten up if you want us to slow down or reduce the pressure we are exerting. We find that our initial examination appears to be less stressful and less painful when our patients know what to expect.

Our description of the first sessions of *Trigger Point Release* may sound formidable. While we can't completely assuage the anxieties of our patients who have never experienced it, it is safe to say that the *Trigger Point Release* we do is nothing to be nervous about. Some patients have likened it to, in the worst case, going to the dentist's office.

Both the examination and the treatment of the inside of the pelvic floor in the male patient are done while the man is lying in the prone position (on his stomach) with pillows under his pelvis. This position is an innovation of Tim Sawyer. Occasionally the man will be examined and treated in the lithotomy position (on the back with knees bent and open). Women can be examined either, prone, on their side, or on their back, depending on the area of the pelvic floor that needs to be reached.

We reach the inside of the pelvis with a gloved finger, liberally lubricated to avoid chafing or irritating the pelvic tissue. In rectal-related treatment, we begin by entering the rectum and examining the *sphincter ani* (the rings of muscle at the opening of the rectum), and then moving to the *coccygeus muscle* and then moving to the back, middle and front of the *levator ani muscles.*

We carefully check the *obturator internus muscle* because of its relationship to the *pudendal nerve*, which runs through the pelvis and *posterior ligaments*—compression or pinching of this nerve is sometimes the source of pain in certain patients.

We usually examine the left side of the body using the right hand, and the right side of the body using the left hand. Using the finger as the instrument of treatment requires that the therapist is in a certain position to gain maximum strength in palpating and stretching the trigger points. Using the hand that is opposite the side of the patient's pelvic floor (right hand to left pelvic floor, and left hand to the right pelvic floor) affords maximum leverage and extension inside.

In our digital rectal examination of male patients, we work with the prostate and the trigger points that are often found in the insertions of the muscles into the pelvis around the prostate. We discuss our treatment of women in Chapter 7. As we assess and work with the trigger points on the edge of the prostate we move into the *anterior*, then middle, then *posterior levator ani muscles*, and then move to the *piriformis* and *coccygeus muscles*. In a 90-degree position (with the finger perpendicular), we move to the side-wall of the pelvis to assess the *obturator muscles*.

A session generally starts outside the pelvis, including the *lower abdominal* and *oblique muscles* with the trigger points found, as it helps prepare the patient for internal work. The treatment of the external muscles consists of *Trigger Point Release*, stretching of soft tissue, followed by heat and instructions for the home stretching program if they are applicable. We examine and treat the following muscles: *abdominals, psoas, quadratus lumborum, gluteals, piriformis, adductors, pectineus,* and *paraspinals*. We work on these muscles with the patient lying in different postures to facilitate lengthening of the tissue and to deactivate trigger points during this phase of treatment. We demonstrate and describe that this is what we need to do with the internal muscles so that the patient is fully informed. In our clinic, we devote sessions to training each patient in self-treatment.

In our examination, we use a three point system to identify the levels of pain and tenderness of the trigger points (0 = no pain, 1+ = mild pain, 2+ = moderate pain, 3 = severe pain). When trigger points are pressed, very often the pressure will prompt someone to jump. This is called "the jump sign" and it is one of the tests verifying the existence of a trigger point. When there is a jump response, or a very tender area, we indicate that by using the designation 3+.

Kinds of techniques used inside the pelvic floor

The only way we can control what we do inside the pelvic floor is with the sensitivity of the finger. In a sense, assessing and treating the pelvic floor is like using Braille. We can't see what we are doing and must rely on the information coming through the sensitivity of a gloved finger.

We use several techniques under these conditions. The most common is called the *pressure/release technique*. It has been called the technique of *ischemic compression*. You will understand this method if you apply pressure to the back of your left hand with your right index finger. You will notice that when you press on the back of your hand and then release it, that a little white spot is temporarily created where the blood was momentarily pushed out by the finger pressure. This is what we do inside the pelvic floor.

We feel for the typical "taut band," characteristic of the trigger point, and apply pressure to it to help release it. We hold this pressure for 15-90 seconds, while always staying in communication with our patient about their level of discomfort. Pressing on trigger points like this, especially at first, can be quite uncomfortable. The tolerance a patient has for pressure release of trigger points is improved to the extent to which they feel they can control the duration and intensity of the pressure. We often ask patients to do RSA breathing discussed elsewhere while doing the release. We proceed systematically throughout the pelvic floor to the trigger points we have identified, applying this pressure release technique.

We sometimes use another technique developed by George Thiele in the 1940's, but regard Thiele massage alone as an inadequate treatment technique. His method involves a sweeping motion, stroking the length of the muscle. We sometimes stroke or apply pressure to a trigger point until we feel it lengthen and soften. At that point we ask the patient to tighten the muscle up while we press against it. Then we ask the patient to relax and let go of the tightening. This method helps lengthen and soften certain rigid pelvic muscles.

After a number of treatments, which vary from patient to patient, the activity of the external and internal trigger points tends to diminish, and we are left with certain remaining and often stubborn trigger points. We ask patients, when it is possible for them, to take hot baths before a self-treatment session as a way of helping loosen muscles that are tight and constricted. We often suggest warm compresses to patients or ask them to take a warm bath after treatment as well.

Flare-ups from treatment

We tell patients that they will have flare-ups throughout treatment. This is a very important communication, because if the patient's expectation is that there will be a steady and unflagging improvement in symptoms, the flare-up after treatment can feel like a defeat and an invalidation.

Flare-ups from self-treatment or treatment by a professional are inevitable and frequent. In stretching tissue that has been shortened for many years, it is not possible to avoid pain and flare-ups as the result of such stretching. It is as if the tissue is saying: *"I am not used to being so lengthened and stretched. I have been tight and rigid for a long time and you are breaking my grip and holding. That hurts."* The *flare-up can be seen as a good thing* because it tends to corroborate our diagnosis and it tells us that we are in the right place. As self-treatment and physical therapy continue, pain and discomfort associated with it tend to diminish, although very uncomfortable flare-ups that hearken back to the level of the original symptoms do happen from time to time and are not a bad thing.

Frequency of treatment

There is no formula determining the minimum or maximum number of treatments required to achieve success with the physical therapy method used in the *Wise-Anderson Protocol*. Some patients respond immediately and require only minimal rehabilitation of the internal and external pelvic-related musculature coordinated with good *Paradoxical Relaxation* practice. Some patients need extensive treatments because of a tendency to return to a baseline tension level. We encourage patients to do self-treatment regularly until painful and constricted tissue softens and stops being painful when stretched or pressed.

Trigger Point Release and the release of emotions

Sometimes during the course of internal *Trigger Point Release* deep emotions related to the tightness in the pelvis come to the surface. These emotions are often related to feelings that have been suppressed in relationship to some kind of trauma or significant emotional event. Grief, fear, and anger sometimes arise and these can occur at home or in the office.

It is important to understand that the release of these emotions (they don't always occur) is part of the resolution of the condition being treated. It should be looked upon positively. Understanding that the expression of these emotions is a good thing, the partner or therapist present with the patient can be most helpful by just allowing the reaction in a caring and open way. There is nothing to be alarmed about when these emotions arise. People usually feel a sense of relief after these experiences. Sometimes it is appropriate to explore these emotions in psychotherapy as a way of resolving them.

Preparation for and processing *Trigger Point Release*

The self-treatment *Trigger Point Release* sessions are best regarded as special times that need to be protected from the demands of the outside world. It is for this reason that we suggest that, when possible, the patient do self-treatment physical therapy sessions in a relaxed way where the patient has no responsibilities afterward. When possible we suggest bathing and doing a relaxation session focusing on feeling and accepting the sensations that are present after the *Trigger Point Release* session.

When possible, we like to train the spouse or partner of the patient to do the internal and external *Trigger Point Release* in places patients may not be able to reach. *A partner, however, is not essential to the success of our treatment.* Similarly, when a patient does not have a partner it is sometimes useful to see a physical therapist from time to time to reach places the patient may not be able to reach.

A patient's recovery from pelvic pain after learning self-treatment

Below is an essay on self-treatment from one of our patients who came to an early clinic and whose story appears later in Chapter 9. We include his follow up story for the 5th edition that appears below his original essay that we presented in the 4th edition. He is intelligent, articulate, a good student and a good writer, thus his description and insights about his home program of *Trigger Point Release* embodies our philosophy and what we aim to train our patients to do.

One of the most important elements of my recovery from pelvic pain has been for me to develop a conceptual understanding of the science of trigger points and myofascial restriction.

In my experience, such an understanding only came when I became wholeheartedly committed to learning how to work on myself, and not remain dependent on a physical and/or massage therapist, though in the beginning stages of recovery working with a physical and/or massage therapist who really knew their stuff was essential for me.

In other words, understanding trigger points and why and when they caused my pain was crucial for me to manage and eliminate them. I finally had to surrender, at some point, to the fact that my condition was not one where I could just go to the doctor, be given a pill, and never have to think about it again.

In my own experience, I had the fortune of being trained by one of the best trigger point physical therapists for pelvic pain when I attended the Stanford Protocol clinic over 2 years ago. It was there that I received a trigger point map of my pelvic floor during the clinic treatment and my first basic understanding, experience and training with regard to my own trigger points and myofascial pain. The description of locations of pelvic pain trigger points in A Headache in the Pelvis has been very important for me to study, along with the Clair Davies' book The Trigger Point Therapy Workbook. I began working on myself with the assistance of tennis balls, a Theracane©, the grip end of a golf club, and other small trigger point tools guided by the instructions I received at the clinic. I would refer to Davies' book to confirm what I was discovering about my own tender, restricted myofascial areas. Davies' point-by-point approach to trigger points in every muscle of the body was and is a helpful guide, although he understandably does not include much information concerning the pelvic floor, as he was a piano-tuner-turned-massage-therapist and massage therapists are not allowed to work inside the pelvic floor.

By attending the Stanford Protocol clinic and committing myself to a home treatment program, I have learned much about trigger points and myofascial tissue. I now conceptually understand the nature of the muscle tissue that I treat with pressure/release and stroking techniques. The most important thing I learned about working on myself was that I could control how much pressure I was applying, and at the same time, unlike the therapist, actually feel the referral of the trigger point inside my own body.

The more I have become familiar with and have come to understand my own tissues and how they feel when I press on them, the more I have been able to maintain my recovery strides away from the therapist for extended periods of time. At this point, over two years from the beginning of my journey, I feel that I have become essentially free of professional help altogether, although I have no hesitation in seeking competent help if I need to.

Myofascial tissue is fascinating. It actually disturbs me that we do not teach children in school what I have learned over the last two and a half years. I have learned that the muscles of my body want to be warm and supple. They want to be stretched often and relaxed constantly to relieve unhealthy levels of tension that build up in them during the course of my daily events and movements. I am a busy professional and know this all too well.

As I look back on my own experience of pelvic pain, it seems that what occurred to me was a sort of muscular breakdown of a particular region of my body. The muscles simply said "no more." The muscles themselves had become hard like concrete and became painful all of the time. The worst areas in my case were exquisitely painful when palpated and stroked.

It was important for me to realize that the knotted up muscles were not solely the reason for my pain...I think about the central nervous system being like the flame on a gas-cooking stove or wall heater. Everyone has seen a gas flame - when the flame is very low, it is soft-colored and blue and puts off very little heat and seems harmless; when the flame is very high, it is a hot, white-orange color, puts off a great deal of heat, and seems quite formidable. Everyone on earth has a default central nervous system level. Like myself, many type A personalities, or people with extreme ambition who live super fast lifestyles, probably have a very elevated central nervous system default level; and by the same token, I would imagine that monks living in a monastery and meditating most of the day would have a very low central nervous system default level.

Now the picture I hold in my mind about this is that every trigger point or area of restricted myofascial tissue has its own little gas flame within it - thus, if you are extremely anxious and stressed and living furiously, your trigger point flame will be white-orange and firing on all cylinders and you will find yourself in a firestorm of pain. If you are calm, relaxed, not threatened, and at peace about your life (whatever your lot), you can have numerous physical trigger points and feel very little pain because the flame within your trigger points is a soft-blue and hardly putting out any heat (i.e. pain).

By my learning how to treat my trigger points at home and doing daily relaxation sessions, I feel I created the optimum environment for the myofascial tissue to release and become supple and pain-free again. The lower you keep your "flame" through Paradoxical Relaxation, the easier it is for the actual physical tissue to open up. Repetition of the home trigger point work and the Paradoxical Relaxation I believe has allowed my muscles to remember their old, relaxed pain-free state.

The process by which I had to learn to treat myself at home took time. At first, I would roll on a tennis ball and not know what in the heck I was looking for; I would dig into my quadratus lumborum with the end of the Theracane© and not have a clue what I was pressing on. But over the course of several months, in conjunction with referring to my clinic training and the Davies' book, I began to feel more comfortable about what I was doing. I began to be able to search out and find tender trigger points and places of restriction almost automatically.

I learned how to gently but firmly apply deep static and stroking pressure to tender myofascial tissue; I have seen the amazing range of motion I have gained in certain muscles immediately after treating them. I have dug deep into my gluteal muscles on the floor with a tennis ball and felt the pain and pressure in my lower back release. Trust me, you will discover the appropriate level of pressure to apply to yourself. Some areas you will find that you can really dig into; other areas will be so tender that you have to go very slowly and work at them over time until you work deeper and deeper, releasing the painful, knotted up tissue.

I found it helpful to consult with a physical/massage therapist who understood trigger points and myofascial pain. While you are learning, I would encourage this. It is really important to find someone who has experience in Trigger Point Release and experience working with pelvic pain. At some point, I found that I could treat certain places even better than the therapist; for others places, I have gone to see my therapist for help.

I haven't had a set regimen. I saw that it was up to me to learn my myofascial map. I think that probably many people, after some brief, helpful trigger point work, find that they can manage their situation with relaxation and other tools, and do not do much trigger point work. Others, like me, become fascinated with the field of trigger points and conduct trigger point "troubleshooting" on themselves all the time. I did a good deal of stretching and took up yoga to further relax and stretch my muscles. You have to find the right balance for yourself. However, in my experience it was necessary to learn my trigger point map and how to explore it in the home environment before I could start to find the right balance for me.

I had to remember that all trigger points are not like "buttons" that I could simply press on to turn off my pain (though I now understand that many times in treatment people with pelvic pain do experience an immediate deactivation of the trigger point and relief from pain). I found in myself, however, that my most deeply ingrained trigger points required a lot of time and repetitive treatment to truly release. I finally understood that it had taken many years, probably decades, of tensing and muscle abuse to create the pain situation that I was in, and that it was not that big a stretch to accept that it would take 2-4 years of rehabilitation to return my muscles to a normal, pain-free state. In fact, I came to appreciate and honor the fact that my body could recover from three decades of abuse in only a few years if I gave it the proper care, rest, and treatment it deserved.

...for me, it has taken over two years, but I was constantly getting better the whole time and actually started to enjoy working on or "milking" the areas of my body that were still tender and knotted up. If you are having pelvic pain, because you are the only one with access to yourself all of the time, I cannot encourage you enough to learn how to perform trigger point work on yourself.

An understandable problem for many pelvic pain patients, as it was for me at first, is their mental attitude towards the internal Trigger Point Release therapy. I had to accept this fact - the muscle tissue of the pelvic floor is no different from the muscle tissue of the shoulder, it's just not accessible on the exterior of your body. Also, pelvic tissue is intimately connected to the organs of the sexual and excretory regions, and thus can create the strangest of symptoms related to going to the bathroom and sexual activities.

But I understand now that my pelvic floor is no less a part of my body than my ear. In fact, every morning I would go into my ear with a Q-tip in order to release any wax or water stuck inside my ear. I thought why is it any different, then, to go inside the anus to release problems with my pelvic floor? Do I love my ear more than my pelvic floor? I realized that no, it's because like everyone else, I was conditioned by society to be embarrassed about the genitals, anus, and rectal areas. You stick your finger in the orifice that is your nose to remove dirt. You stick a toothbrush in the orifice that is your mouth to clean your teeth, gums, and tongue. The anus is simply the orifice you go through to release trigger points in the pelvic floor. It's simply no big deal; I no longer take it so seriously.

One of the major keys for me in becoming comfortable with the internal trigger point work was to learn to work internally on myself. I began getting into a hot shower with a glove and some lubricant and just started by massaging the exterior of the anus. The sphincter itself can have very painful trigger points in it and simply massaging it on the exterior could bring great relief. Later, when I felt ready, I began pushing on inside and massaging the tissue just inside the anus, searching and feeling for tender spots, and going slowly. With the help and guidance of the therapist, and because I am very flexible and with the help of yoga stretching, I have been able to move even further, and do Trigger Point Release on my whole pelvic floor. It is important to understand the anatomy and know the anatomy and trigger point map of your pelvic floor. Being able to treat my own pelvic floor myself has been an amazingly helpful tool in overcoming my chronic pelvic pain. I have tried to maintain a positive attitude and have reminded myself to be thankful that I am learning about an undiscovered area of my body that most people will never have the opportunity to know. What I say is honor your pelvic floor; it has done a whole lot for you through the years.

Of course, these and other descriptions of trigger point work and myofascial tissue will only get you so far because that's all they are, someone else's descriptions. Ultimately, it is up to you to learn and understand the concepts of the Stanford Protocol. No doctor can do it for you. You must surrender to the fact that you have to play the most important part in your healing. The combination of daily trigger point work (through the use of hands, tennis balls, Theracanes©, and anything else you find helpful), deep Paradoxical Relaxation sessions, stretching or yoga, and hot, soothing baths is the most effective way I have found to heal myself and my pelvic pain.

(Follow up report for 5th edition from this patient)

Nearly four years ago I arrived in California at the very end of my rope. I had suffered with chronic discomfort in my urinary tract, frequency, and a few other pelvic pain symptoms for over three years, but had always been able to manage my discomfort and pain as it waxed and waned in my life. But in spring 2004, I literally began to experience every chronic pelvic pain symptom imaginable, and I was in a constant state of pain all day long. Through a mixture of seeming luck and grace, I found A Headache in the Pelvis on the web, and immediately contacted Dr. Wise and signed up for a clinic during the summer of 2004.

These last four years have been quite a journey of healing. In my own experience, long term discipline to the protocol, combined with a deep conceptual understanding of my condition, were the main keys to my recovery. Here are some more specific points that illuminated my way as I took the protocol home with me and made it a part of the core curriculum of my life:

1. *I learned not to impose a false timeline on my healing. I strove to accept that it probably took years (or decades) of protective tensing, stress, and miscellaneous traumas for my pelvis to become symptomatic. When I thought about it, a few years of recovery time for something that has been going on for twenty was not that bad of a deal. I did my best to accept that the combination of flare-ups, waxing and waning, and treatment protocol was my friend for the next few years. With much inner resistance, I invited it into my life. I did my best to allow my body to decide how long it would take to heal, not my ego. When I told myself things like, "I'm going to be fine by Christmas," or "I am not going to have symptoms by summertime," I just made myself anxious. Like the instructions in Paradoxical Relaxation, I did my best to allow my recovery to take whatever pace it needed to*

and tried not to demand results from myself and realized that any arbitrary timeline was not helpful to me. Although I didn't do it perfectly, I saw that the best attitude for me was one of giving myself a psychological space of relaxed patience and discipline.

After dealing with months of anger at my situation, this is how I started to view the project of my pelvic pain healing, and my journey got better immediately. I quit thinking about and demanding results, and only focused my attention on doing the protocol every day in a relaxed, patient way, just like I had brushed my teeth every night of my life. And guess what – by not focusing on results, I started to experience more periods of being free from pelvic pain symptoms. When I was in pain, I just noticed it in a care-free way; and when I was free from pain, I just noticed it and said a calm prayer of thanks, and did not get my ego all tied up in it. The ability to do this psychologically took a long time, and I credit the many sessions of Paradoxical Relaxation and the cognitive therapy in Byron Katie's Loving What Is for giving me the ability to actually do it.

2. *I learned the importance of self-treatment of key external muscles. I saw that the interior pelvic floor is a bowl of muscles that must be treated with proper internal trigger point therapy; but that bowl does not exist by itself. It is intimately attached to the abdominals, psoas, quadratus lumborum, glutes, and supported by the muscles of the front, inner, and back of the thighs. Repetitive treatment of these external muscles, in my own experience, was key in unlocking the entire pelvic region and giving space for the internal pelvic muscles to loosen and relax. I studied the location of these muscles in both A Headache In the Pelvis and Claire Davies' book The Trigger Point Therapy Workbook, and developed creative ways of using the weight of my body to perform proper trigger point holds on these muscles. Here are a few examples:*

- *For the adducters (inner thighs), I would throw the inside of my leg over the back of an old, upholstered chair, and lean my body weight into it;*
- *For the glutes, I would daily get on the floor with a tennis or softball and deeply milk the trigger points out of my gluteal muscles, as taught at the AHIP clinic;*
- *For the psoas, I would lay belly down on the bed, tuck my hands under my belly, and invert my fingers back up, towards the ceiling. This allowed me to perform a deep static hold on my psoas by using my body weight to lean into my fingers. In my experience, releasing the psoas is key in allowing the whole pelvic region to "fall" or relax. Release of the psoas, in my experience, helped my frequency and back stiffness.*

These are just a few examples and are not meant to be exhaustive. I have talked to several other patients who have developed their own creative ways for treating their problem areas. And again, these methods take time to develop. I am still developing new ways to trouble shoot trigger points and keep my muscles supple and relaxed. Learning how to use tennis balls and a Theracane©, as taught at the AHIP clinic and in The Trigger Point Therapy Workbook, is a kind of artistic practice. It is not to be figured out over night, but rather learned over time as you explore your own body and tender restricted myofascial areas. It took me approximately 4-6 months before I became really comfortable using the Theracane© and other tools, and even longer before I began to see how all the external and internal muscles of the pelvic region are interconnected and related. It is not rocket science by any means, but it takes patience, repetitive treatment, and a calm awareness to feel the different sensations that palpation of your trigger points create, which can cover the full range of piercing pain, dull pain, burning, and other pain sensations. In my own experience, deep palpation of the adducters and glutes can sometimes create a deep spacious release referral, rather than a pain referral. Release of the tense torque that your tight, trigger pointed muscles are exerting on the pelvic region is a process that most likely will take months or a few years, not a few days. Give your pelvis permission to take as long as it needs to. I would sometimes actually speak lovingly to my pelvis, and ensure it that it had all the time and space it needed to heal. I think this benefited my recovery greatly.

3. *I had to deal with my discouragement and frustration at times regarding internal self-treatment. I began to think about the sphincter and the perineum as the "home plate" of the pelvic floor, and in my case saw that release of these areas can provide a systemic release throughout the entire region. I tried to be patient, to listen to my body, and not try to heal myself completely with one internal treatment. It never worked that way. For me, it took continuous stretching of the sphincter over many months before it began to easily release and I could maintain that release through Moment to Moment and Paradoxical Relaxation. I think it took years and years of continuous tensing and guarding to cause my pelvis to become tightened and painful, and thus it took a long time to stretch and relax the pelvic floor back into a relaxed, normal state. I had to take responsibility for being the person with the most knowledge of my pelvic muscles and problem areas. I would go back and study A Headache in the Pelvis and the other suggested books. I had to be the doctor I wanted to find.*

I began to experiment with the attitude that my pelvic pain is happening for me, not to me. When I started to see pelvic pain as something that could benefit me, could expand my understanding, patience, compassion, discipline, and acceptance, things got much better for me.

Details of the Physical Therapy used in the *Wise-Anderson Protocol*

There is often confusion among many who wish to follow our protocol about how to tell what is useful physical therapy and training in self-treatment, and what isn't. Our perspective comes from working with many patients who have seen us at Stanford with whom we have used the *Wise-Anderson Protocol* over the years.

We have interviewed many patients who have seen a variety of physical therapists. We have listened carefully to the comparison of their experiences with physical therapists we know are competent in our protocol and their previous experiences. We have looked at the results and want to discuss these comparisons below.

In putting together a brief description of the phenomenon of trigger point activity and myofascial restriction related to the pelvic floor, we are not suggesting that anyone use this information as a substitute for proper in-person physical therapy training, nor are we suggesting that one treats oneself without proper instruction and training. Competently doing our physical therapy protocol is not mastered quickly but comes with the understanding of the trigger point phenomenon, and by experience in successfully working with *Trigger Point Release* in and outside of the pelvic floor after competent instruction.

Physical therapy is one essential part of the equation in our protocol of treating pelvic pain. It is tempting to see an external fix like *Trigger Point Release* as the answer to pelvic pain. When you have pelvic pain of the kind we treat and decide to do whatever it takes to resolve it, you find out there is no quick fix. Results come from committing yourself to the inside job of changing very stubborn inner habits.

More on regular self-treatment

The most exhaustive physical therapy done brilliantly, while essential in our protocol, cannot guarantee that the offending trigger points will behave. Consider that there are 168 hours in a week. Let us say that a person goes to see the physical therapist 2 times a week. That is quite a bit of physical therapy. In the physical therapy session, after a person takes off their clothes, gives the physical therapist a report on their week and begins the physical therapy itself, at the most there is probably 30-45 minutes of hands-on treatment. After the treatment, the tissue is stretched (although sometimes temporarily irritated in the process). At the level of 2 appointments per week that is, at the most, 1½ hours of therapeutic treatment per week. In a good pelvic floor physical therapy session, the pelvic floor tissue has been lengthened, trigger points have been deactivated and life has been made more livable for it.

And then there is what could be called 'the parking lot phenomenon' so typical of modern life. After a physical therapy session, you go down into the parking lot, get into your car, get on your cell phone and get back into your life. Your partner is upset about something on the phone, your work calls with a problem, traffic is bad and your body's same protective guarding and tension, part of your default mode of tension, easily reasserts itself. A good physical therapy session can be reversed in an hour of bad traffic.

After physical therapy twice a week, there are approximately 166 hours remaining in the week to live. The old habit of going 100 miles an hour in one's life and tightening up the pelvis regularly and squeezing and shortening the irritated tissue, as we have discussed, can easily and quickly undo the therapeutic impact of the physical therapy session. A physical therapy treatment that lasts less that 1% of your life is unlikely to work if the old, symptom-provoking habits go on unabated. This is why the ongoing regular relaxation of the pelvic floor and quieting of the nervous system with the relaxation protocol like the one we use, in close connection with regular daily physical therapy self-treatment in which the tissue is repetitively loosened, is necessary. The resolution of the kind of pelvic pain we treat is an inside job of cooperating with the healing mechanism of the body in the short run and the long run. *Trigger Point Release* is an essential and necessary component and for most people not a sufficient one by itself.

Furthermore, pelvic pain syndromes, even when they do go away, tend to be cyclical and often can come back during periods of stress. Knowing how to treat yourself and not having to run to a professional, in our view, makes the flare-up easier to face and deal with. Finally, having the skill to do self-treatment, necessarily including physical therapy self-treatment, on a maintenance basis tends to reduce the frequency of flare-up.

That all being said, we address the issue of what physical therapy we believe works for pelvic pain. *Not all physical therapy for pelvic pain is the same or is effective.* Seeing someone who is a physical therapist and even seeing someone who holds him or herself out as a pelvic floor physical therapist offers no guarantee that the protocol we discuss in this book will be followed. This is critical information for the patient who sees hope for their condition in our protocol and is intent on undergoing it. One can do physical therapy for pelvic pain with a physical therapist who has little understanding and experience in *Trigger Point Release* and receive little benefit. Going to a different physical therapist can make all the difference.

In other words, the experience, understanding and intuitive talent of a physical therapist doing *Trigger Point Release* can make the difference between success and failure of our protocol and the reduction or resolution of one's symptoms or not.

Let us move on to a more detailed discussion of *Trigger Point Release*. Drs. Janet Travell and David Simons introduced trigger points to modern medicine. Travell and Simons published the first edition of *Myofascial Pain and Dysfunction: The Trigger Point Manual* in 1983, which was followed by a second volume in 1992, and a 2nd edition of volume one in 2001. These books were the culmination of research that went back to 1942 when Dr. Travell published her first article on myofascial pain. Janet Travell is well known for the remarkable fact, as we understand it, that she was appointed the White House physician during the Kennedy and Johnson administrations. She had been given this position as an expression of Kennedy's gratitude for her successful treatment of his myofascial pain that so impacted his life and political career. We are fortunate that our senior physical therapist Tim Sawyer, who has been the architect of the physical therapy aspect of our protocol, studied closely with Travell and Simons and then treated patients with them for years.

The concept of trigger points is relatively new to medicine. It is very new to urology. Trigger points are defined as taut bands within a muscle, either at the surface of the muscle or inside the muscle, in the belly or the attachment of the muscle. The trigger point characteristically elicits a twitch response, detectable on ultrasound or via electromyograph (a machine that measures the electrical activity in a muscle in millionths of a volt). The trigger point response can be felt by a trained and sensitive practitioner while palpating the trigger point. When the trigger point is pressed there is often a 'jump' response in the patient, due to the reflexive reaction of the patient to the often exquisite tenderness of the trigger point upon palpation. Furthermore, the trigger point characteristically refers pain/sensation to the site being pressed or to a site remote from it.

A trigger point can be active or latent. An active trigger point is considered able to refer pain and recreate that pain upon palpation when the patient comes in with a complaint of pain. A latent trigger point has the capacity to be the source of pain and under certain circumstances become an active one, but generally the patient does not complain of symptoms from latent trigger points. Trigger points are latent in many people. *Often active trigger points never entirely go away with the best therapy and so the goal of both our physical therapy and Paradoxical Relaxation protocol is to deactivate the trigger points so that they stop creating symptoms.*

The problem that occurs when urologists are asked to consider trigger points as essential ingredients in chronic pelvic pain syndromes is the problem of a 'paradigm conflict'. Our book presents a very different paradigm from the paradigm of conventional medicine. A paradigm is a model of reality. Urologists have little or no training or understanding of the role of trigger points in pelvic pain. The connective tissue and muscles inside and outside the pelvis are the sites in which many offending trigger points are found. This tissue and the trigger points that are found there have rarely been taken seriously as a source of pain by most urologists. This concept of trigger points in urology is poorly understood and not readily accepted.

Where one feels the trigger point pain is often not the source of the pain. For this reason pelvic pain diagnosed by someone unfamiliar with the workings of trigger points are often mistaken because they are unclear that the source of much pelvic pain is not where it seems to be. In other words, pain coming from trigger points often is not coming from where you feel the pain. *While the concept of referred pain is well understood in medicine, the idea that pelvic pain felt in the groin, penis, testicles, vagina, or perineum may originate in a trigger point inside or outside the pelvic floor is far less readily accepted.* Part of the difficulty that doctors have with trigger points is that they have usually received no training in the subject. Furthermore, because there is no objective, litmus paper, gold standard test for evaluating them, the only way clinically to find and treat them is through palpation. This requires training and a sensitive touch. Trigger points do not exist in the reality of many doctors. This is part of the paradigm conflict.

This paradigm conflict has very real consequences to patients with pelvic pain. In a telling example, a woman called us who had very severe rectal pain. She reported that during the course of one of her doctor's pelvic exams, he hit a spot that the woman said, "sent me through the roof." After the exam, the doctor told her that he really did not know what was going on with her, that he couldn't help her and she might simply have to live with the pain. The woman went home despondent, her pelvic floor very irritated and flared up. *The next day she woke up and her pain was almost gone.* It remained so for several days. She called up the doctor's office happily bewildered to share with the doctor what happened. She told the nurse that she thought it was related to the painful spot the doctor pressed. The nurse relayed the news about the woman to the doctor. The doctor then told the nurse to tell the patient she could massage that point herself if it helped her. The patient felt more bewildered.

What probably happened is that the doctor inadvertently pressed and temporarily released a major trigger point for the woman and the woman responded like any of our patients typically respond—with some flare up and then a reduction of symptoms. The doctor, in not understanding anything about trigger point pain and treatment, essentially dismissed this event and the possibility of helping this woman. His ignorance may have had a profound effect on his patient. She remained confused even after we spoke to her.

Trigger points refer pain directly on the trigger point site or to a remote site, which means that where you feel the pain is often not where it actually is coming from. For instance, we find that tip-of-the-penis pain is often referred from trigger points in the anterior portion of the *levator ani muscle* as it attaches to the prostate. This is not obvious and is counter-intuitive. This trigger point is a good 5 inches from the tip of the penis. Who would think that the source of tip-of-the-penis pain would come from a site so far away? To complicate matters further, if you do not have long enough fingers or if you do not understand how the trigger points work in the body, you miss this connection entirely. And if you don't keep pressure on an internal trigger point for the length of time we know is necessary, the trigger point remains active.

The internal muscles that contain trigger points are close to each other and it takes someone who understands the internal pelvic anatomy and is experienced in feeling the muscles inside the pelvic floor, to tell them apart. You can see the location of these muscles in the illustrations to follow. Below is a list of the internal muscles in which most internal trigger points are found. The relationship between symptoms and the location of associated trigger points is described below. Some of the connections reported below have not been published and come from the extensive experience of our senior physical therapist Tim Sawyer.

All of the muscles, both internal and external, must be thoroughly evaluated and treated. When muscles are known to contain trigger points referring pain to an area that the patient is complaining about, they should be examined carefully. The therapist must be trained in identifying trigger points and be able to feel for superficial and deep trigger points located in the belly and the attachments of the muscles. Most importantly, when trigger points are located, they must be held with pressure release which involves pressing on a trigger point with constant pressure, usually for a period of 30-90 seconds.

When appropriate the following techniques are used:

- Voluntary contraction and release/hold-relax/
  contract-relax reciprocal inhibition
- Spray and stretch occasionally with
  stubborn external trigger points
- Deep tissue mobilization including striping, strumming,
  effleurage
- Myofascial release/skin rolling
- Strain-counter-strain/muscle energy release

Anyone who has pelvic pain of the kind we treat should know that specific trigger points in specific pelvic muscles tend to refer specific kinds of symptoms. This knowledge is critical for the physical therapist who is treating pelvic pain and training patients in self-treatment. As we have mentioned, pain in the tip of the penis or the sense of urgency and frequency is typically created by active trigger points in the anterior (front) portion of the *levator ani muscle* as it attaches to the prostate. When the physician or physical therapist does an examination, knowledge of the relationship between symptoms and pelvic trigger points is essential to make the diagnosis of tension/neuromuscular related pelvic pain and dysfunction. We are much more confident in our diagnosis and ability to help the patient when we find relationships between the trigger points and the kinds of symptoms they typically refer.

The illustrations to follow indicate the internal and external pelvic floor-related trigger points and the location of the pain and symptoms they typically refer. Trigger points are sometimes idiosyncratic and not all patients fit all the patterns we describe here and so they must be located manually. Sometimes only one or two trigger points fit the referral pattern we describe below. To reiterate, we sometimes can help people with tight and tender pelvic muscles where we find no discernible trigger points.

Internal Pelvic Floor Trigger Points in Men and Where They Typically Refer Pain and Sensation

In working internally, we generally work with patients in the prone position with a cushion under their stomach, an innovation of the physical therapist, Tim Sawyer. The right hand is used to examine and work the left side of the pelvic floor and the left hand to work the right side of the pelvic floor. Patients tend to feel less vulnerable and more comfortable in this position and it affords the practitioner good access inside and outside the pelvic floor.

The following illustrations show trigger points in the internal pelvic muscles.

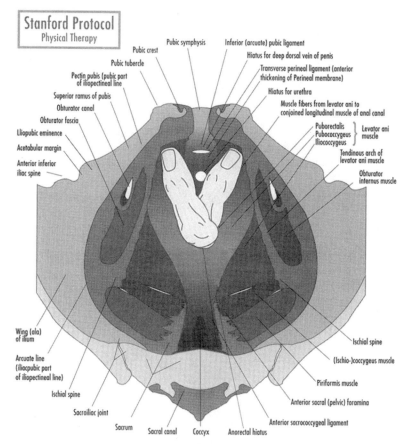

Stanford Protocol
Physical Therapy

Pubic symphysis
Pubic crest
Pubic tubercle
Pectin pubis (pubic part of iliopectineal line)
Superior ramus of pubis
Obturator canal
Obturator fascia
Iliopubic eminence
Acetabular margin
Anterior inferior iliac spine

Inferior (arcuate) pubic ligament
Hiatus for deep dorsal vein of penis
Transverse perineal ligament (anterior thickening of Perineal membrane)
Hiatus for urethra
Muscle fibers from levator ani to conjoined longitudinal muscle of anal canal
Puborectalis
Pubococcygeus } Levator ani muscle
Iliococcygeus
Tendinous arch of levator ani muscle
Obturator internus muscle

Wing (ala) of ilium
Arcuate line (iliacpubic part of iliopectineal line)
Ischial spine
Sacroiliac joint
Sacrum
Sacral canal
Coccyx
Anorectal hiatus

Ischial spine
(Ischio-)coccygeus muscle
Piriformis muscle
Anterior sacral (pelvic) foramina
Anterior sacrococcygeal ligament

Anterior Levator Ani, Superior Portion (or Puborectalis)

This is one of the most important trigger point sites in male pelvic pain, and palpating high enough up and firmly enough is critical in proper treatment. Frequently this area is the site of trigger points that are responsible for the tip-of-the-penis and shaft-of-the-penis pain. Furthermore, trigger points in this area can refer to the bladder, urethra, pressure, and fullness in the prostate.

- *One of the most important trigger point sites for male pelvic pain*
- *Can refer -tip-of-the-penis, shaft of the penis, bladder and urethral pain, frequency and urgency*
- *Can refer pressure/fullness in prostate*

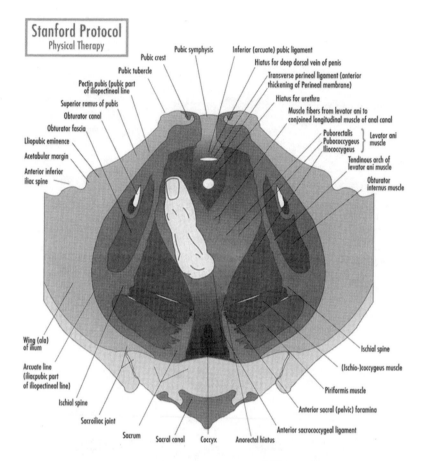

Stanford Protocol
Physical Therapy

Pubic crest
Pubic tubercle
Pectin pubis (pubic part of iliopectineal line)
Superior ramus of pubis
Obturator canal
Obturator fascia
Lliopubic eminence
Acetabular margin
Anterior inferior iliac spine

Pubic symphysis
Inferior (arcuate) pubic ligament
Hiatus for deep dorsal vein of penis
Transverse perineal ligament (anterior thickening of Perineal membrane)
Hiatus for urethra
Muscle fibers from levator ani to conjoined longitudinal muscle of anal canal
Puborectalis
Pubococcygeus } Levator ani muscle
Iliococcygeus
Tendinous arch of levator ani muscle
Obturator internus muscle

Wing (ala) of ilium
Arcuate line (iliacpubic part of iliopectineal line)
Ischial spine
Sacroiliac joint
Sacrum
Sacral canal
Coccyx
Anorectal hiatus
Anterior sacrococcygeal ligament
Anterior sacral (pelvic) foramina
Piriformis muscle
(Ischio-)coccygeus muscle
Ischial spine

Anterior Levator Ani, Middle Portion (or Levator Prostatae)

- Trigger points in this area can refer pain and pressure to the base of the penis, prostate, bladder and pelvis and recreate frequency and urgency

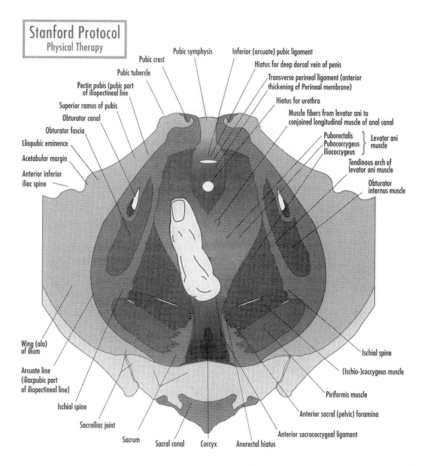

Stanford Protocol
Physical Therapy

Pubic crest
Pubic tubercle
Pectin pubis (pubic part of iliopectineal line
Superior ramus of pubis
Obturator canal
Obturator fascia
Iliopubic eminence
Acetabular margin
Anterior inferior iliac spine

Pubic symphysis

Pubic symphysis
Inferior (arcuate) pubic ligament
Hiatus for deep dorsal vein of penis
Transverse perineal ligament (anterior thickening of Perineal membrane)
Hiatus for urethra
Muscle fibers from levator ani to conjoined longitudinal muscle of anal canal
Puborectalis
Pubococcygeus } Levator ani muscle
Iliococcygeus
Tendinous arch of levator ani muscle
Obturator internus muscle

Wing (ala) of ilium
Arcuate line (iliacpubic part of iliopectineal line)
Ischial spine
Sacroiliac joint
Sacrum
Sacral canal
Coccyx
Anorectal hiatus

Ischial spine
(Ischio-)coccygeus muscle
Piriformis muscle
Anterior sacral (pelvic) foramina
Anterior sacrococcygeal ligament

Anterior Levator Ani, Inferior Portion (or Puborectalis)

- Can refer pain and pressure to the perineum, the base of the penis and the prostate.
- This is one of the most common and important trigger points in male pelvic pain

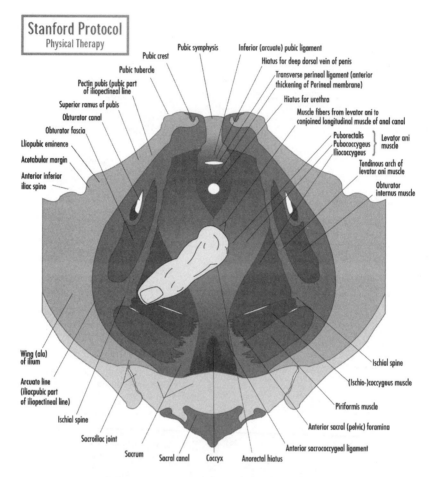

Middle Levator Ani - (Iliococcygeus)

Trigger points in the middle levator ani (iliococcygeus) typically refer lateral wall pain, perineal pain and anal sphincter pain. Trigger points can refer forward toward the anterior levators and the prostate. Trigger points here can refer discomfort associated with a sense of prostate fullness.

> • *Can refer lateral wall, perineal, anal sphincter, prostate fullness pain/discomfort referral pattern toward the anterior levators and prostate*

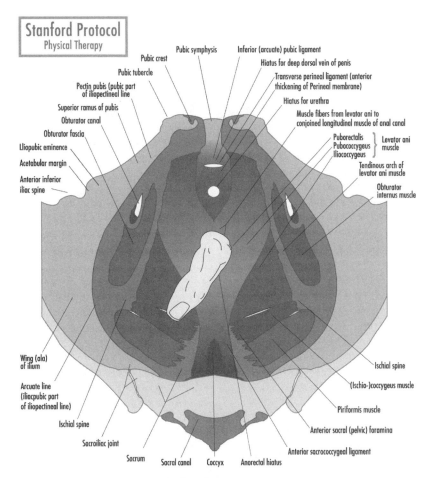

Coccygeus/Ischio-coccygeus

Trigger points in this muscle typically refers pain and pressure associated with the sense of have a golf-ball-in-the-rectum, pain to the coccyx and gluteus maximus. Pre or post bowel movement pain is often associated with the sense of having a full bowel.

- *Can refer symptoms to coccygeus, coccyx, gluteus maximus, pre or post bowel movement pain/full bowel sensation and discomfort*

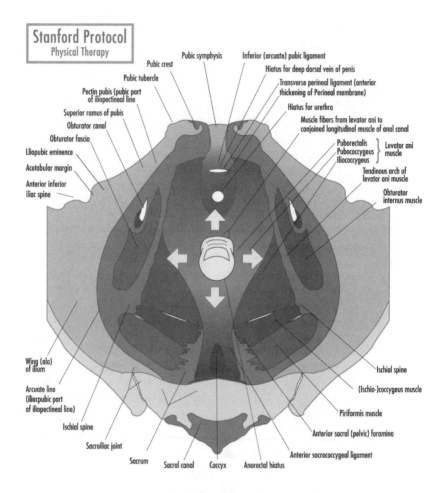

Sphincter Ani

Trigger points in this area may cause anal pain in the anal sphinter itself as well as pain going toward the front and back part of the anal sphincter. Treatment is done by gently stretching the sphincter upward in the 12 o'clock position, sideways in the 3 o'clock position, downward to the 6 o'clock position and sideways toward the 9 o'clock position.

- *Can refer pain in the anal sphincter itself as well as radiating to the front and back from the sphincter*

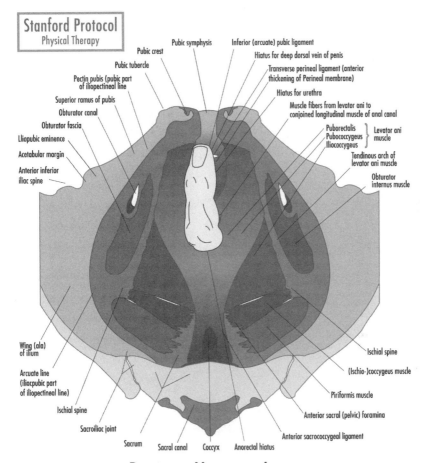

Stanford Protocol
Physical Therapy

Pubic symphysis
Pubic crest
Pubic tubercle
Pectin pubis (pubic part of iliopectineal line)
Superior ramus of pubis
Obturator canal
Obturator fascia
Iliopubic eminence
Acetabular margin
Anterior inferior iliac spine

Inferior (arcuate) pubic ligament
Hiatus for deep dorsal vein of penis
Transverse perineal ligament (anterior thickening of Perineal membrane)
Hiatus for urethra
Muscle fibers from levator ani to conjoined longitudinal muscle of anal canal
Puborectalis
Pubococcygeus
Iliococcygeus
} Levator ani muscle
Tendinous arch of levator ani muscle
Obturator internus muscle

Wing (ala) of ilium
Arcuate line (iliacpubic part of iliopectineal line)
Ischial spine
Sacroiliac joint
Sacrum
Sacral canal
Coccyx
Anorectal hiatus

Ischial spine
(Ischio-)coccygeus muscle
Piriformis muscle
Anterior sacral (pelvic) foramina
Anterior sacrococcygeal ligament

Prostate Massage Area

- Traditionally urologists massage the prostate to extract prostatic fluid in order to examine it under the microscope or to drain the prostate of inflammation or infection. The massage of the prostate in the Stanford Protocol is not done for this purpose. We massage the prostate when the physician specifically prescribes this massage or we do it to stretch the associated connective tissue. While some physicians do prostate massage vigorously or roughly, we do not. Especially if the prostate is tender, we are very gentle at first and our purpose is to desensitize the sensitivity of the prostate so that with repeated ongoing massage over a period of a number of massages, the prostate becomes less painful. Our method of prostate massage is as follows. We locate the prostate and do lateral sweeps from outside to inside when the finger is on one side (lateral to medial) of the prostate. And then from the other side with same hand, we do lateral to medial (outside to inside) sweeps ...always going from the outside to the center of the prostate. We then go from top to the bottom (superior to inferior). If the prostate is excrutiatingly painful, we are particularly gentle. The duration of the entire massage is approximately one minute.

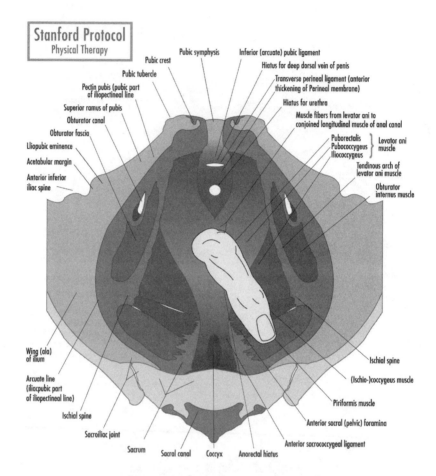

Stanford Protocol
Physical Therapy

Pubic symphysis

Pubic crest

Pubic tubercle

Pectin pubis (pubic part of iliopectineal line

Superior ramus of pubis

Obturator canal

Obturator fascia

Iliopubic eminence

Acetabular margin

Anterior inferior iliac spine

Inferior (arcuate) pubic ligament

Hiatus for deep dorsal vein of penis

Transverse perineal ligament (anterior thickening of Perineal membrane)

Hiatus for urethra

Muscle fibers from levator ani to conjoined longitudinal muscle of anal canal

Puborectalis
Pubococcygeus   } Levator ani
Iliococcygeus   muscle

Tendinous arch of levator ani muscle

Obturator internus muscle

Wing (ala) of ilium

Arcuate line (iliacpubic part of iliopectineal line)

Ischial spine

Sacroiliac joint

Sacrum   Sacral canal   Coccyx   Anorectal hiatus

Ischial spine

(Ischio-)coccygeus muscle

Piriformis muscle

Anterior sacral (pelvic) foramina

Anterior sacrococcygeal ligament

Piriformis (internally accessed)

Trigger points here can refer to the sacroiliac joint, the hip girdle and hamstrings. Patients can feel increased pain at the palpation site.

> - *Can refer to sacroiliac joint, hip girdle, hamstrings and increased pain at palpation site*

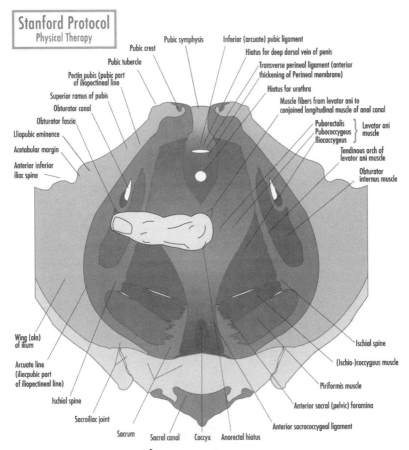

Labels in figure:

Stanford Protocol
Physical Therapy

Pubic symphysis
Pubic crest
Pubic tubercle
Pectin pubis (pubic part of iliopectineal line
Superior ramus of pubis
Obturator canal
Obturator fascia
Lliopubic eminence
Acetabular margin
Anterior inferior iliac spine

Inferior (arcuate) pubic ligament
Hiatus for deep dorsal vein of penis
Transverse perineal ligament (anterior thickening of Perineal membrane)
Hiatus for urethra
Muscle fibers from levator ani to conjoined longitudinal muscle of anal canal
Puborectalis
Pubococcygeus
Iliococcygeus
Levator ani muscle
Tendinous arch of levator ani muscle
Obturator internus muscle

Wing (ala) of ilium
Arcuate line (iliacpubic part of iliopectineal line)
Ischial spine
Sacroiliac joint
Sacrum
Sacral canal
Coccyx
Anorectal hiatus

Ischial spine
(Ischio-)coccygeus muscle
Piriformis muscle
Anterior sacral (pelvic) foramina
Anterior sacrococcygeal ligament

Obturator Internus

Trigger points in the obturator can refer pain to the perineum, outward toward hip, to the whole pelvic floor both anteriorly and posteriorly. The obturator is intimate with the pudendal nerve and can refer a dull ache and burning in the pelvic floor on the side that it is being palpated. Trigger points in the obturator can refer the golf-ball-in-the-rectum feeling, symptoms to the coccyx, hamstrings and posterior thigh. In women, trigger points in the obturator can refer to the urethra, the vagina, and specifically the vulva and is a very important point in the treatment of vulvar pain.

- *Can refer dull ache on the side palpated, golf-ball-in-the-rectum sensation, coccyx, hamstrings, posterior thigh, urethra, vagina, vulva (important in vulvodynia)*

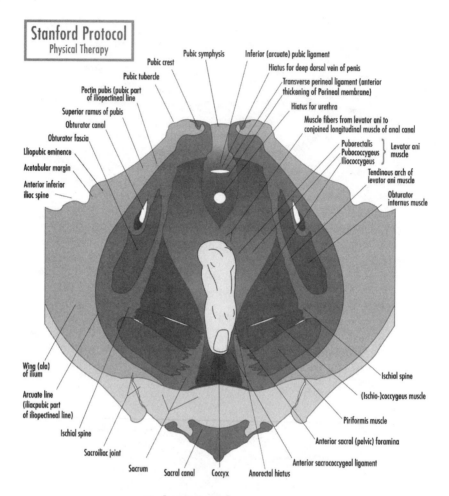

Stanford Protocol
Physical Therapy

Pubic symphysis
Pubic crest
Pubic tubercle
Pectin pubis (pubic part of iliopectineal line)
Superior ramus of pubis
Obturator canal
Obturator fascia
Iliopubic eminence
Acetabular margin
Anterior inferior iliac spine

Inferior (arcuate) pubic ligament
Hiatus for deep dorsal vein of penis
Transverse perineal ligament (anterior thickening of Perineal membrane)
Hiatus for urethra
Muscle fibers from levator ani to conjoined longitudinal muscle of anal canal
Puborectalis
Pubococcygeus } Levator ani muscle
Iliococcygeus
Tendinous arch of levator ani muscle
Obturator internus muscle

Wing (ala) of ilium
Arcuate line (iliacpubic part of iliopectineal line)
Ischial spine
Sacroiliac joint
Sacrum
Sacral canal
Coccyx
Anorectal hiatus

Ischial spine
(Ischio-)coccygeus muscle
Piriformis muscle
Anterior sacral (pelvic) foramina
Anterior sacrococcygeal ligament

Palpating the coccyx

This is a bony palpation. In treating pelvic pain, if the coccyx is immobile, it can be a factor that perpetuates trigger points that cause pelvic pain.

- *An immobile coccyx can perpetuate pelvic pain*

External Pelvic Floor Trigger Points and Where They Typically Refer Pain and Sensation

External trigger points can be as important in perpetuating a pain cycle as internal trigger points. For example we treated a man for whom significant groin pain came from his *quadratus lumborum muscle*, located on the side of the body. Again, this trigger point was relatively far away from where the pain was felt. When this trigger point was treated, the man experienced tremendous relief. Every doctor that this man saw in the years he suffered with this trigger point missed this. We have treated people who have had abdominal trigger points that refer excruciating pain into the pelvis.

To the therapist experienced in *Myofascial/Trigger Point Release*, the patient's symptoms, as well as the physical examination give the essential clues as to the location of the trigger points. We are grateful to Dr. David Simons, coauthor of *Myofascial Pain and Dysfunction: The Trigger Point Manual*,* and his publisher for allowing us to use the original drawings in his book. We have taken the liberty of adding a pointing finger on each drawing. The tip of the pointing finger marks the location of the trigger point likely to be causing the pain patterns illustrated in the shaded areas.

The following illustrations show trigger points in the external muscles that can contribute to pelvic pain.

---

* The identification under each drawing of external trigger points related to pelvic pain herein provides easy reference to the volume number and figure where the drawing originated in *Myofascial Pain and Dysfunction: The Trigger Point Manual,* 2nd edition by Janet G. Travell and David G. Simons, published copyright held by Lippincott, Williams & Wilkins, (October 1, 1998). Original drawings by Barbara Abeloff. Proofreading and editing by Lois S. Simons. Copyright 1989, Lippincott, Williams & Wilkins.

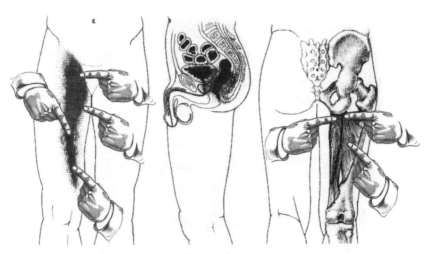

ADDUCTOR MAGNUS MUSCLE
v.2 Fig. 15.2

Pain felt in shaded area
Finger tip locates trigger point

ADDUCTOR MAGNUS

- *This muscle is missed by many clinicians*
- *The adductor magnus is a critical muscle to check for trigger points which can refer pain throughout the pelvic floor including perineum, bladder and prostate*
- *When trigger points continue to be active internally, the culprit may be unresolved trigger points in the adductor magnus*
- *Trigger points in the adductor magnus can refer the sensation of having a golf ball in the rectum*

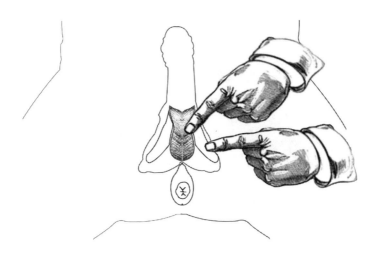

Pain felt in shaded area
Finger tip locates trigger point

BULBOSPONGIOSIS AND ISCHIOCAVERNOSIS

- *Trigger points in the bulbospongiosis and ischiocavernosis can refer pain and sensation to the base of the penis and the perineum*

A Headache in the Pelvis

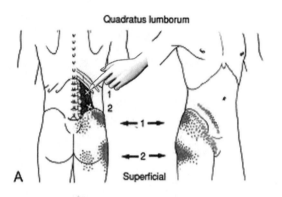

Quadratus lumborum

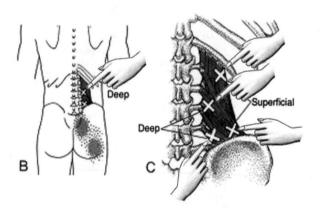

Pain felt in shaded area
Finger tip locates trigger point

Quadratus Lumborum is best palpated
with the patient lying on the side.
These trigger points are found between
the last rib and the crest of the ilium
and between the lateral obliques
and the lumbar paraspinals.

Quadratus Lumborum

- Crest of the ilium and the lower quadrant of the abdomen
- Outer aspect of the groin (can refer to labia in women, testicle or lateral penis in men)
- Greater trochanter (hip) and to lateral upper thigh
- The sacral iliac joint
- The lower buttock

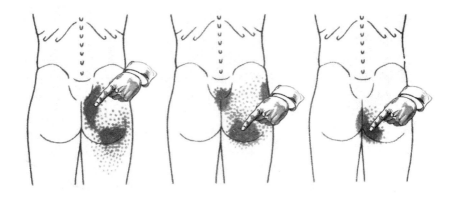

GLUTEUS MAXIMUS
v.2 Fig. 7.1

Pain felt in shaded area
Finger tip locates trigger point

GLUTEUS (MAXIMUS)

- *Trigger points in the gluteus maximus can refer pain and sensation into the hip buttocks, tailbone, sacrum and hamstrings*

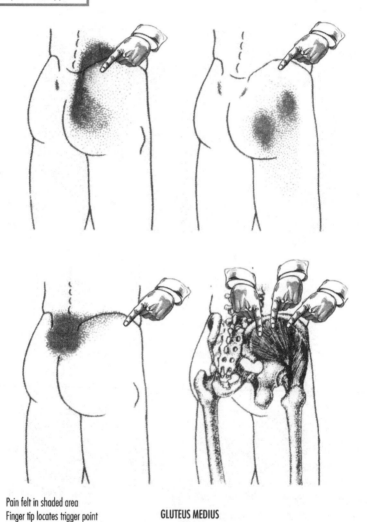

Stanford Protocol
Physical Therapy

Pain felt in shaded area
Finger tip locates trigger point

GLUTEUS MEDIUS
v.2 Fig. 8.1

GLUTEUS (MEDIUS)

- *Trigger points in the gluteus medius can refer pain and sensation around the buttocks, hip girdle and down the leg as well as into the testicles*

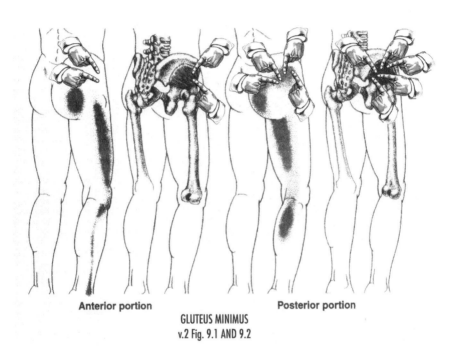

Stanford Protocol
Physical Therapy

Anterior portion   **Posterior portion**

GLUTEUS MINIMUS
v.2 Fig. 9.1 AND 9.2

Pain felt in shaded area
Finger tip locates trigger point

GLUTEUS (MINIMUS)

- *Trigger points in the gluteus minimus can refer pain and sensation down the leg and sometimes into the testicles*

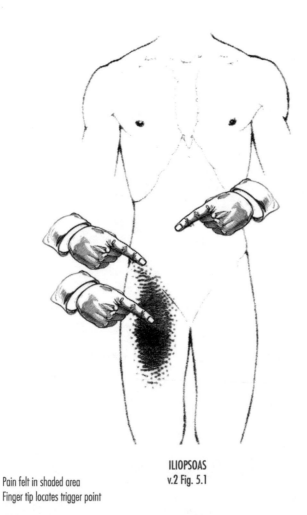

Pain felt in shaded area
Finger tip locates trigger point

ILIOPSOAS
v.2 Fig. 5.1

ILIOPSOAS

- *Trigger points in the iliopsoas can refer pain to the groin, anterior (front part) thigh and low back*

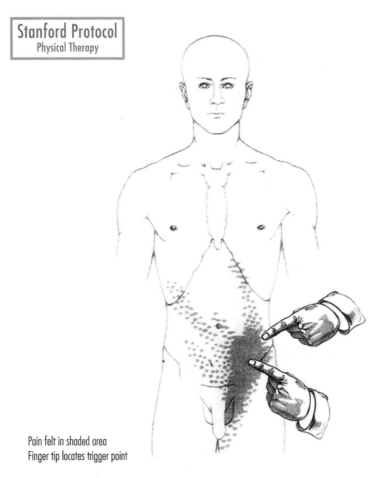

Stanford Protocol
Physical Therapy

Pain felt in shaded area
Finger tip locates trigger point

LATERAL ABDOMINALS OBLIQUE
V.1 Fig. 49.1

LATERAL ABDOMINALS OBLIQUE

- *Trigger points in the lateral abdominals can refer pain to the whole stomach, up into the ribs, down the groin and into the testicles... this is an important source of testicular pain*

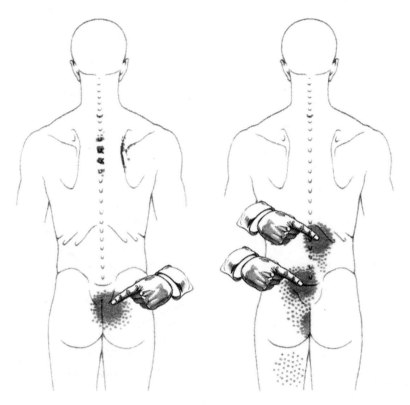

Stanford Protocol
Physical Therapy

MULTIFIDI
v.1 Fig. 48.2

Pain felt in shaded area
Finger tip locates trigger point

PARASPINALS and MULTIFIDI

- *Trigger points in the paraspinals tend to refer pain and sensation into the low back however this is pain that doesn't tend to fan out but is tightly contained in a specific area*

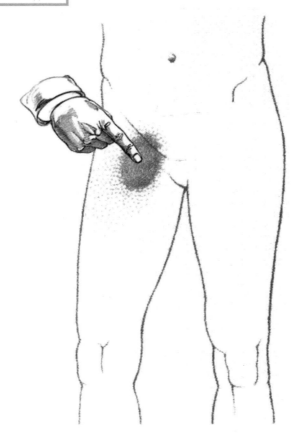

Pain felt in shaded area
Finger tip locates trigger point

PECTINEUS
v.2 Fig. 13.1

PECTINEUS

- *Trigger points in the pectineus can refer pain and sensation to the groin… this is a major trigger point for groin pain*

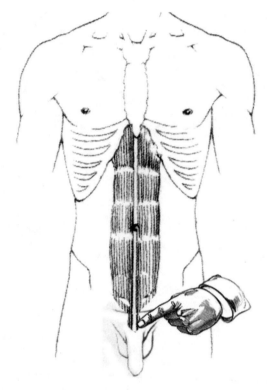

PYRAMIDALIS
v.2 Fig. 13.1

Pain felt in shaded area
Finger tip locates trigger point

PYRAMIDALIS

- *The pyramidalis is not present in some individuals but when it is present and has trigger points, they can refer pain and sensation to the bladder, pubic bone and urethra*

Modern medicine can be likened to Christianity and schools of thought in medicine to the different denominations like the Baptists, Unitarians, and Episcopalians. In the world of physical therapy, there are different churches or schools of thought about how, for instance, you do *Trigger Point Release*. Our protocol closely follows the methods of Travell and Simons. Many patients that we have seen have been treated previously by physical therapists using different methods. They have shared their experiences and compared them to our protocol and the others they have used. *We are convinced that the methodology we use is by far the most effective in the treatment of patients with trigger points.*

Here are some important points about the Stanford Protocol for physical therapy of the pelvic floor. If the trigger point is not palpated vigorously and specifically enough, the trigger point can simply resist deactivation. Yet there is danger of injuring the tissue if the pressure is inappropriately vigorous. Experience and talent in feeling the tissue and sensing how much to palpate is imperative. Physical therapists that are not experienced in dealing specifically with pelvic pain and training patients in self-treatment can err in several ways—most importantly, they do not find the trigger point, and they are not vigorous enough in palpating when the trigger point is found, or they do not use pressure release on the trigger points for 30-90 seconds.

Our general rule of thumb is that the trigger point should be pressed for 30-90 seconds. This is no small feat especially when a physical therapist with delicate hands is working on a muscle inside the pelvic floor of a large and strong man or woman. A large stress is put on the physical therapist's finger in every *Trigger Point Release* session and the therapist's finger is prone to injury unless the finger is used properly and the therapist is endowed with a certain level of strength and a certain kind of finger. Doing *Trigger Point Release* therapy can put your fingers at risk of injury and it is why some physical therapists choose to not or are not able to follow our protocol.

Flare-up of symptoms is common especially after the first number of *Trigger Point Release* sessions. These flare-ups usually abate as treatment continues although they can recur in times of a flare-up. Without their knowledge, we have seen some inexperienced therapists back off from treatment after a patient's flare-up out of fear that they did something wrong. This concern is immediately gotten across to patients who become concerned that they are going down the wrong road. Doubt about physical therapy and the whole course of treatment arises and it is not uncommon for patients to stop treatment. This is all because the therapist did not have enough training and experience to see the big picture of treatment and the common occurrence of flare-ups after treatment.

When people do trigger point release it is best, when possible, to not immediately go back into a situation of demand and tension. If you think about the physical therapy that we do as stretching and lengthening of contracted tissue that can allow it to rest and heal, taking time after a therapy session to remain quiet and rest the pelvic floor is important. A tightened pelvic floor is usually the physical expression of a psychologically defended state and releasing the pelvic tissues can trigger emotional release and psychological insight during and/or after the physical therapy session. In our view, both the therapist and patient need to be aware of this possibility and regard such reactions as positive signs of healing. Abreactions should be allowed and not suppressed or denied.

The management of expectations in *Trigger Point Release* is essential and both patient and therapist must clearly understand that flare-ups are common and to be expected and progress often occurs over the period of many months. Often treatment can feel like three steps ahead and two steps back for quite a while. The idea that there should be a quick fix, and that the therapist is responsible for making it all happen often results in the failure of treatment.

There can be multiple trigger points either inside or outside the pelvic floor that refer to the same area of pain and if not all of them are treated, then the pain can persist. There is sometimes a very perplexing network of trigger points that are involved in pelvic pain to the inexperienced

Trigger Point Release therapist. At this time there are few physical therapists that we refer patients to who we believe are competent in our protocol. If any inexperienced therapist is motivated to learn and the patient is willing to be patient with the therapist, a therapist new to this work can learn it. Seeing someone with little experience whose work is not being supervised by someone trained and experienced can result in disappointment and abandonment of the protocol.

We have defined what we include in our protocol and what we do not. A summary is provided.

- The emphasis of our physical therapy work with pelvic pain is on *Trigger Point Release*. We consider a thorough examination of possible interior and exterior trigger points to be essential in our protocol. Our protocol is most promising when we can find internal or external trigger points that tend to recreate a patient's symptoms. It should be said that while we have the most consistent success with people in whom we can find trigger points that recreate their symptoms, sometimes we have helped people with no clear trigger points but with a much contracted pelvic floor.

- At this point, as a rule we do not use pelvic floor biofeedback therapeutically in which an anal probe is inserted and patients are asked to do EMG–monitored Kegel exercises. Also, we consider unremarkable pelvic floor biofeedback readings a poor measure of what is going on in the pelvic floor or whether our protocol is indicated. We have written about these subjects elsewhere in this book.

- Generally, we do not use electrical stimulation either at the office or for home treatment and generally have not found it useful.

- Reiterating, the physical therapy emphasis for pelvic pain is on *Trigger Point Release*. If postural and/or mechanical factors appear related to the pelvic pain, we treat the most important perpetuating factors found, including postural obliquities. We treat posture and pelvic obliquities often, and instruct patients in relevant home stretches and/or stabilization exercises. If the postural perpetuating factors is large, we then refer the patient to a physical therapist closer to their home.

- *Skin rolling or connective tissue massage* can be a very important self help tool which many of our patients are encouraged to use. This method is explained below.

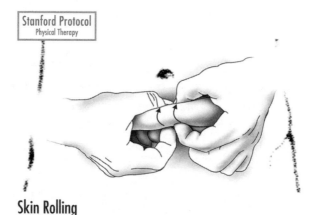

Skin Rolling

We sometimes recommend skin rolling or connective tissue massage. This method is explained below. It is difficult to explain how to do skin rolling. It is not simply a pinching of the skin and rolling it in place but rolling the skin while moving the roll of skin downward just as a wave moves from off shore to the shore. Skin rolling is rolling the skin down or up in a moving wave. The point is that in skin rolling, you roll the skin downward, sideways or vertically but the skin roll isn't stationary-- it moves. In other words you alternately walk the fingers along the skin by continuously pushing down with the thumb and up with the index and third finger and thereby move downward, rolling the skin as the skin rolls moves downward just as a wave moves from off shore to the shore.

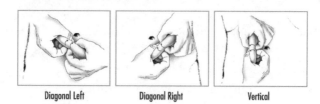

Diagonal Left   Diagonal Right   Vertical

- We encourage patients to do home trigger point release using a *Theracane*, a tennis ball and/or *knobber*.

- We only do prostate massage when prescribed by a physician and when the prostate is tender. It is not done routinely. From our perspective, the purpose of prostate massage is for stretching the associated connective tissue especially where it attaches to the prostate, and is not done for prostatic fluid drainage.

- While we appreciate the efficacy of Feldenkrais, craniosacral manipulation, the Alexander method, internal Thiele massage and other modalities for many kinds of problems, we generally do not use or recommend these methods for the pelvic pain we treat.

- Before and after treatment, we use gentle, moderate or deep effleurage or Swedish type massage on the external areas (gluteals, back, leg and stomach).

- Our physical therapy protocol is based on the knowledge that multiple trigger points can refer to one place and each trigger point must be evaluated and treated.

- We use pressure release of trigger points applying pressure for 30 to 90 seconds.

- We encourage patients to self-treat both internally and externally after proper supervision.

- When possible and with the patient's permission, we train the individual's partner to do our method of *Trigger Point Release*.

- We believe that the success of a patient, appropriate for our protocol, depends on regularly doing the home practices that we prescribe. We do not advise taking up these activities unless one is properly supervised.

The muscles of the pelvic floor are easily contracted but stretching them in the way that you can stretch your shoulders or arms is not so easily accomplished. However, they can be stretched to some degree. We consider it essential to train patients in relevant stretches. They include:

- Adductor/pectineus posture
- Lateral rotators and piriformis posture
- Cobra posture
- Pelvic tilt posture
- Knee pull posture
- Iliopsoas posture
- Quadratus lumborum posture
- Squat posture
- Adductor posture

We sometimes deem it appropriate to train the patient in the use of an experimental self-administered myofascial/trigger point wand. We are inclined to use this especially when there is no physical therapist available near the patient's home. We are still in the experimental stage using this kind of wand.

We hope that this discussion helps to shed some light on the physical therapy that we recommend. The physical therapy discussed here is what we have seen be most helpful in alleviating the pelvic pain and symptoms we treat.

Home stretching program

We ask patients to do certain stretches several times a day throughout the week. These stretches include a stretch of the *psoas* muscle, stretching of the abdomen (which can be thought of as a trunk extension), a partial cobra stretch; a side bend stretch and sometimes pressing a tennis ball against a wall to deal with trigger points and tightness in the *quadratus lumborum*.

Stretches are also done with *adductor* and *pectineus muscles*. We educate our patients in doing diaphragmatic breathing while doing these stretches. When possible, we encourage patients to take a hot bath before stretching.

Home Stretches

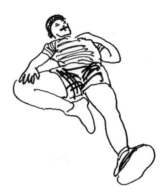

1. Stretching the adductors (pectineus)

This stretch is done while lying down on a firm surface and first bending one knee while the other unbent leg is resting on the floor. The hand on the same side as the bent knee is placed on the inside of the knee and then slowly pushes the bent knee outward toward the floor. The bent knee is held down toward the floor by the hand for between 15 to 30 seconds and then return the bent leg is returned to the upright position or slide leg down to rest on the floor. This is repeated with the other leg. This is done 3 times or as needed during the day.

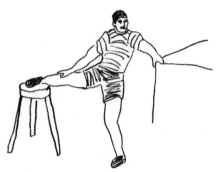

2.   Adductor stretch

In this stretch, the knee that is supporting you is bent slightly in order to increase or decrease the stretch on the inner thigh. The leg that is stretched out is placed on a stool. This should be held for 30 seconds or longer. Change leg after one adductor is stretched to stretch the other adductor. This stretch should not be done if there is any pain experienced in the knees.

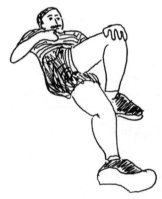

3.   Stretching the lateral rotators and the piriformis

This stretch is done lying down on a firm surface and like stretch #1, one knee is bent while the other leg is resting unbent on the floor. The hand that is opposite the bent knee is placed on the outside of the bent knee and pulled down toward the floor as illustrated in picture. The stretch is held for 15 to 30 seconds. This stretch is repeated three times and done as needed during the day.

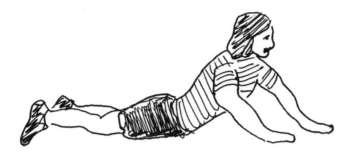

4. The Cobra

This is a well known yoga stretch and is done lying stomach down while slowly pushing upper body upward by straightening the arms and bending back the lower back. This is held for 15-30 seconds. For those with low back pain, this can be a partial cobra with the arms partially extended rather than fully extended. This stretch is repeated three times and done as needed during the day.

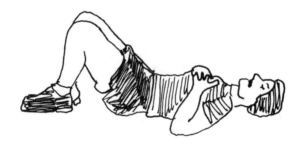

5. Pelvic tilt

This stretch is done on a firm surface, face up with both knees bent. The abdomen and buttocks are tightened with the result of rocking the pelvis and putting the lower back flat against the floor. The lower back is held for 5-10 seconds against the floor and then rested. This is done three times and done as needed during the day.

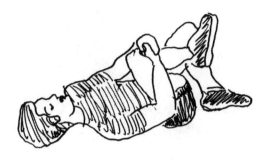

6. Knee pull

This exercise is done on the back on a firm surface. Both knees are bent with feet resting comfortably on the floor. One leg is taken below the knee and pulled back toward the chest and held between 15-30 seconds. This is done three times and done as needed during the day.

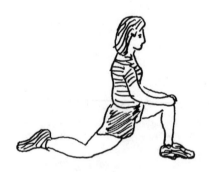

7. Kneeling stretch of the iliopsoas

This exercise is done kneeling on one leg with the other leg pulled back. With the upper body vertical and erect, without bending the head forward, the body is shifted forward stretching the thigh and groin for 5-20 seconds. This is repeated 5-20 times twice a day.

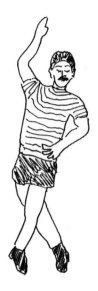

8.   Stretching the quadratus lumborum and hip abductors

This exercise is done standing with hands on the hips. One leg is crossed in front of the other rests on the floor. The hips are bent forming a "C" and stretching the other side of the body. This is done three times and repeated as needed during the day.

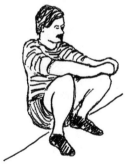

9.   Squat stretch

This stretch opens up the pelvic floor. Squatting on both feet with the back supported against the wall without your 'sit-bones' touching the floor. When there is no discomfort, this pose can be done for 1 + minutes or longer depending on the advice of your physical therapist or physician. This stretch should not be done if there is any pain in the knees.

Sawyer self-administered *Trigger Point Release* technique

We teach people how to do both internal and external *Trigger Point Release* on themselves. An instrument called a *Theracane©* can help in releasing trigger points outside the body. The *Theracane©* looks like a funny kind of cane with balls at both ends and small two perpendicular rods coming out of the straight end. A tennis ball can also be used to assist in some *Trigger Point Release*. In the last few years we have been fortunate to be able to give our patients a specifically designed internal trigger point wand for them to treat their own internal trigger points.

Instruction for external *Trigger Point Release* is typically done on the *abdominals* or muscles above the pubic bone, the *adductors* or the muscles of the inner thigh and around the *perineum, gluteal* muscles (*minimus, medius* and *maximus), quadratus lumborum*, and other external trigger points associated with pelvic pain. The program of self-administered external treatment for pelvic pain was developed by Tim Sawyer, our senior physical therapist. One should not rely on the instructions for the kind of *Trigger Point Release* described here, but on the instruction and supervision of a physical therapist knowledgeable in this technique.

Patients are instructed to sit comfortably on the floor or in a chair. This makes it easy to reach their *adductors, abdominals*, and *perineum. Abdominals* can also be reached lying down. Patients are shown how to locate the taut bands of trigger points or tender points on the *abdominals* and *adductors* by systematically feeling these muscles for any tender or painful spots. These tender spots may or may not refer pain into the pelvic floor.

When a tender spot is found, gentle but firm pressure is applied for between 15-90 seconds, or less if the trigger point releases earlier, then skin rolling on the areas can be performed, followed by massage. Sometimes the patient is shown how to do skin rolling in which the skin above the inner thigh and above the pubic bone is systematically held in a gentle pinch and rolled or kneaded like kneading dough.

Using the Theracane© and tennis ball

On the following pages we illustrate the use of the tennis ball and Theracane© in working with some external trigger points related to pelvic pain.

Using a tennis ball (or sometimes a larger ball)

The beauty of a tennis ball (or sometimes a larger ball like a soft, softball) for *Trigger Point Release* is that one simply lies on the ball at the site of the trigger point and gravity does the rest. In our instruction we suggest patients rest lightly at first on the ball for 30-90 seconds (or less if the trigger point releases earlier) and then put more weight on the ball as the area becomes less sensitive. Sometimes trigger points can be extremely painful. Care must be taken to rest lightly on the ball and only to the extent that one can easily tolerate the discomfort. Generally speaking, as the trigger point releases, the discomfort of the trigger point abates and eventually one can fully rest on the ball with little discomfort. It is useful to do RSA breathing throughout the work with the ball or Theracane©, as we discuss later.

Patients sometimes lean against the wall with the tennis ball separating their trigger point from the wall. This often puts less vigorous pressure on the trigger point than lying down on the ball.

Before using the tennis ball to do *Trigger Point Release* it is very important for the physical therapist instructing patients in treatment to show them where the *pudendal nerve* is so that they do not irritate it.

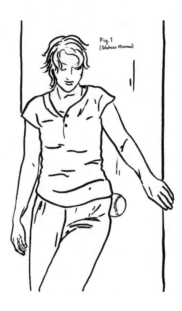

Fig. 1

Releasing trigger points in the *gluteus minimus, medius* and *maximus* by resting on a tennis ball against a wall.

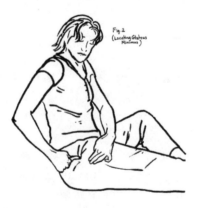

Fig. 2

Identifying the *gluteus minimus*

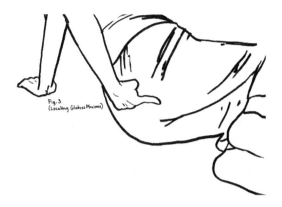

Fig.3

Identifying *gluteus maximus*

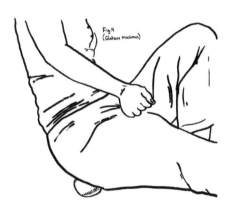

Fig. 4

Using a tennis ball to release *gluteus maximus* trigger points

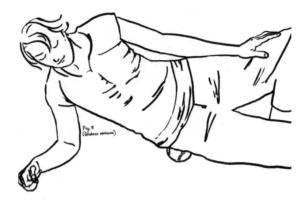

Fig. 5

Using a tennis ball to release *gluteus medius and minimus* trigger points

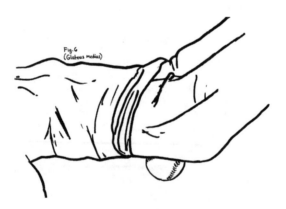

Fig. 6

Using a tennis ball to release *gluteus medius* trigger points

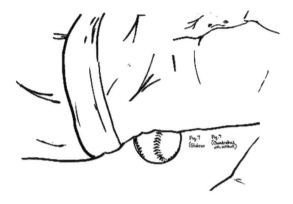

Fig. 7

Releasing trigger points in the *quadratus lumborum* by lying on a soft, softball

Using the Theracane©

The best leverage we have found in using the Theracane© is holding it at its very ends when using the short protrusions. In doing abdominal *Trigger Point Release*, we put a small cross cut into a tennis ball with a knife, in order to be able to put it on the protruded end of the rod coming out of the straight end. This softens the knob that is being pushed against the trigger point. When doing abdominal *Trigger Point Release* it is very important not to put undue pressure against the aorta in the middle of the abdomen and the instructing and supervising physical therapist should show the patient where this is in the mid section a little to the left in the abdomen and how to avoid putting undue pressure onto it. Sometimes the knobs on the Theracane© can be used without a tennis ball and the supervising physical therapist can make suggestions about when this is appropriate.

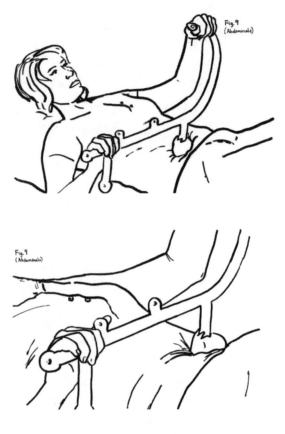

Fig. 9

Releasing trigger points in the abdomen with a Theracane© end, softened by a scored tennis ball. As we discuss in a later chapter, this abdominal *Trigger Point Release*, when following the path of the ascending, transverse and descending colon, anecdotally has been helpful for some patients with irritable bowel syndrome in reducing or stopping abdominal pain and for some patients with esophageal reflux in reducing or stopping sensations of heartburn. While these are very interesting findings and merit scientific investigation, we are not advising readers to treat their abdominal pain or heartburn this way.

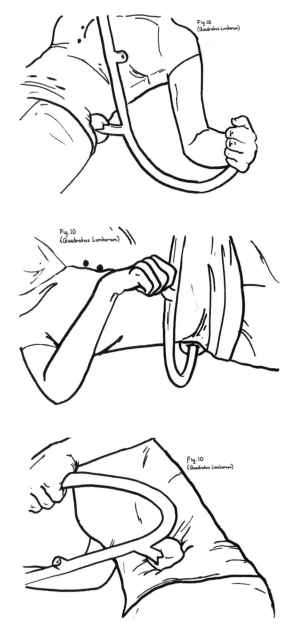

Fig. 10

Releasing trigger points in the *quadratus lumborum* using a Theracane©
end, softened by a scored tennis ball

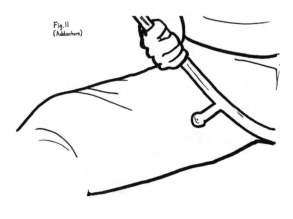

Fig. 11

Releasing trigger points in the *adductors* using a Theracane© end, with no tennis ball.

Many pelvic pain patients have increased muscle tension and trigger points in the large muscles of the hip girdle. These areas can be treated by stretching, leaning on a tennis ball against the wall or carefully rolling on a tennis ball placed on the floor. Tim has noticed that many therapists and patients, however, overlook important potential trigger points in the middle and lower areas of the buttocks around the greater trochanter and the 'sit bones' (or ischial tuberosity). These muscles include the lower part of the gluteus maximus, piriformis, and other short lateral rotator muscles of the hip (gemelli, quadratus femoris, and the obturators and the proximal insertion of the adductors and hamstrings.

Patients who continue to struggle with different aspects of sitting pain, tail bone, rectal and perineal pain, visceral pain some describe as deep prostate pain, back of leg pain and hip pain, may be overlooking the role that trigger points can play in these muscles. We encourage our patients to develop the confidence to use their fingers and sometimes a convenient trigger point tool (tennis ball, theracane, or small knobber) and explore these small, important muscles for painful trigger points and areas of tenderness and restriction, and then treating these areas repetitively with either gentle massage using olive oil or massage lotion, a 10-15 minute milking/strumming technique, or a 60-90 second pressure-release technique. Often trigger points and areas of restriction and tenderness in these lower buttocks muscles can feel "nervy" or "tingly" or very sensitive to the patient and it can prevent or scare the patient from treating these areas. If any of these sensations are experienced during our clinic or after, we ask our patients to check in with our physical therapist before proceeding.

Trigger points in these lower hip girdle and upper leg areas, however, have been known to cause troubling types of pain and uncomfortable sensation. Having the confidence to return to them again and again, with appropriate pressure and proper treatment often enables the release of the trigger points and restriction in these muscles. When these muscles are untreated they can play a perpetuating role in both external and internal pelvic pain and dysfunction.

When teaching patients self treatment techniques for these areas we encourage them to first massage gently around the 'sit bones', along the perineum, around the outside of the anus, along the gluteal folds and down along the medial aspect of the inner thigh along the adductor muscles and behind the leg along the hamstrings. Gentle massage allows the patient to feel his or her own body while learning to detect tense and potentially sore trigger pointed areas. Once these areas are located, the patient can proceed with more vigorous techniques than those described above. All of this requires a certain amount of interest, enthusiasm and diligence from our patients to continue to be their own best therapist and explore these areas on a repetitive basis during the course of their work with our protocol.

Why physical therapy is necessary but usually not sufficient to provide resolution of muscle related pelvic pain

Our viewpoint, very simply, is that pelvic pain is the result of a chronic hypertonicity in the pelvic floor, fed by protective guarding, anxiety and tension. This chronic tension can be the source of the bewildering symptoms experienced by those who suffer from pelvic pain of a neuromuscular origin. Heightened anxiety and nervous system arousal become the default emotional and nervous system modes feeding the tension, pain anxiety cycle. This is why the cycle seems to take on a life of its own even after the initiating situation goes away.

The aim of the *Wise-Anderson Protocol* is twofold: one, to regularly help dissolve the tension and two, to change someone's inner habits that feed it. It is our experience that without changing the habit of tightening up the pelvis and then feeding the resultant tightness with anxiety and heightened arousal, the body tends to revert back to the chronic tension in the pelvic floor.

In the *Wise-Anderson Protocol*, physical therapy and *Paradoxical Relaxation* are different sides of the same coin

Physical therapy done periodically, typically cannot change the default mode of the body that produces the trigger points, spasm and chronic vigilance, which is their origin. We believe that for most patients we see, it is essential that they regularly practice moving from a chronically vigilant state, to a state of relaxation and flexibility of the muscles of the pelvic basin. In a nutshell, the *Wise-Anderson Protocol*, in order to be successful, must teach patients *both* to regularly dissolve the chronically tight pelvic floor and modify the habits of body and mind that bring it about and keep it going. Physical therapy and *Paradoxical Relaxation* are two sides of the same coin—each is necessary but not sufficient for a long-term solution to pelvic pain.

More Notes on the *Wise-Anderson Protocol* Physical Therapy

Trigger point technique

We have received calls from physical therapists and patients asking questions about various aspects of the *Trigger Point Release* we use.

One of the questions that has arisen from both therapists doing *Trigger Point Release* and from our patients to whom we teach self *Trigger Point Release* is how hard to press on the trigger point. This is an important question which we hope to clarify below.

In our experience, in order to deactivate the trigger point, it has to be pressed to the point of being uncomfortable/painful but not overwhelmingly painful. This is a fine line. If we were to quantify this on a scale of 0-10, where 0 is no pressure and 10 is the most extreme pressure, in general, the trigger point should be pressed at the level of approximately 5-7. Not less and not more unless the person has hyperirritable trigger points which we discuss below. In other words, if the trigger point is not pressed with sufficient pressure, it does not seem to deactivate and so the timid therapist or the timid patient doing self-treatment physical therapy who is afraid to cause any discomfort to the client or him or herself, is wasting his or her time. Without appropriate pressure applied, the trigger point, even if it is accurately found (which is no small thing), will not release.

Similarly, if the trigger point is pressed with great force causing an overwhelming amount of pain triggering protective guarding, the trigger point will tend not to release. This kind of forced *Trigger Point Release* is sometimes done by men and women who think that they have to power through their pain and bear the consequences of this kind of forceful, aggressive self-treatment. This kind of overly forceful and aggressive treatment, in our experience, is counterproductive and usually fails.

So the middle path of sufficient pressure to produce a level of discomfort/pain of between 5-7, but not more or less, is the kind of guideline we use. For best results, the patient must feel sufficiently safe and trusting to at least begin to relax during the pressure. Pressing on a trigger point and the patient resisting the pressure instead of relaxing with it, isn't a good idea. Furthermore, it is better to start the *Trigger Point Release* at the lower end of the scale and work up to a higher level with one's full understanding, expectation and cooperation.

Some patients have reported that if they can't relax with the pressure, either when they do it to themselves or when being treated by their partner or a therapist, then their trigger point usually doesn't let go. This is telling and intuitive. We want to be firm but gentle and sensitive with ourselves in all ways. *Trigger Point Release* has to be a cooperative and relaxed dance between the recipient of the trigger point pressure and the one who is pressing on the trigger point.

Using RSA breathing during *Trigger Point Release*

Recently we have introduced the innovation of asking patients to begin doing RSA breathing, just prior to and during the *Trigger Point Release* session. RSA breathing is described in Chapter 5. The practice of RSA breathing aims to coordinate heartbeat and respiration, bringing the respiration rate down to approximately six breaths per minute and specifically slowing down the activity of the nervous system. There are some reports that the breathing that facilitates a quieting of nervous system arousal also potentiates the therapeutic effects of *Trigger Point Release*.

Hyperirritability

In this vein, we want to discuss the phenomenon of pelvic floor hyperirritability. There are some patients who are so sensitive and have such a high level of discomfort in their pelvises and in the areas related to them, that one cannot touch their anal sphincter or vagina or even lightly press on any related trigger points without causing excruciating pain. This hyperirritability is crucial to understand and work with.

When hyperirritable patients work with themselves, they have to proceed carefully. We instruct patients to do gentle skin rolling on their abdomen, inner thighs and perineum preceded and followed by long soothing strokes, massaging these muscles. We encourage this to be done before they do any work close to the genitals or anus. Putting warmth on these areas or taking a warm bath is useful in conjunction with the skin rolling and the long stroke massage of the abdomen and the inner and outer thighs and buttocks. Sometimes we encourage patients to do *Trigger Point Release* in a warm bath. This is by way of relaxing the pelvic floor muscles and making the *Trigger Point Release* easier and less painful.

When someone is hyperirritable, we suggest they start simply touching and gently skin rolling over the trigger points. During *Trigger Point Release*, if their level of discomfort reaches a 5-7, which may be a 1 or 2 of someone not hyperirritable, they need to not press harder. *Trigger Point Release*, done by patients trained in self-treatment or *Trigger Point Release* done by a health care practitioner must not be a torture.

Hyperirritability resulting in exquisite pain will usually accommodate to increasingly greater pressure on the trigger point if the level of pressure is very gradually increased over a period of a number of weeks or months. This has to be done with an attitude of kindness toward the body and trust that the body wants to get better and be free of the pain. Hyperirritable patients need to do very gentle stretching, very gentle massage and very gentle *Trigger Point Release* at first. There is no race here. There must be no urgency to get rid of the pain. One must be patient and bring the body along with graduated levels of stretching and discomfort in pressing on trigger points. We are quite happy if the patient trained in self-treatment has to take 3-12 months or longer of regular skin rolling, self *Trigger Point Release* and stretching to calm down their hyperirritability. Any other attitude that contains urgency and insensitivity in doing the physical therapy component of our protocol is counterproductive and tends to stall treatment. Hyperirritability may also be caused by an underlying perpetuating factor that only a skilled therapist or MD who understands and treats myofascial pain can evaluate.

Exercise, weight lifting and bicycle riding

In the world of pelvic pain, it has become a kind of biblical injunction among certain practitioners that no one with pelvic pain should lift weights, ride a bicycle, drink coffee, tea, alcohol or eat spicy foods. We think these kinds of prohibitions are sometimes unnecessary. If there are no tests that indicate problems in the bladder or urethra and if the patient does not notice any untoward effects in drinking coffee, alcohol or in eating spicy foods, or doing weight lifting or bicycle riding, in our view there is no reason to give them up. If on the other hand, a patient has irritation or inflammation/ulceration in their bladder or urethra or experiences flare ups after bicycle riding or weight lifting, then it is a different story and obviously one needs to be selective about one's food and drink or mode of exercise. We discuss the effect of food and drink in more detail in Chapter 7.

Many individuals who come to see us to feel that exercise might hurt them. We have had patients who have stayed in bed for months because of their idea that exercise would hurt their condition. *We encourage people to do aerobic exercise that is the least irritating to them.* Again, we do not make a blanket pronouncement about bicycle riding either. One of our patients with pelvic pain reported that bicycle riding actually made his pelvis feel better. If bicycle riding does not exacerbate one's symptoms, or if one's symptoms in the area of sitting have cleared up, we think it entirely reasonable for someone who loves bicycle riding to experiment with bicycle riding to see if is workable for him or her. If he or she notices symptoms related to this activity, then common sense says to curtail such an activity. If no symptoms occur, we see no reason to banish bicycle riding or other activities that have been routinely discouraged by some who treat pelvic pain.

The Internal Trigger Point Wand

In the course of our work giving patients with pelvic pain the tools to help themselves, we have explored different home treatments that allow patients to reach and deactivate trigger points and areas of restriction related to their pelvic floor. In this book we have described and illustrated what we consider to be the most useful of external self-treatment methods for trigger point release and myofascial release. To this end we describe the use of the finger, theracane, tennis ball and certain kinds of stretching to help deactivate trigger points and release areas of myofascial restriction. We also have devoted a significant section to describe where internal trigger points are typically located in individuals who have pelvic pain.

Doing internal trigger point release and internal myofascial release is not simple and we do not recommend someone doing this without competent instruction and supervision. Over and over again, we have seen people who have had no instruction attempt to improvise with some tool for internal self treatment, and wind up flaring themselves up and scaring themselves. Although it is unusual and is an extreme example, someone we heard of was not able to get the device they were using out of their rectum and had to go the emergency room.

While internal self treatment is not rocket science, you have to know what you're doing and usually someone needs to show you how. When you have questions about your internal trigger point release you need to be able to talk to someone who can advise you. Once instructed and you know what you're doing, it can often make a major difference.

We have had reports of numerous physical therapists prescribing sex toys in the form of dildos to do internal work. These devices have been designed for masturbation and are not meant for medical treatment. They are typically clumsy and imprecise in terms of the goal of locating and releasing internal areas of pain.

Early on we explored the world of sex toys to see if there was anything appropriate to be used for internal trigger point release and to our dismay we could find nothing appropriate. We experimented with a relatively large number of designs for a tool that would be able to do internal trigger point release. Over the years we developed a design for an internal trigger point wand with safety features and treatment features that have heretofore been unavailable.

We began the use of our wand in 2008 in an Institutional Review Board supervised clinical trial. At the time of the writing of this book, this wand is being used by over 200 individuals with pelvic pain. To date, the safety effectiveness of our wand has been remarkably high.

The purpose of the *Wise-Anderson* Internal Trigger Point Wand is to provide an 'extended finger' that is easily navigated inside the pelvic floor and easily used to palpate trigger points with the end of helping to reduce trigger point sensitivity, soreness and discomfort in the muscles of the pelvic floor. The conventional method of doing internal trigger point release is done by a physical therapist who inserts a gloved and lubricated finger vaginally or rectally while the patient is lying down. In the *Wise-Anderson Protocol*, the physical therapist locates an internal trigger point and then typically holds pressure on it for approximately 15- 90 seconds. The aim of the method is to reduce the sensitivity of trigger points, and sore, painful myofascial tissue within the pelvic basin.

The *Wise-Anderson* Internal Trigger Point Wand makes it possible for someone suffering from painful internal trigger points and pelvic floor muscle pain to be taught to reduce or resolve painful trigger point sensitivity. This can be done without the inconvenience or expense of having to see a physician, physical therapist, or other appropriate healthcare professional on an ongoing basis.

The importance of having time to do relaxation after internal treatment

Here is an example of someone's experience in the conventional treatment of pelvic pain. This is the experience of one of our patients before and after he began doing self administered internal trigger point release:

"I would leave work to go to the physical therapist, drive the hour or so to her office that was located in a hospital setting, park the car, and go in. Once inside I would be ushered into a room where I would change into a gown, lie on a therapeutic bed and my physical therapist would work on me. Usually we would talk for a while during treatment. I would talk about how my week was and how my symptoms were doing.

The actual hands on work lasted between 20 and 40 minutes depending on how much we talked. She was a good physical therapist and knew her stuff. When we were finished I would get dressed, get back in the car and start the long drive back to work.

Going for treatment was a stress for me because I would easily miss 3 hours of work from the time I left until the time I got back. For most of the drive my mind would be focused on all the phone calls and emails I was missing and all the work I'd have to catch up on when I got back. I'd worry about how much time I was missing. Even when I had a very good physical therapy appointment, the whole process was stressful. If there was any kind of real stress happening on top of it, by the end of the day it was as if I hadn't even had the treatment at all.

When I started treating myself I had so much more freedom. I could treat myself in the privacy of my own home at night once my day was over. The best part is that I can relax afterward. It feels like my pelvic floor has a chance to stay relaxed without having to tighten up again right after internal treatment."

The importance of resting the internal tissue after internal trigger point release

The value of being able to do internal self treatment with the wand is that after treatment you have the ability to rest the tissue that has been sore and contracted after it has been lengthened and released from its constriction. In pelvic pain syndromes, the tissue in and around the pelvic floor gets used to being shortened, contracted, and painful. We've had numbers of patients who have had to drive long distances for internal physical therapy and by the time they made the 1-5 hour trip back home, much of the value of the session was reversed because of the car ride and stress of the trip.

Contracted and sore tissue inside the pelvic floor must be repetitively released. The body has to get used to pelvic muscles that are not sore and contracted. To release the pelvic floor muscles and then soon after go back into the default contracted mode, can sometimes be like taking 2 steps forward and then 2 steps back. With the internal wand the patient can routinely give the pelvis a chance to remain released for an extended period of time after treatment.

Self treatment and the flare ups that typically come with stress

Even if people are successful in stopping their pelvic pain symptoms at one point in time, these symptoms typically reoccur during periods of stress. If you have confidence in a way of treating these symptoms, they usually stop being the kind of major suffering that they are when you feel helpless to do anything about them. In other words, knowing that you can reduce or stop your symptoms if they do reoccur tends to make their reoccurrence a far less significant event. The wand is an essential component in gaining this confidence in treating yourself.

Knowing how hard to press inside

The nerves inside the pelvic floor provide different feedback than the nerves, for instance, in your hands or arms, especially if you are anxious or unwittingly guarded inside the pelvic floor. In those cases, your experience of how hard you may be pressing inside may be compromised. In other words, it's sometimes difficult to discern how hard you are pressing inside. Sometimes individuals who are very anxious and desperate to stop their pain can press too hard and too long on the tissue inside the pelvic floor, and may create significant flare up of symptoms or worse.

It is for this reason that one of the most important features we incorporated into our Wand, allows for the remote measurement of the pressure being exerted at the tip of the Wand. Whether you accurately sense how hard you are pressing, the Wand gives you an objective measure of the amount of pressure you are exerting inside. This is an important safety feature.

The Wand also has in its design, a moveable stop that limits how deeply the Wand can be inserted. This is both a safety feature, and one that more accurately allows the user to locate the areas to be treated. We designed the Wand to have a diameter that is small enough to cause little disturbance to the orifice in which it is inserted so that the sensation of pressing the tissue with the tip of the Wand is more easily and accurately felt.

Doing internal self trigger point release

It usually takes a couple of months to become familiar with internal trigger point treatment. Doing internal trigger point release can be thought of as being dropped in the middle of Tokyo when you don't know Japanese or the customs of the country. At first, you have very little idea of where you are or how to locate yourself or move around. But as time goes on, you get to familiarize yourself with the various structures and signs. These landmarks can allow you to orient yourself. After remaining in this once unfamiliar neighborhood, it gets to become familiar.

Often people learning internal trigger point release with the Wand can get to know and treat their own pelvic floor like the best of therapists. In our protocol, we often suggest that people do physical therapy 3 or 4 times a week. For some, this is prohibitive in terms of time and expense. The savings related to cost and convenience, not to mention the beneficial issues of efficacy, are considerable.

In order to use the Wand, a physician or physical therapist competent in internal trigger point release is essential. The physician or PT must find the trigger points and areas of restriction internally and then ask the person using the Wand to find the same trigger points with the Wand. This process needs to be done enough times to allow the user of the Wand to become comfortable in using it. In this way the physician or PT is an instructor and guide to the patient in being able to use the Wand independently. While ultimately it is our view that it is beneficial in all ways for patients to take responsibility for, and be able to treat their internal trigger point sensitivity themselves, competent consultation with a physical therapist is essential. There certainly are situations in which a person may not be able to do internal self treatment and treatment with a physical therapist is the best option.

Given the option, most of us would choose to be able to take care of our own health without having to rely on anyone else. The *Wise-Anderson* Internal Trigger Point Wand was designed to give the user the ability to become independent of professional help and treatment. The Wand has safety features which give feedback about the depth of insertion and assistance with easily navigating the wand internally. It can mitigate the impact of flare ups after symptoms have abated by empowering the user to calm down sore and tight myofascial tissue when flare ups do arise. The use of the Wand can be reduced, or need not be used, once symptoms begin to abate.

CHAPTER 7

PELVIC PAIN IN WOMEN

We have been able to help a significant number of women with pelvic pain using the *Wise-Anderson Protocol.* We regularly evaluate and treat women diagnosed with various named conditions such as *interstitial cystitis (IC), urethral syndrome, painful bladder syndrome, pelvic floor dysfunction, levator ani syndrome, pelvic floor myalgia, dyspareunia, vulvodynia,* and *chronic pelvic pain* among other diagnoses. We believe most of these conditions are related with chronic tension or spasm in the muscles of the pelvic basin and fed by anxiety, protective guarding and the habitual tendency to tighten the pelvic muscles--essentially the same circumstances seen in our male patients.

Women with pelvic pain often complain of one or more of the following kinds of symptoms (very few women have all symptoms):

- vaginal pain
- rectal pain
- pain around or above the pubic bone
- discomfort with sitting
- discomfort or pain with intercourse or sexual activity
- exacerbation of pelvic pain related to menstruation
- exacerbation of symptoms with stress and anxiety
- urinary frequency

- urinary urgency or hesitancy
- pain during or after urination
- pain during or after bowel movements
- pain related to childbirth

Bladder Pain Syndrome or Interstitial Cystitis

A majority of women who have participated in our program for pelvic pain have been diagnosed with the disorder of interstitial cystitis or bladder pain syndrome (IC/BPS). From epidemiological studies the prevalence of IC is estimated to be 300 cases per 100,000 women. While men also have this condition, it is 5 to 10 times more prevalent in women. IC is a chronic disease of unknown cause that is characterized by pelvic pain in multiple sites and bladder dysfunction including urinary frequency and urgency, nocturia (desire to urinate during the night) and increased symptoms of urinary urgency with intercourse. Patients with IC may only have bladder symptoms and no other pain. While suprapubic pain or pain felt above the pubic bone is a prominent feature, additional pain sites include the urethra, genitalia and others such as the groin, low back, thighs and buttocks. This condition may coexist with other disorders such as irritable bowel syndrome, fibromyalgia, vulvodynia, vulvar vestibulitis, pelvic floor dysfunction, Raynaud's syndrome, and migraine headache among others.

Recently an international consultation of scientific experts met and voted to use the new term "bladder pain syndrome" (BPS) for the disorder commonly called interstitial cystitis or painful bladder syndrome. BPS is a clinical diagnosis encompassing the pattern of multiple symptoms as described above. For our discussions herein we retain the IC terminology, although that name IC focuses narrowly on inflammation within the wall of the bladder and may not accurately describe the majority of patients with the syndrome. The trend at the present time is to identify the characteristics or phenotypes of the chronic pelvic pain syndrome in women. Analyzing these categories may help narrow the focus of treatment.

The purpose of this chapter is to present a more comprehensive understanding of IC. We cannot provide all of the research on IC or consider all theories but do include those approaches that best correspond to our experience in treating patients with IC. It is important to understand that IC remains a controversial diagnosis. There are many clinicians who think that this is a catch-all diagnosis, a diagnosis of exclusion, and that its existence is not well substantiated, while others feel strongly that it is a definite condition with demonstrable pathology.

Descriptions of pain associated with interstitial cystitis

In a recent survey of 264 women with IC conducted by physicians at the University of Maryland and Johns Hopkins University, it was found that the respondents were quite precise in identifying multiple sites of pain with pain sensations described as throbbing, tender, piercing or aching. For genital pain sites, burning, stinging and sharp were the pain descriptions. The order ranking of the most frequently reported sites of pain were suprapubic, urethral and genital areas, and then followed by other non-genitourinary sites. Suprapubic and urethral pain were reported as worsening either with bladder filling or just before urination in 50% or more of the women. Approximately 80% of survey respondents also indicated pain worsening in these areas after consumption of certain food and drinks.

Theories to explain interstitial cystitis

IC may arise from a triggering event. A patient may have experienced a urinary infection, surgery, childbirth, a viral illness, or a physical or psychological trauma. Sensations of bladder pain then become a prominent feature. There is some evidence, as espoused by Dr. Tony Buffington, that an imbalance between the cortisone-producing endocrine system and a hyper activated nervous system is responsible for the disorder. However, considerably more research is required to sort out the complexities involved.

One theory is that IC is a result of a neurovascular insult, and that the symptoms of pain and urinary dysfunction are secondary to an ongoing process affecting the bladder. Drs. Erwin and Galloway at Emory University have treated many patients with painful bladder disorders by blocking nerves in the lumbar area of the spinal cord to stop the natural adrenaline-producing nerve activity in the bladder. They suggested that IC may be due to over stimulation of the nerves to muscles and blood vessels in the bladder which then results in spasm of the vessels and deprivation of oxygen to the organ. This phenomenon has been shown to cause capillary blood vessel fragility in other parts of the body. The nerve-blockade treatment that they employed temporarily improved the pain in many patients.

Physicians understand IC/BPS to be pelvic pain associated with urinary urgency and frequency. However, many women are incorrectly diagnosed as having a urinary tract infection (UTI), analogous to the misdiagnosis of chronic bacterial prostatitis with men, and thus are treated with a myriad of antimicrobial agents. Ironically many women drink copious amounts of cranberry juice as it is thought to benefit a UTI although cranberry juice actually may irritate IC symptoms. Some clinicians believe that the old diagnosis of urethral syndrome, associated with symptoms of urinary urgency, frequency, dysuria, suprapubic or low back pain and voiding difficulties may be related to bladder pain syndrome.

Diagnosis of IC

A common diagnostic procedure for IC involves cystoscopy under anesthesia with bladder hydro-distension. The bladder is like a collapsed balloon when empty. The cystoscopic procedure involves filling the bladder with water to full capacity at relatively high pressure, then visualizing the wall of the bladder and the underlying blood vessels with a mini-camera attached to a catheter inserted through the urethra into the bladder. A bladder that appears inflamed or even ulcerated and has small capillary vessel bleeding is thought to be indicative of IC. The bleeding results from fragility of blood vessels when the bladder is stretched. As the bladder is emptied the tiny vessels rupture, creating small micro-hemorrhages and formation of a characteristic bloody pattern in the surface of the bladder. The relevancy of the diagnostic test has been challenged. Some critics say that if you stretch anyone's bladder strongly enough, you can probably make it bleed. However, the diagnostic test is only meaningful if the patient has all the rest of the hallmarks of chronic pelvic pain and urinary symptoms.

Bladder distention (stretching) under anesthesia is also currently used as a therapeutic tool to manage IC. About 30% of patients, a relatively small and unimpressive proportion, note a sustained improvement after undergoing this procedure. Biopsy of the bladder is rarely necessary as no serious diseases are uncovered, although superficial bladder cancer needs to be ruled out.

One finding related to IC is that the mucosal lining of the bladder, known as the glycosaminoglycan (GAG) layer, may not be providing an adequate barrier function for the bladder. Defects in the integrity of the GAG layer may allow micro pores or tiny gaps in the mucosa to develop, allowing urinary metabolites or toxins, especially potassium to penetrate the lining through to the sub mucosal receptors of nerves and blood vessels. When a physician introduces potassium solutions into the bladder of someone suffering from IC, this causes pain and some believe that this observation serves to confirm the leakage of noxious stimuli into the submucosa layer of the bladder. This commonly used diagnostic test for IC aims to determine whether the potassium solution causes more pain than water when introduced into the bladder. One of the questions about this test is whether there is any association between the sensitivity of the bladder to potassium and the finding of the blood vessel fragility on stretching of the bladder. Dr. Gergeoire from Quebec, Canada showed no difference in blood vessel fragility in those who had positive potassium tests and those who did not. The merit of the potassium test as a diagnostic indicator for IC may be called into question.

Neurogenic inflammation in the bladder

IC is a bladder condition generally involving inflammation. Dr. Ragi

Doggweiler and others have discussed the theory of neurogenic inflammation as it relates to the bladder. This theory is compelling. Neurogenic inflammation is an inflammatory process that is induced through stimulation of nerve receptors.

In this conceptual model of neurogenic inflammation an insult to the bladder or pelvic floor, which may be physical, such as post delivery trauma or frequent urinary tract infections) or a psychological stressor, such as intense anxiety or physical stress, may be initiating factors in the development of IC symptoms. This stressful perpetrator in the bladder and pelvic floor is thought to send messages to the part of the spine that controls bladder and pelvic floor function. These intense signals to the spinal cord from the pelvic muscles produce what is called *neural windup,* the activity of the nervous system in the spine becomes strongly aroused.

This *windup* of the activity in the spinal nerves (initiated from signals from the pelvis) is thought to cause a high level of nervous activity in the pelvis and bladder. The *neural windup* is believed to create a cascade of events which results in inflammation. In this *neural windup* model, we have a self-feeding cycle of increased pain, increased anxiety, which continues to support the arousal and the *windup* of the nervous system. This then supports inflammation causing more pain and contraction and leads to more inflammation and anxiety. This is a difficult cycle to break. The *Wise-Anderson Protocol* described in this book attempts to intervene in this cycle.

Anxiety and interstitial cystitis

Oemler and associates in Germany reported that people with IC had a higher level of life adversities than normal subjects without IC (controls) based on a survey of accumulative childhood experiences. Survey results from IC patients revealed a tendency to have a poor emotional relationship with their parents, a more difficult and anxiety-laden childhood, and indications of physical abuse. IC patients had higher scores for dysfunction than the controls.

Anxiety can produce and exacerbate inflammation

Numerous studies have shown that stress and anxiety impair the healing of wounds. Broadbent and co-workers in New Zealand recently reported that psychological stress is associated with slower wound healing. They suggest that reduction of psychological stress can improve wound repair following surgery. Pitsavos and his team in Greece showed that anxiety increases inflammation in healthy people. In Sweden, Johansen and colleagues found a positive relationship between the occurrence of gum inflammation and anxiety.

Grossi and his team in Sweden found that stress in women tends to result in increased inflammation. In Israel, Melamed and colleagues found that the fear of terrorism promoted increased levels of low-grade inflammation in apparently healthy adults. Song and his team in British Columbia reported that increased anxiety and stress produced an inflammatory response in laboratory rats. Liu and associates in Wisconsin found that anxiety during examination-taking exacerbated the inflammatory response in asthma.

Although it appears that anxiety is pro-inflammatory and interferes with the body's natural healing mechanisms there is little current evidence on the effect of lowering anxiety and general nervous system arousal and the improvement of IC.

Anxiety and mucous membrane inflammation , a common denominator: Interstitial cystitis, irritable bowel syndrome, colitis, gum disease, burning mouth syndrome, anal fissures, gastritis, idiopathic dyspepsia

The bladder is lined with mucosa (a mucous membrane). In this section we will discuss the similar effects of anxiety on inflammation of the mucosa in other body areas in order to gain insight about inflammation and the bladder.

Mucosa lines all the cavities of the body that open externally, including the nose, mouth, esophagus, stomach, intestines, bladder, vagina and lungs. Inflammation, ulceration and pain can occur in all body locations lined with mucous membranes. Anxiety has been associated with onset and exacerbation of inflammation in mucosal tissues. Thus, the strong effect of anxiety on bladder conditions is not unexpected, nor should reduced anxiety be unexpected to have an equally powerful healing effect.

Wolf and Wolff found that "sustained hyper function" of the bowel was associated with increased fragility of the bowel's mucous membrane such that even minor stresses resulted in hemorrhage or ulceration. This was particularly evident in individuals with ulcerative colitis. While these patients appeared outwardly calm and superficially peaceful, underneath this apparent placid demeanor, the person often sat on "a powder keg" of intense hostility, resentment and guilt. These long standing, unrelieved feelings were associated with hyper function of the colon with increased motor activity, increased vascularity, turgescence and small hemorrhagic lesions.

If you speak to dentists, they will tell you that patients who are anxious or significantly stressed often have gums that are puffy and inflamed. This observation is supported by the research of Johannsen in Sweden and Vettore in Brazil which indicate the adverse effect of anxiety on gum inflammation.

Irritable bowel syndrome, a very common condition of pain, bloating and disturbed bowel habits, is associated with mucosal inflammation. Numerous studies support the association between anxiety and bowel mucosal inflammation. Wolf and Wolff in their classic book *The Colon*, documented the change in color and mucous secretion of subjects who became anxious or agitated.

Inflammation of the esophagus mucosa, called gastro-esophageal reflux disorder (GERD--commonly called heartburn) and esophagitis (inflammation of the esophagus), nausea, functional idiopathic dyspepsia, gastritis, stomach ulceration, burning mouth syndrome, and even anal fissures are associated with anxiety.

With the *Wise-Anderson Protocol*, we utilize a two-pronged approach of 1) deactivating the offending muscular trigger points that create pain in the pelvis and 2) teach patients to relax a painful, contracted pelvis in order to lower anxiety and the arousal of the autonomic nervous system.

Depressive symptoms and quality of life in interstitial cystitis patients

A recent publication by Dr. Nan Rothrock, University of Iowa, indicates that IC patients have poor functioning in various life domains, and that with increased severity of symptoms there is further deterioration in quality of life. It is always difficult for the physician, friends and acquaintances to appreciate the extent of disability and suffering resulting from a chronic pain disorder. IC adversely affects leisure activities, family relations, and travel in 70 to 94% of patients.

Depression and fatigue are common experiences for these patients as are difficulty concentrating and insomnia. The University of Iowa study involved only IC female patients who completed questionnaires for psychological assessment including depressive symptoms. Bladder biopsies also were examined. A comparative control group of 40 age-matched women without IC completed the depression questionnaires. The study showed that the IC patients with more severe disease had significantly greater limitations in their physical and social functioning, as well as a greater impact on their mental health. Of interest is that bladder biopsies revealed the absence or only mild inflammation in 80% of the patients and no ulceration in 80%. However, 80% of patients had moderate to severe capillary fragility with petechial hemorrhages (pinpoint bleeding). No specific IC symptom was associated with depression. The positive note in this study is that although IC patients had proportionally more depression than healthy controls, there was very little severe depression and patients were able to cope with their normal life experiences.

Intervening in the possible self-feeding cycle of IC

The constellation of pelvic trauma, chronic pelvic pain, protective guarding against pain, chronic pelvic tension including pain-referring trigger points, a predisposition toward anxiety and catastrophic thinking that feeds anxiety and inflammation in the bladder may all be part of a self-feeding, self-perpetuating cycle in women and men with IC. As with male pelvic pain, the goal of our *Wise-Anderson Protocol* is to interrupt this cascade of events.

In our view, the focus on quieting nervous system arousal needs to be done regularly, especially because IC patients may have a greater predisposition toward anxiety or have relatively more anxiety as a result of their condition. While patients may become discouraged when hearing this, we are not, and simply feel that it takes more effort and intention to reduce the general level of nervousness in order for patients to help themselves. Quieting anxiety in our protocol includes both regular practice in profound relaxation, the management of thinking that tends to spin off into catastrophic thinking, and dealing with lifestyle issues and one's relationships. Importantly, anxiety is almost always significantly reduced in IC patients when they feel they can do something to help themselves.

Trigger points and IC

We have found there are often a large number of trigger points in the pelvic floor in individuals with IC and they are often very painful. These trigger points can be accessed and manipulated by a physical therapist. However, we strongly believe that it is important that IC patients also be taught how to identify and work on the trigger points themselves.

Research on diet and IC

Unlike other conditions of pelvic pain where there is no clear association with foods that may induce symptoms, in IC the management of one's diet may be important. If one continually eats foods and drinks beverages that irritate the bladder, this practice will undermine other aspects of treatment. Physicians have suggested caffeine, alcohol, spicy, acidic or tomato-containing foods, carbonated drinks, and even multivitamins as possible aggravating factors for IC. Many patients can identify other foods that presumably create difficulty.

However, strict dietary directives may not be useful and are often unnecessarily restrictive. It only makes sense to eliminate foods that one knows will affect their bladder, if painful bladder symptoms occur. An ongoing evaluation is useful as sensitivities to specific foods may vary from time to time. We strongly suggest keeping a diary to identify the food or drinks that appear to be associated with subsequent increased pain or urinary frequency and urgency.

In a recent study Robert Moldwin, Barbara Shorter and colleagues at Long Island University examined the effect of foods, beverages and supplements on IC patients. Study results suggested that elimination of coffee, tea, alcoholic beverages, citrus fruits and juices, spicy foods, hot peppers, and certain artificial sweeteners may have a positive effect on reducing a patient's symptoms. This is in agreement with much of the conventional wisdom among IC patient advocate groups. However, some studies have found little difference in ingesting substances that alkalinize the urine. In general, monitoring of diet probably has a role in controlling IC symptoms but elimination of possibly offending foods has not been shown to be curative.

Current management and treatment of IC

Several therapeutic approaches are currently being used to manage the symptoms of IC. These include oral medications, injection of agents directly into the bladder lining or instillations of agents into the bladder through a catheter.

Several pharmaceutical drugs have been used to manage IC symptoms. There is only one oral drug approved by the U.S. Food and Drug Administration (FDA) for the specific indication of IC. However, its usefulness as we discuss further is questionable. The drug pentosan polysulfate sodium (Elmiron®) is intended to improve the GAG layer of the bladder. In multiple clinical trials of this drug, 28-40% of all patients were reported to have had significant improvement. The drug must be used for an extended periods of three to six months to achieve the greatest benefit. In an NIH-sponsored clinical trial the effects of Elmiron® and the antihistamine called hydroxyzine used as single agents or in combination and compared with a placebo were evaluated. Thirty-four percent of patients had a response (reduction of symptoms) with Elmiron® compared to 18% of patients on placebo. With the antihistamine alone, 31% of patients had a response as did 20% on placebo. When both drugs were taken together, 40% of patients obtained a response. *The overall conclusion was that neither of the drugs, either used alone or in combination, resulted in significant improvement of IC symptoms to warrant further study.*

It is a consensus of the NIH research groups that amitriptyline (Elavil®), a long-term traditional antidepressant, might be beneficial in reducing painful bladder syndrome. National trials are underway to determine the effectiveness of this agent versus placebo.

Instillation of drugs into the bladder such as steroids, anesthetics and antibiotic solutions are treatment approaches to ease pain and frequency in IC patients. Dimethylsulfoxide (DMSO) has been approved for this purpose and reports have indicated that up to 70% of IC patients experience some relief of symptoms. Often physicians will create a "cocktail" with DMSO adding hydrocortisone, alkalinizing sodium bicarbonate, Lidocaine® or Marcaine® (a topical anesthetic) and heparin to act as a surface sealant. Initially there also was hope that immune modulation of the bladder surface by instillation of a tuberculosis vaccine (BCG) would provide some benefit for IC. However, when this approach was tested against a placebo in national clinical trials no meaningful benefit was achieved. Hyaluronic acid (Cystostat®) has not been approved in the United States, but reports of benefit after placement in the bladder have come from Canadian studies.

Botulinum toxin A or Botox® which has been used extensively in dermatology to smooth skin wrinkles by creating a temporary nerve paralysis has also been injected directly into the bladder lining to relieve pelvic floor spasms, pelvic pain and overactive bladder. A new experimental approach, only so far tested in animals, uses liposomes as a drug carrier for Botox®. The Botox® is encapsulated into liposomes which are instilled into the bladder. The liposomes are tiny fat-like bubbles which themselves may coat and soothe the irritated bladder and protect the bladder from the potentially irritating effects of the Botox®. This approach allows the medication to be delivered where it is needed without injection. Furthermore, in the first and recent study in a small number of actual patients with IC, installation of liposomes alone without any drugs was compared with oral Elmiron. At 4 weeks after beginning treatment, frequency and nocturia decreased significantly in both groups. Patients who were treated with liposomes also had a significant decrease in pain and urinary urgency. These approaches with Botox® and/or liposomes require large placebo-clinical trials and further comparative studies to evaluate safety and effectiveness for IC patients.

Approximately 5 to 10% of patients with IC have lesions called Hunner's ulcers on the bladder wall. Removing the ulcers with fulguration or "burning" them off with electrical cautery or laser treatment, or excision to cut off the lesion and surrounding tissue can bring relief. The ulcers can reoccur and repeat treatment is recommended when symptoms reappear. A new treatment under evaluation involves injection of a steroid. Some patients just live with their ulcers and attempt some to gain symptom relief by removing acid food and drinks from their diet, if indeed they appear to aggravate their condition.

Bladder conditioning, namely stretching the bladder with timed voiding is a non-pharmacological and patient-directed approach. This conditioning helps to desensitize IC patients to the sensation of needing to void. They are taught to gradually stretch the bladder by deferring urination for several minutes each day, attempting to increase the total volume voided. It is important to do this throughout the day with increased fluid intake and voiding by the clock rather than succumb to the urgency they feel. When needed, we teach techniques to suppress the urgency. However, if their discomfort is more than 6 or 7 on a scale of 10, then they need to give in to the urge to urinate.

Pelvic floor muscle management, particularly of pelvic floor and bladder related trigger points, usually benefits this group of patients. In a California study, Weiss reported that treatment of urgency/frequency syndrome with intrapelvic myofascial release treatment resulted in reduced symptoms. The study involved both men and women. Of the 42 patients who had urgency/frequency (with or without pain) for 6 to 14 years, 83% had moderate to marked improvement or complete resolution. He postulated that the bladder is not completely responsible for the symptoms and that the pelvic floor and the sphincter muscles play a major role. These patients typically have tender spots in the pelvis on palpation and it is consistent with the trigger points we have described. Many patients with the diagnosis of IC describe difficult voiding in childhood and may have had previous trauma contributing to their dysfunction, even triggering events that appear so trivial as to not be recognized as a cause.

Anatomically the pelvic floor myofascial trigger points may influence the bladder. This occurs because their nerve nuclei or origins lie in close proximity within the spinal cord to incoming nerve endings from bladder autonomic nerves. Flare-ups of IC, including pain and urinary urgency, can be activated by stress, dietary indiscretions, improper exercise or movement, trauma, sexual activity, cold weather, hormonal shifts, and viral infection. Details of the actual neurophysiologic changes within the nervous system and within the muscular tissue have yet to be worked out by the basic scientists, but clinicians continue to seek the relationships that may guide basic investigation.

A recent national clinical trial utilizing manual pelvic physical therapy to treat women with IC revealed that 81 women treated at 11 different centers showed 59% of them improving to a moderate or markedly improved status.

Potential therapeutic approaches for IC under evaluation

Attention is being drawn to the potential of gene therapy for IC bladder pain. While in the early stages of research in animal bladders, scientists are using the herpes simplex virus as a "carrier" for a gene for a substance that participates in the synthesis of a natural painkiller in the body. When animals with bladder irritation got the gene, there was lower bladder hyperactivity and less-pain-related behavior. Laboratory analysis showed that the gene had been incorporated into the bladder and the nerve roots that receive pain impulses from the bladder.

Researchers are exploring new drug targets to ease bladder pain and hypersensitivity. They are focusing on receptors or protein molecules embedded in the outside surface (plasma membrane) or within cells (the cytoplasm). Drugs can be designed to bind to the receptors and specifically block processes that excite bladder activity. One such experimental agent blocks a prostaglandin receptor in the central nervous system and may help control bladder over activity and pain. Another drug targets spinal corticotropin-releasing factor (CRF) which is released when animals are stressed, resulting in hypersensitivity to pain. This last study supports the role of stress in making bladder pain worse and implicates spinal cord CRF-like compounds and their receptors in the process. Yet another approach is targeting the sensory nerves in the bladder and their receptors. When ATP (adenosine triphosphate), a major source of energy for cellular reactions, or similar compounds attach to the nerve receptors they become more sensitive to noxious or irritating stimulation. Blocking of the ATP receptors fully blocked certain types of chronic inflammation and neuropathic pain.

Another innovative and experimental approach utilizes forms of electrical stimulation for symptom relief in patients with IC. Similar to the process of acupuncture, the electrical pulses are targeted to nerves sending signals from the pelvis to the spinal cord. Electrode leads may be implanted into the sacral nerves, near the pudendal nerve or the tibial nerve in the ankle. The more common therapy involves sacral neuromodulation to alleviate over active bladder. Pudendal nerve stimulation has been used but when sacral stimulation stops working or does not work. Dr. Ken Peters and colleagues at William Beaumont Hospital in Michigan recently treated a group of patients, most had prior sacral neuromodulation; 71% of the 84 patients had 50% symptom improvements described as significant for frequency, voided volume, incontinence and urgency. Some of the patients had complications requiring revisions in 7 and reoperations in 4 others. The effectiveness of electrical nerve stimulation of the tibial nerve near the ankle has been compared with extended release tolterodine (Detrol LA) for treatment of overactive bladder. While objective measurements showed similar improvements in both groups, more patients who got the nerve stimulation said they were cured or improved than those on drug. These nerve stimulation procedures have been approved by the Food and Drug Administration for treatment overactive bladder, they may have potential in IC but have not been specifically evaluated nor approved for pain relief in patients with IC.

Vulvodynia

Vulvodynia or hypersensitivity of the vulva and vaginal opening was first described in the 19th century. It includes disorders named *vulvar vestibulitis* and *essential vulvodynia*. The incidence and prevalence of these conditions is not definitively known. Some estimates suggest that up to 15% of women with IC also have vulvar pain. Typically 50% of women with vulvodynia experience dyspareunia which is pain during or right after sexual intercourse. They feel pain during penile insertion into the vagina, as well as pain while inserting tampons. *Vulvar vestibulitis* is defined as inflammation of the tissue at the vaginal entrance with a pronounced redness and exquisite sensitivity when touched even lightly. Sharp pain occurs when this delicate skin is rubbed, and this pain often prohibits or limits normal sexual intercourse. Even clothing such as pantyhose or tight fitting lingerie may be irritating.

This disorder commonly occurs in sexually active young women, and can even develop after previous normal, non-painful sexual intercourse. It is not unusual for these women to have a coincident occurrence of IC with their vulvodynia. Many women are misdiagnosed as having fungal vaginitis, lichen planus, or contact dermatitis, and are treated with anti-fungal agents and other topical medications; these may even worsen some of the inflammatory responses. Some have suggested there is coinciding sub-clinical infection of the human papilloma virus or genital wart virus, but there is no scientific proof.

Patients are frequently treated with medications such as antidepressants (e.g., Elavil®) for neuropathic pain, topical estrogens, and cortisone creams. *Surgical or destructive manipulations of the tissues typically have a disappointing outcome.* There is some evidence that injections of botulinum toxins (usually Botox®) into the vulva may help for a period of 3 to 6 months in women with vulvar vestibulitis. Retreatment appears to be successful and side effects are limited. More research needs to be done to confirm the value of this therapy.

Hormones and menstruation

Today girls are reaching menarche at younger ages. The extreme pain and spasm experienced by some very young women before and during their menstrual flow may be related to the tightness developed in their pelvises because of earlier conditioning. Normalizing pelvic muscle tone and function, or even simply adding an aerobic component to her exercise program is sometimes helpful for a more comfortable menses.

Pregnancy and pelvic pain

Hormonal changes during pregnancy cause a softening of connective tissue. Poor posture, slouching or sitting with pressure on the coccyx (tail bone) could predispose it to strain and pain. This is an ideal time to learn to sit without pressure on the coccyx. Ideally sitting erect with a normal concave curve in the lumbar spine and transmitting weight through the ischial tuberosities (sitting bones at the bottom of the pelvis) may go a long way in preventing coccydynia/coccygodynia (tail bone pain) during the childbearing years. Once this condition develops, it may be necessary to sit on a cushion to reduce pressure on the coccyx and thereby transmitting weight through the thighs and ischial tuberosities.

Round ligament pain

Round ligament pain sometimes occurs in pregnant women. It is a sharp stitch-like pain in the lower abdomen and groin often lasting up to 20 minutes and caused by sudden changes in posture, such as rolling over in bed or standing from a sitting position. The round ligaments are fibromuscular cords which help support the uterus and extend into the labia majora. These ligaments can become hypertrophied or enlarged and more vascular during pregnancy to support the increased weight of the baby. Gently pulling in the belly and tilting the pelvis backwards to support the baby before changing position is sometimes suggested to help this problem. Occasionally a support belt may be useful with a large baby or multiple pregnancies.

Urinary urgency and frequency during pregnancy

Urinary urgency and frequency can occur as normal sensations during early and late pregnancy. In the first trimester, the uterus becomes heavier and presses on the bladder and does not allow it to expand as usual. In the last trimester, the pressure of the baby's head moving into position for birth often makes a woman feel like she has a constant urgency to urinate.

Symphysis pubis pain and pregnancy

This is also caused by ligamentous laxity during pregnancy which causes increased movement of the joint holding the pelvis together in front. Avoiding unilateral weight bearing or exercise, wearing a sacroiliac belt and consulting with a physical therapist for stabilizing postural exercise and activities of daily living can be helpful.

Diastasis of the rectus abdominus

What is referred to as the belly of the rectus abdominal muscles tends to separate during pregnancy due to both hormonal and anatomical changes. As the abdominal muscles play a key role in posture and good body mechanics (which directly relate to pelvic pain) it is important to be aware of ways of minimizing muscle separation during any exercise program.

Labor and delivery

The physical efforts of labor and delivery can greatly affect a woman's pelvic floor, and can set the stage for a number of pelvic pain syndromes. Even in ideal birthing situations, the pelvic floor muscles can stretch up to one and a half times their normal length, sometimes resulting in overstretched nerves or even rupture of some muscle fibers.

In Western civilizations, birthing women are predisposed to other problems as well. In collaboration with health care providers, couples are more prone to request induction of labor for their convenience instead of allowing nature to take its course. Rupturing of membranes artificially or use of hormones like pitocin to speed up the labor process can make labor and delivery much more painful and difficult for a woman. This often necessitates the use of more pain medications, the resultant loss of control, and the need for larger episiotomies and even instrumentation. A gentler, more natural process, even if longer, is kinder to the pelvic floor. Of course, there are conditions which necessitate intervention for the health of the baby or mother; choosing an obstetrician sensitive to these issues is important.

Birthing in more difficult anti-gravity positions is unfortunately still common, as are the use of analgesic or anesthetic agents which decrease or nullify active labor and delivery participation by the mother. Instrumentation in the form of forceps delivery, when employed, sometimes results in large episiotomies and tears.

Unfortunately, it is not unusual to hear some women complain of pelvic pain or dysfunction after childbirth. Pain or dysfunction persisting for six weeks or more after delivery necessitates professional care. Most complaints are of weakness, stress or urge urinary or bowel incontinence. A program of graduated pelvic floor exercise and behavioral training is usually sufficient to correct these problems. However, dyspareunia (pain during and/or after intercourse) or difficulty and pain during or right after a bowel movement can be the result of poor healing or scar tissue formation, and rarely, even the vaginal opening being too tightly sutured during episiotomy repair.

With a very large baby or a difficult presentation like posterior, face, or breech, the pelvic bones sometimes separate, especially if instrumentation like forceps or suction is used. The mother may have pain or may not be able to turn over in bed or get up to walk. She also may have vaginal, suprapubic, sacroiliac and groin pain. Bowel movements may increase her pain, and urinary pain, urgency and frequency are often present. A timely rehabilitation is possible with a disciplined program of non-weight bearing pelvic stabilization with a belt and appropriate exercise combined with *Myofascial Release* and *Trigger Point Release*. However, this can be a difficult task for a new mother. Occasionally, injections into the pubic symphysis and sacroiliac joints are necessary to enhance stability (prolo-therapy).

Reducing the risk of pelvic pain after childbirth

Conventional wisdom is not always wise. The conventional wisdom in the past endorsed midline episiotomies, turned an indifferent eye to prolonged 2nd stage labor, and to large weight gain during pregnancy among other practices. The current obstetrical understanding with regard to childbirth has changed in recent years. Below are some important considerations when making plans about childbirth. These are even more important if there is an existing pelvic pain condition.

The facility chosen in which to give birth is an important decision, particularly in terms of it having a sympathetic gentle birthing philosophy and methodology. A relaxed birthing atmosphere that is as homelike and comfortable as possible is important because it enables the laboring mother to be more relaxed and at ease.

We also consider it important to choose a health professional empathetic to the ideals of natural gentle birthing. This could be a midwife or physician who is comfortable with a woman laboring and delivering in different positions; someone who sincerely endorses this and is not simply giving lip-service to these ideas, but is committed to and has had experience in the practice of them.

Obviously there is a place for medical monitors and intravenous drips in difficult or complicated deliveries. However, in the absence of the need for monitoring and medical intervention, we think it important that a woman be free to walk around, get down on all fours and gently rock, rhythmically 'dance' moving her pelvis from side to side (there are reports that belly dancing originated as a child birth ritual) or bounce gently on a big birthing ball. A birthing ball is a large, sturdy and inflatable ball that a mother sits, and can rhythmically bounce on. It is sometimes recommended in order for a mother to help her baby to find the best position to travel down through the pelvis and birth canal.

The subject of birthing is far beyond the scope of this book. Suffice it to say that we prefer natural birthing in as home like an environment as possible. This is in contrast to turning birthing mothers into hospital patients and transforming a beautiful and natural human process into a medical procedure.

Many birthing experts support the idea of a mother staying home as long as possible. A good childbirth educator and/or *doula* (a specially trained labor assistant) may be consulted to help with the decision of when, during the final stages of labor, to go to the birthing facility. The importance of staying as long as possible in a comfortable and stress free environment is illustrated in studies on mice. When the birthing environment of mice is disturbed, by gently lifting the laboring mother and placing her in another location, her delivery is significantly delayed, the equivalent of many hours in a human being.

It is recommended to find the most experienced childbirth educator available. Someone in private practice may feel freer to teach you about all the choices available. A hospital, or physician employed educator of the hospital, may be more likely to direct you toward their facility. Some have said that employing the services of a *doula* who can navigate the system is a good investment. The *doula* usually has the time, patience, and the physical and emotional skills needed to support a natural and mother-centered birthing experience.

It is obviously important to get in good physical shape with a good exercise program that helps stretch the muscles necessary for birth, to train endurance, proper relaxation, and posture.

It is important to learn how to contract and especially how to release pelvic muscles to facilitate birthing. Daily massaging, warming the vaginal muscles and stretching the vaginal opening with a natural oil like almond, sesame or olive, may be helpful to avoid tearing during childbirth. It is important to note that while we consider that yoga can be helpful in preparation for childbirth, overly vigorous yoga can overstretch ligaments (which are already softened with the hormone relaxin). A yoga teacher who understands the kind of gentle stretching that is helpful for childbirth is essential.

The second stage of childbirth has to do with the cervix dilating to about 10 centimeters. The popular image of this stage is that of the soon to be mother, with cheering from others in the room, pushing hard for a long time to release the baby. There is more and more agreement, however, that strong, prolonged pushing during the second stage of childbirth is not a good idea. Gentle pushing is imperative as is a not-too-prolonged second stage of labor. If one has ever watched a calf or puppy being born, one will observe how the mother pants gently, pushes a little, and then goes back to panting. When a woman co-operates with her body, her uterus is usually able to do its work, and it is the uterus which does most of the work in expelling a baby. Many natural birthing advocates consider a mother's position at birth to be important.

Many women in third world countries, who are used to squatting, typically give birth squatting. In a squatting position the pelvic outlet widens. Some birthing consultants report that when women are given the opportunity to choose any position during the second stage of labor, most will opt for being supported in a half squat. This way the birth is gravity assisted.

As we have mentioned, prolonged pushing and a prolonged second stage of labor is considered by many obstetricians a part of childbirth to be avoided as it raises the risk of tissue tearing and postpartum pain and incontinence. Additionally, it can cause stretching of the nerves and muscles which can result in weakness, pelvic prolapse and incontinence (especially when hormonal changes during menopause occur).

Related to this is the current trend to avoid episiotomy which is the cutting of the perineum to permit a wider opening for the exit of the child. Both medialateral episiotomies, in which the cut is made laterally into the perineum, or a medial episiotomy, in which the incision is straight down toward the perineum are not recommended by many obstetricians as these can facilitate a larger tear. Again, the exception is when the life of the child or the mother is at stake.

The case against episiotomy can be understood from experience in the fabric store. Typically, to more easily tear a fabric, you make a small cut at the beginning of the tear which facilitates an easy cutting or ripping of the fabric. In the same way, the episiotomy tends to facilitate more tearing in the tissue than the natural and spontaneous tearing that might occur during childbirth. A skilled professional is important at the birth to help make the appropriate decision about episiotomy, as a severely torn perineum or pelvic floor is a major problem and not easy to repair.

Also, contrary to the indifference of conventional wisdom with regard to weight gain, many obstetricians suggest to limit weight gain to not more than 20 to 30 pounds. More weight tends to mean bigger babies, which tends to mean more risk of trauma in getting them out.

Exercises that tighten the abdomen are often not friendly to easy childbirth. Some doctors report, that dancers for example, tend to have more difficulty in childbirth because their pelvis and abdomen have been trained to remain tight and constricted. What has emerged in recent times is that weight-control, stretching and relaxation techniques tend to make childbirth easier and diminish the likelihood of trauma.

Finally, relaxation has been universally appreciated in facilitating childbirth. In the same way as we support patients to not be afraid of pain and to relax with pain, so the mother giving birth does well to relax with discomfort and pain instead of contracting against it. The mother who has practiced appropriate stretching and relaxation even in the presence of discomfort has a better chance of an easier birth.

Dyspareunia (painful intercourse)

Women with dyspareunia are sometimes diagnosed as being "frigid," an often unkind and ignorant diagnosis intimating that they have a psychological problem with intimacy or simply hate sex. Appropriate treatment for painful intercourse is necessary no matter what the cause. This problem can manifest at a very young age when teenagers find that inserting even a small tampon during menstruation is too painful. These are often the same women who find it difficult to have a gynecological exam, because insertion of a speculum into the vagina causes pain. Sometimes they are not even able to tolerate the physician's examining finger. Mostly these problems stem from chronic muscle tightness or guarding but there are instances where the hymen may be thicker than normal and can result in more of a physical barrier. Most patients respond well to vaginal massage and stretching, *Trigger Point Release* and pelvic floor relaxation. Rarely does this condition require surgery.

A young woman with dyspareunia comes to mind. She came to see us after having had two children. Her marriage was never consummated. Instead, she was artificially impregnated with her husband's sperm and had a cesarean birth for both children. In her mid thirties, both she and her husband finally decided to confront her inability to have intercourse. After one consultation, where they were taught the techniques of vaginal massage and *Paradoxical Relaxation*, the couple was finally able to have sexual intercourse. Most often, however, there are more factors involved in the vaginismus (or spasm and tightness of the vaginal muscles) requiring more extensive *Myofascial Release* and *Trigger Point Release*, as well as psychological and sex counseling.

Vaginismus

Vaginismus refers to a usually instantaneous, painful tightening/spasm of the muscles around the entrance of the vagina. The normal state of these vaginal muscles is closed. Typically when relaxed the vagina is able to open, allowing the woman to engage in sexual intercourse, the insertion of a tampon, or the insertion of a finger during a medical examination. This abrupt vaginal spasm can derive from experiences earlier in life relating to cultural conditioning, sexual trauma or a negative sexual experience. Aside from being painful and usually out of the woman's control, it can profoundly affect a woman's life by interfering with the normal development of an intimate relationship, allowing her to be sexual or to bear children. It is a difficult situation for any woman to be physically unable to develop an intimate sexual relationship because of this condition.

The difference between someone with vaginismus and the pelvic pain that we have treated is that typically a woman with vaginismus only has vaginal pain and constriction in anticipation of or during sexual activity, during medical examination or tampon insertion. The *Wise-Anderson Protocol* is usually able to help a woman overcome this condition by teaching her to do self *Trigger Point Release*, *Paradoxical Relaxation*, and vaginal stretching, sometimes with the use of graduated sizes of vaginal dilators.

In our view, vaginismus is not simply a physical problem of tight or spastic muscles, but as with many pelvic pain conditions it may involve negative past conditioning and attitudes.

Menopause

As women approach menopause and hormone levels drop, less mucous is secreted and the vaginal tissue can become more fragile. Painful intercourse, urinary urgency, frequency, or even incontinence can attend this time of life. Estrogen replacement therapy (ERT) or local estrogen replacement inserted into the vaginal opening can be helpful. This augments vaginal tissue health and can even help with stress incontinence if the problem is mainly urethral tissue thinning. A program of pelvic floor muscle exercises, using both slow and fast contractions (even doing six 5-10 second contractions followed by 10 quick vaginal muscle flicks after each urination) can make a difference. This can be helpful in combination with vaginal stretching and gentle *Trigger Point Release* and *Myofascial Release* and is often all that is necessary.

Not getting lost in one's symptoms and keeping the big picture

It is easy to "medicalize" the subject of pelvic pain in general and women's pelvic pain in particular. In doing so one can lose sight of the larger picture that *a woman who has pelvic pain is more than her pelvic pain*. In our view, there are often other important factors involved in female pelvic pain aside from specific symptoms conventional medicine takes into account. A woman's pelvic pain is present along with her anxiety and general level of nervous system arousal, early conditioning, the quality of her relationships, her skill in relationships, and the level of her insight into her thinking, emotions, and her past. Pelvic pain, as we understand it and describe it in this book, may be the consequence of, or may be exacerbated by how some women (and men) express their fears and suppress their feelings in order to maintain equilibrium in their lives. In discussing this we are not in any way negating the fact that there also may have been a provoking trauma or medical reason for the initiation of the pain syndrome.

An archetypal illustration of the relationship between emotions and pelvic pain

During the writing of the fourth edition of our book, a physical therapist with whom we work closely, reported doing a session with a woman with pelvic pain who had experienced an intense flare-up of her symptoms after having a substantial period of being pain free after practicing our protocol. She began seeing the therapist in an attempt to reverse the flare-up.

During the course of the physical therapy session a remarkable event occurred. It was remarkable not because it was uncommon (indeed it is the most common of events) but because the event was witnessed in a therapeutic setting. This is what happened.

During the physical therapy session, while the therapist had her finger inside the patient's vagina, the patient began to talk about something about which she was very upset. As the woman shared her upset feelings, the therapist felt her finger being crushed in a vise-like grip of the woman's pelvic muscle contraction. The patient was middle-aged and the physical therapist was amazed at the strength of contraction of the muscles of this woman's pelvic floor while she shared her upset feelings—a strength of contraction not even felt in the pelvic strength of substantially younger women. We emphasize that the pelvic contraction that appeared suddenly in this patient was huge.

"Did you feel that?" the physical therapist asked her patient. "Did I feel what?" replied the patient. "Can't you feel the spasm that your pelvis has gone into right now while you are talking about these upsetting things?" asked the physical therapist. The patient was dumbfounded. "I don't feel anything" replied the patient. She had no sense of the relationship between her emotions and the reaction of her pelvic muscles. Only after a number of attempts on the part of our colleague to help the patient recreate her upsetting feelings and simultaneously feel her pelvic muscles contract, was the patient able to appreciate what was going on inside her pelvis when she was upset.

This story also relates to the phenomenon of colonic spasm seen in the study we have described, discussed by researchers in the 1950's. To recall, they discussed an experiment in which a group of army recruits having a rectal exam were deliberately exposed to the discussions of the doctors while the recruits were being examined with a rectal scope. One doctor said to the other, "Look at that cancer in his colon." Upon each recruit hearing this catastrophic news, his rectum almost always went into spasm. When hearing that there was no cancer, and that these comments were part of an experiment (an experiment that would never be allowed today), the rectal spasms immediately released.

The story of this woman and the study on the colonic spasm of the army recruits are examples of what we believe are everyday occurrences in the lives of women and men with pelvic pain. Furthermore, like the woman in our story, at best most pelvic pain patients are only dimly aware of the connection between their worry, anger, anxiety, and general emotional reactivity, and the strong and ongoing contractions of their pelvic muscles. We believe that patients who are not sensitive to the signals of their body, usually see no connection between anything that has gone on in their lives and the flare-ups they are having.

The tendency to chronically contract the pelvis under stress or as an emotional reactivity response we believe are general conditions that underlie pelvic pain. We are proposing as shown by the examples provided and the research done by Gevirtz and Hubbard (on stress-related increase in electrical activity of the trigger points) that the source of pelvic pain comes both from trigger point activity and chronic tension in the pelvis potentiated by nervous system arousal.

The pelvis, for those with pelvic pain, can be thought of as the site of their "gut reaction." Perhaps what could be called a gut reaction in some people could be called a pelvic reaction in those with pelvic pain. We believe that whenever someone with pelvic pain is upset or concerned, without any training to abort this, pelvic floor contraction is a component. This is particularly true when a pelvic floor is sore or hyperirritable and its contraction is set off by very small events that otherwise would have no effect on the person if the pelvis was not sore and irritated. Consequently our protocol emphasizes teaching patients the skill of profoundly relaxing their pelvic muscles and regularly lowering their level of anxiety.

Internal and External Pelvic Floor Trigger Points in Women and Where They Typically Refer Pain and Sensation

On the following pages we have compiled the internal and external trigger points most frequently implicated in pelvic pain in women, along with a description of their referral patterns.

The illustrations on the following pages show trigger points in the internal and external pelvic muscles.

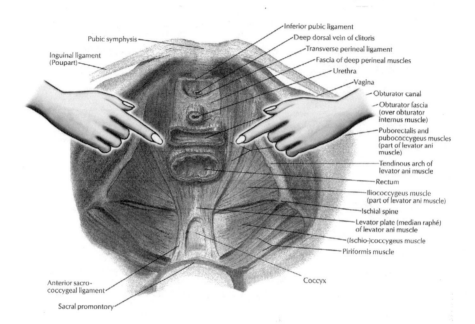

Stanford Protocol
Physical Therapy

Inferior pubic ligament
Deep dorsal vein of clitoris
Pubic symphysis
Transverse perineal ligament
Inguinal ligament (Poupart)
Fascia of deep perineal muscles
Urethra
Vagina
Obturator canal
Obturator fascia (over obturator internus muscle)
Puborectalis and pubococcygeus muscles (part of levator ani muscle)
Tendinous arch of levator ani muscle
Rectum
Iliococcygeus muscle (part of levator ani muscle)
Ischial spine
Levator plate (median raphé) of levator ani muscle
(Ischio-)coccygeus muscle
Piriformis muscle
Coccyx
Anterior sacro-coccygeal ligament
Sacral promontory

Anterior Levator Ani (Inferior Portion)

This is the part of the muscle closest to the back of the pubic bone.
Trigger points can refer to the bladder, urethra, clitoris, mons pubis,
vaginal lips (labium majus and minus) or vestibule (entrance)
of vagina. Trigger points referred discomfort to the bladder can be
associated with a sense of urinary urgency.

> • Can refer lateral vaginal wall, perineal, anal
>   sphincter or referral pattern toward the anterior
>   levators, bladder and urethra.

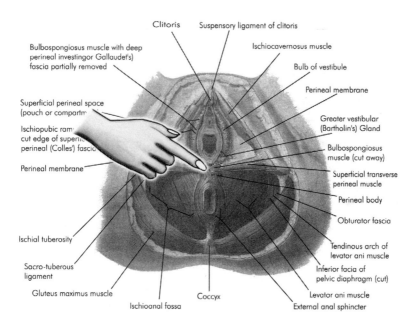

Stanford Protocol
Physical Therapy

Clitoris · Suspensory ligament of clitoris

Bulbospongiosus muscle with deep perineal investingor Gallaudet's) fascia partially removed

Ischiocavernosus muscle

Bulb of vestibule

Perineal membrane

Superficial perineal space (pouch or compartm

Greater vestibular (Bartholin's) Gland

Ischiopubic ram
cut edge of superi
perineal (Colles') fascic

Bulbospongiosus muscle (cut away)

Perineal membrane

Superficial transverse perineal muscle

Perineal body

Obturator fascia

Ischial tuberosity

Tendinous arch of levator ani muscle

Sacro-tuberous ligament

Inferior facia of pelvic diaphragm (cut)

Gluteus maximus muscle · Coccyx · Levator ani muscle

Ischioanal fossa · External anal sphincter

Perineal Body

> • *Trigger points in the perineum can refer pain and sensation to the rectum, vagina, and site of palpation*

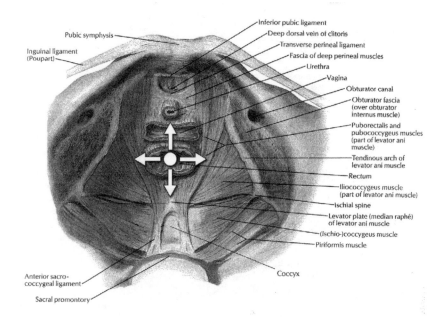

Sphincter Ani (Stretch)

Trigger points in this area may cause pain in the anal sphincter as well
as pain going toward the front and back part of the anal sphincter.
Treatment is done by gently stretching the sphincter upward in the 12 o'clock
position, sideways in the 3 o'clock position, downward to the 6 o'clock
position and sideways toward the 9 o'clock position.

- *Can refer pain in the anal sphincter itself as well as
  radiating to the front and back from the sphincter*
- *This technique helps stretch the levator ani muscle*

Stanford Protocol
Physical Therapy

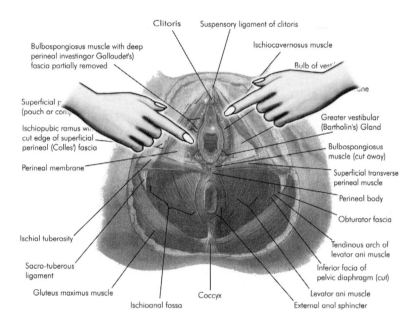

Clitoris   Suspensory ligament of clitoris

Bulbospongiosus muscle with deep
perineal investingor Gallaudet's)
fascia partially removed

Ischiocavernosus muscle

Bulb of vest'

Superficial p
(pouch or con

une

Ischiopubic ramus wi
cut edge of superficial
perineal (Colles') fascia

Greater vestibular
(Bartholin's) Gland

Perineal membrane

Bulbospongiosus
muscle (cut away)

Superficial transverse
perineal muscle

Perineal body

Obturator fascia

Ischial tuberosity

Tendinous arch of
levator ani muscle

Sacro-tuberous
ligament

Inferior facia of
pelvic diaphragm (cut)

Gluteus maximus muscle

Coccyx

Levator ani muscle

Ischioanal fossa

External anal sphincter

Bulbospongiosis and Ischiocavernosis

- *Trigger points in the bulbospongiosis and ischiocavernosis can refer pain and sensation to the perineum and vagina*

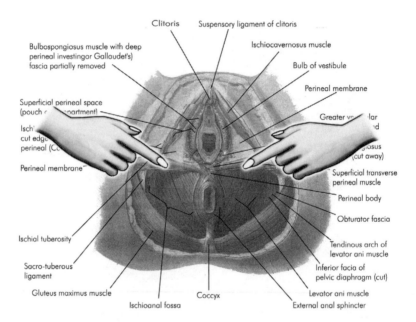

Stanford Protocol
Physical Therapy

Clitoris　　Suspensory ligament of clitoris

Bulbospongiosus muscle with deep
perineal investingor Gallaudet's)
fascia partially removed

Ischiocavernosus muscle

Bulb of vestibule

Perineal membrane

Superficial perineal space
(pouch of ompartment)

Greater v   lar
         d

Isch
cut edge
perineal (C

osus
(cut away)

Perineal membrane

Superficial transverse
perineal muscle

Perineal body

Obturator fascia

Ischial tuberosity

Tendinous arch of
levator ani muscle

Sacro-tuberous
ligament

Inferior facia of
pelvic diaphragm (cut)

Gluteus maximus muscle　　Coccyx

Levator ani muscle

Ischioanal fossa

External anal sphincter

Superficial Transverse Perineal Muscles

- *Trigger points in the superficial transverse perineal muscles
  can refer pain and sensation to the vagina and on the site
  of palpation*

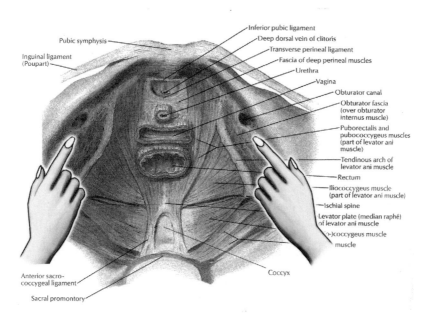

Pubic symphysis

Inguinal ligament (Poupart)

Inferior pubic ligament

Deep dorsal vein of clitoris

Transverse perineal ligament

Fascia of deep perineal muscles

Urethra

Vagina

Obturator canal

Obturator fascia (over obturator internus muscle)

Puborectalis and pubococcygeus muscles (part of levator ani muscle)

Tendinous arch of levator ani muscle

Rectum

Iliococcygeus muscle (part of levator ani muscle)

Ischial spine

Levator plate (median raphé) of levator ani muscle

(o-)coccygeus muscle

muscle

Coccyx

Anterior sacro-coccygeal ligament

Sacral promontory

Obturator Internus

Trigger points in the obturator can refer pain to the perineum, outward toward hip, to the whole pelvic floor both anteriorly and posteriorly. The obturator is intimate with the pudendal nerve and can refer a dull ache and burning in the pelvic floor on the side that it is being palpated. Trigger points in the obturator can refer the golf-ball-in-the-rectum feeling, symptoms to the coccyx, hamstrings and posterior thigh. In women, trigger points in the obturator can refer to the urethra, the vagina, and specifically the vulva and is a very important point in the treatment of vulvar pain.

> ● *Can refer dull ache on the side palpated, golf-ball-in-the-rectum sensation, coccyx, hamstrings, posterior thigh, urethra, vagina, vulva (important in vulvodynia)*

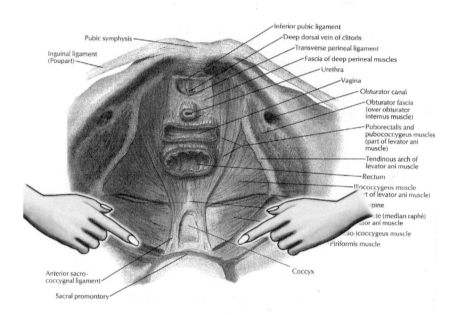

Inferior pubic ligament
Pubic symphysis
Deep dorsal vein of clitoris
Transverse perineal ligament
Inguinal ligament (Poupart)
Fascia of deep perineal muscles
Urethra
Vagina
Obturator canal
Obturator fascia (over obturator internus muscle)
Puborectalis and pubococcygeus muscles (part of levator ani muscle)
Tendinous arch of levator ani muscle
Rectum
Iliococcygeus muscle (part of levator ani muscle)
spine
te (median raphé)
tor ani muscle
(ilio-)coccygeus muscle
Piriformis muscle
Anterior sacro-coccygeal ligament
Coccyx
Sacral promontory

Piriformis (Internally Accessed)

Trigger points here can refer to the sacroiliac joint, the hip girdle and hamstrings. Patients can feel increased pain at the palpation site.

> • Can refer to sacroiliac joint, hip girdle, hamstrings and increased pain at palpation site.

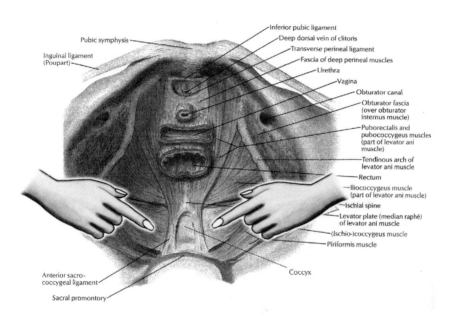

Inferior pubic ligament
Deep dorsal vein of clitoris
Pubic symphysis
Transverse perineal ligament
Inguinal ligament (Poupart)
Fascia of deep perineal muscles
Urethra
Vagina
Obturator canal
Obturator fascia (over obturator internus muscle)
Puborectalis and pubococcygeus muscles (part of levator ani muscle)
Tendinous arch of levator ani muscle
Rectum
Iliococcygeus muscle (part of levator ani muscle)
Ischial spine
Levator plate (median raphé) of levator ani muscle
(Ischio-)coccygeus muscle
Piriformis muscle
Anterior sacro-coccygeal ligament
Coccyx
Sacral promontory

Coccygeus - Ischiococcygeus

Trigger points in this muscle typically refers pain and pressure associated with the sense of having a golfball or stick in the recturm, pain to the coccyx, anus and gluteus maximus. Pre or post bowel movement pain is often associated with the sense of having a full bowel.

> ● Can refer symptoms to coccygeus, coccyx, gluteus maximus, pre or post bowel movement pain/full bowel sensation and discomfort.

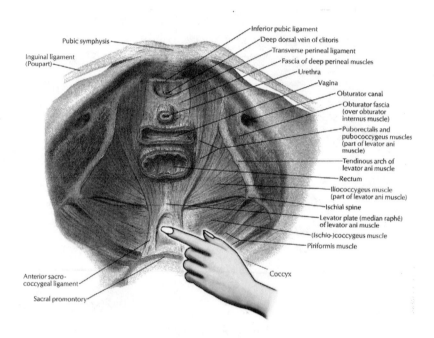

Inferior pubic ligament
Deep dorsal vein of clitoris
Transverse perineal ligament
Fascia of deep perineal muscles
Urethra
Vagina
Obturator canal
Obturator fascia (over obturator internus muscle)
Puborectalis and pubococcygeus muscles (part of levator ani muscle)
Tendinous arch of levator ani muscle
Rectum
Iliococcygeus muscle (part of levator ani muscle)
Ischial spine
Levator plate (median raphé) of levator ani muscle
(Ischio-)coccygeus muscle
Piriformis muscle
Coccyx
Pubic symphysis
Inguinal ligament (Poupart)
Anterior sacro-coccygeal ligament
Sacral promontory

Palpating the Coccyx

This is a bony palpation. In treating pelvic pain, if the coccyx is immobile it can be a factor that perpetuates trigger points that cause pelvic pain.

> • *An immobile coccyx can perpetuate pelvic pain*

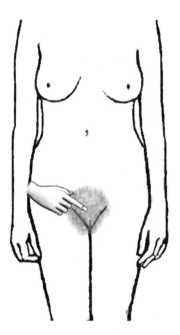

Pain felt in shaded area
Finger tip locates trigger point

Pyramidalis

- The pyramidalis is not present in some individuals but when it is present and has trigger points, they can refer pain and sensation to the bladder, pubic bone and urethra

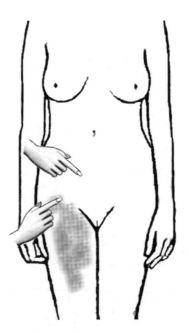

Stanford Protocol
Physical Therapy

Pain felt in shaded area
Finger tip locates trigger point

Iliopsoas

- *Trigger points in the iliopsoas can refer pain to the groin, labia, anterior (front part) thigh and low back*
- *When constipated, passage of stool can trigger pain*

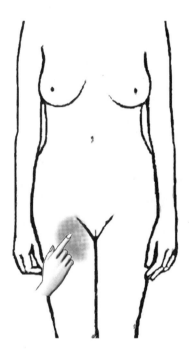

Pain felt in shaded area
Finger tip locates trigger point

Pectineus

- *Trigger points in the pectineus can refer pain and sensation to the groin... this is a major trigger point for groin pain*
- *Sexual activity that involves vigorous squeezing of the thighs can activate these trigger points (especially in women)*

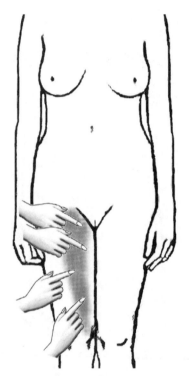

Stanford Protocol
Physical Therapy

Pain felt in shaded area
Finger tip locates trigger point

Adductor Magnus

- *This muscle is missed by many clinicians*
- *The adductor magnus is a critical muscle to check for trigger points which can refer pain throughout the pelvic floor including perineum, rectal or vaginal pain (and less often bladder pain)*
- *Deep groin pain, which is sometimes described as generalized internal pelvic pain.*
- *Patient has difficulty indentifying pain in any specific pelvic structure*
- *Pain over the pubic bone*
- *Pain sometimes described as shooting up inside the pelvis*
- *Sometimes symptoms occur only during sexual intercourse*
- *When trigger points continue to be active internally, the culprit may be unresolved trigger points in the adductor magnus*
- *Trigger points in the adductor magnus can refer the sensation of having a golf ball in the rectum*

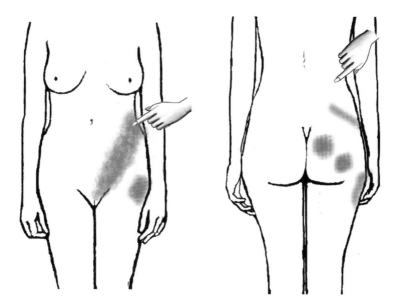

Stanford Protocol
Physical Therapy

Pain felt in shaded area
Finger tip locates trigger point

Quadratus Lumborum

- Trigger points in this muscle are one of the most commonly overlooked muscular sources of pelvic pain. It is a complex muscle made up of both deep and superficial fibers which refer pain to the sacro-iliac region, hip, buttock, abdomen, and groin
- In the female patient, pain can also be referred to the anterior thigh, labia and vagina

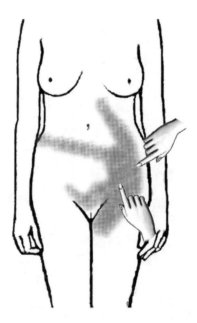

Stanford Protocol
Physical Therapy

Pain felt in shaded area
Finger tip locates trigger point

Lateral Abdominals Oblique

- *Trigger points in the lateral abdominals can refer pain to the whole stomach, up into the ribs, down the groin and into the vagina and labia... this is an important source of vaginal and labial pain*

Stanford Protocol
Physical Therapy

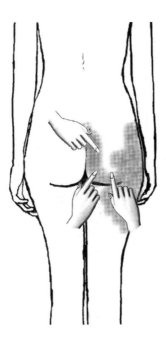

Pain felt in shaded area
Finger tip locates trigger point

Gluteus (Maximus)

- *Trigger points in the gluteus maximus can refer pain and sensation into the hip, buttocks, tailbone, sacrum hamstrings*
- *Can refer pain to the entire buttock and tenderness deep within the buttock*
- *Can refer pain that covers the entire lower sacrum*
- *Sitting on a hard seat can feel like a nail is pressing into the sitz (or sitting) bone*
- *Pain in the coccyx (coccyxgodynia)*
- *Restlessness or pain on prolonged sitting (more than 15 - 20 minutes) and increased pain when walking uphill or swimming crawl stroke*
- *Needs to sleep with pillow placed between knees; sit upright on soft surface (not donut or in slouching position)*

Stanford Protocol
Physical Therapy

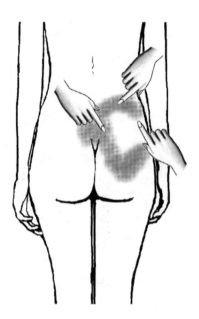

Pain felt in shaded area
Finger tip locates trigger point

Gluteus (Medius)

- *Trigger points in the gluteus medius can refer pain and sensation around the buttocks, hip girdle, and down the leg as well as into the vagina*
- *Sometimes is the cause of hip pain in later stages of pregnancy*
- *Needs to sleep with a pillow placed between knees and in side-lying on unaffected side (rather than on back); sit upright on soft surface (not donut or in slouching position)*

Stanford Protocol
Physical Therapy

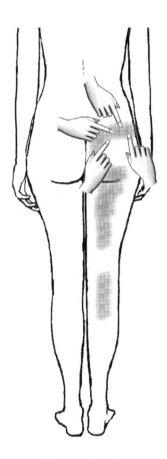

Posterior Portion

Pain felt in shaded area
Finger tip locates trigger point

Gluteus (Minimus)

- *Trigger points in the gluteus minimus can refer pain and sensation down the leg and sometimes into the vagina*
- *Some of these trigger points are found through deep palpation*

Stanford Protocol
Physical Therapy

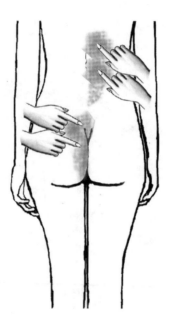

Pain felt in shaded area
Finger tip locates trigger point

Paraspinals and Multifidi

- *Trigger points in the paraspinals tend to refer pain and sensation into the low back, however this is pain that doesn't tend to fan out but is tightly contained in a specific area*

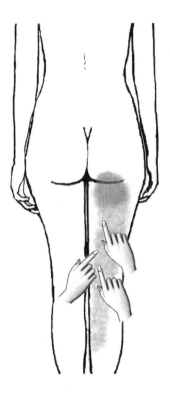

Stanford Protocol
Physical Therapy

Pain felt in shaded area
Finger tip locates trigger point

Hamstring Muscles

- *Trigger points in hamstring can refer pain to back of leg down to the back of the knee*
- *The gluteal crease and the ischial tuberosity (may cause difficulty sitting)*
- *Can be associated with trigger points in the obturator internus, piriformis and gluteals*
- *Can also be confused with sciatica*

CHAPTER 8

FREQUENT CONCERNS

There are certain questions, among others, that patients ask about issues including sex, work, relationships, exercise, pain medication, psychotherapy, and alternative treatments, as well as what loved ones can do. In this chapter we will address them. In addition, we share a perspective that we believe is most helpful while you are in the midst of dealing with pelvic pain and dysfunction.

Keeping Your Perspective and Helping Yourself

Pelvic pain is not your enemy

The more severe your symptoms the more your life tends to revolve around them. One study reported that dealing with pelvic pain had the same impact on one's life as dealing with heart disease or chronic inflammatory bowel disease. Most patients are anxious and depressed and consider their pelvic pain an alien condition that has invaded their lives. It is one of the intentions of this book to deal with pelvic pain from a number of different perspectives including a larger existential one. In this section we will discuss the larger view.

Pelvic pain usually does not occur in someone who feels balanced, relaxed, and happy. It tends to be the expression of what is out of balance, fearful, and out of sorts. Viewed this way, you can consider your pelvic pain and dysfunction an intimate advisor about your life. *Pelvic pain is not your enemy. Consider that pelvic pain is part of the main curriculum of your life and not a distraction from it.* Perhaps your curriculum has to do with learning to listen to your own body, to face and manage your anxiety, to manage your thinking so that you don't get angry and frustrated so easily, to soften your general tendency to become emotionally reactive, to permit your love and tender feelings, or to express yourself instead of holding things in. Whatever the lessons that are there for you, we believe their resolution can positively influence your healing.

You really do have a choice about how you view your condition

A young man with pelvic pain called us from the New York area. He was greatly distressed about his pain and other symptoms. More than anything, he wanted his sexual interest to return, an interest that had waned since the onset of his condition. His anxiety revolved around numerous theories he read about on the Internet that would condemn him to a life in which he would never get better.

"Do you think this is an autoimmune disease?" he asked, as he quoted some information he had read on the Internet. This young man, like many of our patients, attempted to discover a solution for his problem by reading the literature and the conflicting views and information on the web. This is a subject for which we offer some advice below.

The theories he read about implicating autoimmunity, occult organisms, nerve entrapment, and neurological pathology tended to offer little supporting evidence or effective treatment. They were largely speculative.

The result of his reading made him more anxious and uncertain than before. The more he read that scared him, the more his pain increased.

He didn't know what to believe and yet his thinking interpreted his condition from the most hopeless of perspectives, a fear-producing view that offered nothing to him, while making his condition worse.

Once starting our protocol, a number of our patients decided to stop reading about ideas regarding pelvic pain. "All these theories and speculations about my condition scare me," said one patient. "I have decided not to read any more for now and instead focus on the constructive action I am taking by choosing to begin this treatment." In this way, they were choosing to take charge of how they looked at their condition.

The pain is not the worst suffering

It is not the pain that is the deepest source of suffering when someone struggles with chronic pelvic pain syndrome. If we knew for sure that we were going to get better, most pelvic pain and discomfort, while not being something we would choose, would be okay. We would most likely put up with it without the kind of angst that attends most people who suffer from pelvic pain. *It is the meaning you give to the symptoms that causes the real suffering.*

Indeed, it is the catastrophic meaning one gives to the symptoms and how the impact of this meaning interacts with the pain and tension that is so difficult in dealing with pelvic pain. Consider the following young man who called us in a great state of anxiety about his condition. He was handsome, accomplished, wealthy, and admired by his peers. Women fell in love with him regularly. His friends loved him. He was successful in his profession. He had it all.

For three years, he had experienced pain at the tip of his penis along with some post-ejaculatory discomfort and urinary frequency and urgency. The doctors he was fortunate enough to see told him that they could find nothing wrong and there was nothing to worry about. He believed them. He characterized these symptoms to himself as an insignificant annoyance and went on with his life with little concern.

He then happened to go on the Internet and started reading the scary stories of those who suffer from pelvic pain and see no light at the end of the tunnel, and scary theories about what some speculate about pelvic pain. His pain became much worse quickly and he spiraled into a dark and deeply upset state. His sleep became disturbed. He withdrew socially. He began to worry about others abandoning him because of his condition. His pain, from being a minor annoyance, sometimes became unbearable. His life became a living hell.

This went on for quite some time. Then he found our book and as quickly as he spiraled into his dark night of the soul, he came out of it. He became clear about what was wrong with him and both his symptoms and his attitude improved dramatically. He came to one of our clinics and his condition further improved. He began having days of no symptoms. Instead of a negative spiral downward, which we describe as the tension-anxiety-pain cycle, he began a positive spiral out of his hole. His view of his condition and its meaning changed. He stopped his catastrophic thinking and saw the possibility of becoming free of symptoms. The ups and downs of his physical pain and dysfunction were greatly influenced by his view of what his symptoms meant.

In his classic book, *From Death Camp to Existentialism,* psychiatrist Victor Frankl observed that while he was in a Nazi concentration camp during World War II, he discovered the one thing that the Nazis could not take from him was his choice about how to view things. Frankl was clear in his belief that the way he chose to see things helped him survive. Below we will discuss a strategy to deal with the potpourri of theories and remedies offered to deal with chronic pelvic pain.

In Chapter 3, we discuss the nocebo effect—the effect of believing something harmless can hurt you. Theories on the Internet that paint your symptoms as hopeless, if believed, can be seen as a nocebo. Many people with pelvic pain walk around miserable for years believing theories that paint a catastrophic picture about their symptoms.

A pessimistic view of your condition can literally cause more pain

We have shown that there is scientific evidence demonstrating that your perspective directly affects your pain. Dr. Richard Gevirtz, one of the investigators who discovered that stress increases the level of electrical activity (and pain) in trigger points, put it this way in a telephone call. He said, "Where people have a clear cut model of what is wrong with them and understand that there is something they can do to help themselves, they de-catastrophize what is going on within them. This changed view may physically lower their pain by reducing the effects of sympathetic nervous system arousal inside their trigger points. *The source of their pain is not independent of their thoughts and feelings.*"

A school of psychology called cognitive therapy focuses on helping anxious and depressed individuals identify their habitual negative thinking that triggers or aggravates their depressed or anxious states. From the viewpoint of cognitive therapy, when there is a choice, you are going to feel better when you see the glass is half full instead of half empty. A slew of aphorisms illustrate this point.

- *The only difference between a stepping stone and a stumbling block is what you make of it*

- *A glass full to the middle with water can equally be seen as half full or half empty*

- *When being chased out of town, raise a flag and pretend you are leading a parade*

- *When life gives you lemons, make lemonade*

An optimist and a pessimist

A psychologist wanted to study identical twin children, one of whom was considered to be an optimist and the other a pessimist. The pessimistic child was placed in a room full of toys. The optimistic child was placed in a room filled with horse manure. When the psychologist returned after several hours, he found that the pessimistic child had not moved from his chair. Upon inquiring about why the child had not moved to play with the toys, he replied that he was afraid he might break them. When the psychologist entered the room with the optimistic child, he was surprised to see the child covered with manure and digging through it. "What are you doing?" asked the psychologist. Without hesitating, the optimistic child said, "With all this horse manure, there has got to be a pony somewhere."

When we have no physical symptoms, we often can tolerate habitual negative ways of thinking. With a condition like a headache in the pelvis that is so intimately tied up with our nervous system arousal and the thinking that triggers it, our habitual, negative ways of thinking are less benign. They actually increase our level of pain and suffering.

Catastrophic thinking only makes you more miserable and is usually not true

Catastrophic thinking is a name given to a pessimistic and negative way of interpreting an event in which you always imagine the worst. The following example of catastrophic thinking illustrates our point. Imagine you feel a little more rectal discomfort than usual when sitting. From this awareness you think that perhaps the doctor has missed a tumor that might be cancerous. You then imagine having surgery in which they have to remove the tumor. Eventually you die despite the removal of the cancer. You imagine that during your dying no one wants to take care of you and you die alone.

This kind of thinking is not uncommon in many patients that we see. When you tend toward catastrophic thinking, such thinking often feels unremarkable. The catastrophic thinker has rarely considered that there is an alternative to this way of seeing things. When you think catastrophically, you usually are only dimly aware of the contents of your thoughts, and only become fully aware of them and their effects after further examination.

In catastrophic thinking, fear always arises. The thought that something serious is wrong with you sets off an alarm in your body that releases emergency substances like adrenaline and cortisol, readying your body for fight or flight. All of a sudden, your thinking creates a physical event inside of you.

When you began "catastrophizing" about the rectal pain, as we described above, you unwittingly told yourself a story. You jumped from the present moment to four or five steps in the future when you are diagnosed with cancer. When you have pelvic pain of the kind we describe, these steps that you simply assume would lead you to a diagnosis of cancer are extremely unlikely.

Catastrophic thinking is rarely true and creates needless suffering. The fear of cancer or some other problem that has remained undiagnosed is common with individuals we see who have pelvic pain. This common process of catastrophizing pelvic pain and dysfunction can spin someone into an anxiety state in which the tension-anxiety-pain cycle makes the pain worse and adds misery to the already existing pain and dysfunction. We believe that many visits to the emergency room for pelvic pain occur when catastrophic thinking strongly triggers the tension-anxiety-pain cycle which then spins out of control.

Ironically, during the writing of this section of our book, we received a call from someone on the East Coast who was in the kind of anxiety state we have been describing. He described himself as "going crazy" as he read the accounts of sufferers of pelvic pain on the Internet who had not been helped and were wretched and desperate. He said his "pain was through the roof." The day after we had an opportunity to discuss our protocol and understanding about the treatment for chronic pelvic pain syndromes, he reported that not only was he feeling relieved emotionally, but also he expressed his puzzlement because he said his pain diminished substantially since our conversation with him. It is not uncommon for patients we have seen to report a reduction in pain simply from the reassurance they feel that perhaps something can be done to help their condition. To one degree or another, most of our patients not only suffer with pelvic pain and dysfunction but also a viewpoint that intensifies their symptoms.

The core treatment we use is aimed at rehabilitating the pelvic muscles and the habit of tensing them. However, it is very important to deal with the negative and anxiety producing thinking that is so typical in patients who have chronic pelvic pain syndromes. People with pelvic pain that we treat tend toward catastrophic thinking, even prior to the onset of symptoms. Changing this tendency is a major life event and is essential. Below we discuss issues relating to dealing with the kind of negative thinking that aggravates this condition.

Managing catastrophic and anxiety/pain producing thinking: the use of cognitive therapy

How do you stop the kind of thinking which unnecessarily produces anxiety and feeds the cycle of tension, pain, and anxiety? You must first of all see the real connections between your symptoms and your thinking and entertain the idea that it is possible to change catastrophic thinking. What generally can be called cognitive therapy labels and identifies negative thinking and helps a patient evaluate the credibility of this thinking so that he or she is not a victim of it. For example, using principles of cognitive therapy a person will think, "I can never do anything right" in response to a frustration they are having or an error they have made. When the person who wishes to gain control of catastrophic thinking becomes aware of the triggering of this kind of thinking, he or she will reflect, "Let me look at the statement 'I can never do anything right' and evaluate whether there is truth in it." Below we share some exercises and processes we use with patients.

Negative thought inventory

The negative thought inventory below is an assessment process that you can use to become aware of the effect of your thoughts on your condition. Choose a three-hour period of time when you tend to feel the worst and pay attention to your thoughts. Use a small tape recorder to record any negative thoughts that occur to you on a minute-by-minute basis. After the thought, choose a number from 0 to 10 as to your level of pain. Some examples of the relevant thoughts could include:

- What is wrong with me?
- The pain is worse (maybe it will never get better)
- Am I ever going to get better?
- How can I go on?
- It just does not stop
- What is going to happen to me?
- Here it is again
- I can't understand why it is worse
- Why me?
- Why am I different than so-and-so?
- Will I ever be normal?
- I am never going to get better
- How can I live my life this way?
- No one will love me like this
- Maybe I have cancer
- Maybe I have a sexually transmitted disease and they have not found it yet
- Maybe I have bacteria or fungus they will never find
- If I only had not had sex with so-and-so
- What if I won't be able to function?
- What if I get fired?
- Maybe I won't be able to support myself

Do your best to record your negative thoughts and their effect on your symptoms. This may not be the most enjoyable exercise, but we believe it is instructive in helping you see the frequency of certain thoughts and their effect. When you have recorded fifteen minutes of these thoughts, listen to them at the end of a relaxation period. Notice the level of your pelvic symptoms when hearing these thoughts. Record your reactions and insights after this exercise.

Inquiring into negative and catastrophic thoughts with understanding

Our body responds to the conditions in which we find ourselves. Our body tends to respond to our thoughts as if they were real whether they are or not. A person sees a rope, which triggers the thought that the rope is a snake. This person will likely respond with alarm and anxiety as the body instinctually prepares for the danger of a snake. When he sees the rope and releases himself from the idea that it is a snake, his state of alarm stops and his body relaxes because he discovers there is no danger.

Cognitive therapy is not new. It is a general term that refers to the understanding that thinking, in large part, creates the reality we live in. The basic principles of cognitive therapy are found in an ancient document, *The Dharmapada*, which states that we create the world we see with our thoughts. If we think we are victims, we ruin our lives. When our view does not see ourselves as victims, our lives transform.

Cognitive therapy is found in the work of Albert Ellis in his *Rational Emotive Therapy*, and in the work of Aaron Beck, former president of the American Psychological Association and others. *A Course in Miracles*, which we have mentioned earlier, is an existential textbook and a powerful form of cognitive therapy. For instance, in one of the beginning lessons in *A Course in Miracles*, it is taught that meaning is not inherent in anything. Instead, we give meaning to everything we see. The year long course offers daily lessons to help students of the Course take back control over what they think.

The best form of cognitive therapy, in our opinion, is offered in the work of Byron Katie who provides an approach to disarming catastrophic thinking by means of a process that one can do oneself. This is the approach we recommend. Her method, which we have adapted to dealing with the negative thoughts around pelvic pain, offers a way of loosening the grip of habitual negative and catastrophic thinking.

Step One: Finding the core thought

The key to disarming the catastrophic thinking related to pelvic pain and dysfunction, involves first identifying the core thought that your fear and anxiety rest on.

Most physicians rarely have the time or inclination to delve into the kinds of thinking that are common to people with pelvic pain. Typically, the person with chronic pelvic pain syndromes lives in a dark world of negative thoughts that is rarely shared with anyone. Each negative thought is taken to be real by the body as it contracts against the scary world created by the thought. These scary thoughts are like gasoline on the fire of the pelvic pain, inflaming the pain and the cycle of tension, anxiety and pain.

Formulating the core thought as a statement and not a question

The negative thought inventory is a rich source of the core thoughts fueling much suffering in pelvic pain syndromes. The cognitive therapy process works best with core thoughts that are simple declaratory statements. It is useful to write down these thoughts in the form of sentences. Instead of the thought "Will I ever be normal?" the reformulation of the thought turns out to read, "I will never be normal." Instead of the thought, "Will I ever be able to enjoy sex again?" the reformulated sentence is "I will never be able to enjoy sex again."

It is also useful to take the catastrophic thoughts that appear tentative and make them definitive. The thought "Maybe I'm going to be in pain for the rest of my life" then becomes "I'm going to be in pain for the rest of my life."

Both making the negative thinking into statements and making them as if they are stating a certainty are framing them in the way in which the body hears them. This reformulation makes the sting of these thoughts easier to identify and deal with when their validity is questioned by this process.

Step Two: Face the core thought with openness and curiosity

Like the pain, the negative thoughts are not your enemy. They come from a frightened person's struggle to protect him or herself. The thought of consciously facing one's negative thinking can appear daunting and depressing. This approach, however, in clearly formulating the core negative thoughts and then examining their validity, usually lightens their impact. In learning to face and evaluate the validity of the negative thinking, it is often possible to soften or neutralize this kind of thinking. It's best to face negative thinking with curiosity and an interest in seeing whether the thoughts are true.

How to evaluate the validity of the core thoughts from your heart

It is sometimes useful to experiment with bringing attention to the feeling in your chest and heart area. Feel the breath and the sensation in your chest as the air comes in and out. With your eyes closed and your attention on your heart and chest area, say your name and feel the feeling in the chest. For example you might say, "My name is John" or "My name is Lindsey" and then you feel the sensation in your chest of truthfully saying your name.

Now keep your attention in your chest area and finish the sentence, "My name is _____" but with a false name. If your name is John, see how it feels in your chest to say that your name is Walter or Dennis. You will probably feel a little tightening or strangeness in your chest. Experiment with feeling your chest as you say your true occupation (e.g., I am an engineer) and then notice the feeling in your chest when you don't tell the truth (e.g., I am a baker or kindergarten teacher).

The point of this exercise is to feel your body's reaction to what is true and what is not true. The body can help you address the validity of your negative thoughts. Refer to the sensation in your body as you address the questions below.

Examining the validity of the core thought

After you have identified the core thought (it is useful to write the thoughts and the answers to the questions down on paper), ask the following questions to yourself about the thought. Feel the area in and around your chest and respond to the questions from this area. In other words, your answers should agree with the feeling in your chest area.

Question your core thought as follows:

1. What is the evidence I have for this core thought?
2. Using this evidence, can I say for sure that this thought is true?
3. What happens physically inside me when I believe that this thought is true?
4. What happens to my self esteem when I believe that this thought is true?
5. What happens to my experience of my life force, my generosity, and love when I believe this thought?
6. What has been the effect of this thought or this kind of thought on my life in the past?
7. What would happen to my life if I simply were incapable of thinking this thought or this kind of thought?
8. What is the opposite kind of thought to this one?

We ask our patients to notice the effect of this questioning on their mood and the impact that this thought has upon them. Catastrophic and negative thinking has usually been practiced for a long time. This questioning process needs to be done often during the day as these kind of thoughts arise very often. It is possible for this process to help reduce the level of suffering that attends pelvic pain and dysfunction.

Our description of this process is rarely sufficient to become proficient at it. We discuss this method in our monthly 6-day clinics.

Information specifically about this cognitive therapy work can be found at www.thework.org and in the books of Byron Katie.

The advanced use of *Paradoxical Relaxation*: distinguishing between what fearful thoughts arise and the tensions related to such thoughts

Cognitive therapy focuses on the content of what you are thinking. Edmund Jacobson discovered that each negative thought has its own characteristic muscular posture. This means, for example, that when you think the thought, "Maybe I will never get over this pain," it would not be unusual for your shoulders to rise, your diaphragm to pull in, your jaw to tense and your anal sphincter to contract, your forehead to furrow, and your eyes to look down. All anxiety-producing thoughts tend to recruit their own characteristic muscle tensions.

While each negative thought tends to have its own characteristic set of muscle tensions, in general, each thought tends to elicit a certain visual mental picture that causes the eyes to tense and to look in a certain direction. For example when you have the thought, "Maybe I will never get over this pain," you may repeatedly have a picture of yourself disabled in bed or all alone as an old person. This mental picture is a key to the negative thought and has its own subtle tensions of the small muscles of the eyes.

As someone advances in *Paradoxical Relaxation*, we begin training and identifying these patterns of muscle tension associated with thinking. We practice relaxing these tensions.

The woman we described earlier who compulsively imagined killing her child learned this procedure of identifying and letting go of muscle tensions associated with this horrific thought. In doing so she freed herself from the guilt and fear that was stimulated by this thought.

It is important to become aware of and to gain control over negative thinking, especially the thinking that is part of a habit of tensing the pelvic muscles. For some individuals, it can be life-changing to be able to do this.

Cognitive therapy in and of itself, is usually limited in its ability to calm down catastrophic thinking when one's symptoms continue unabated and out of our control. When we are able to do something that clearly reduces or stops our symptoms, catastrophic thinking about the symptoms typically disappears.

What to do about the conflicting (often scary and disheartening) information on the Internet about your condition

We are often asked about other theories regarding the nature of chronic pelvic pain, a subject we touched upon earlier. Many individuals who ask questions about other theories are already in an anxiety state and are looking for some kind of reassurance or guidance as to the nature of their condition and the best course of treatment. When they go on the Internet, they read about various theories contending that chronic pelvic pain may be an autoimmune disorder, a condition caused by a trapped nerve, a condition in which occult bacteria are yet to be discovered, or a deteriorating neurological pelvic condition. These theories often tend to promote fear and helplessness in the sufferer.

When you have pelvic pain, it is deeply disturbing to read theories which promote fear, helplessness, and confusion or hear stories of people who are not doing well with their pain or dysfunction. When you have pain and dysfunction, you usually feel some degree of anxiety and helplessness which is often exacerbated by these kinds of theories. Some of our patients have asked us whether they should ignore the ideas that they read on the web or simply avoid the Internet websites devoted to pelvic pain. Others have asked us if there is some way to find out if in fact they have the problem that these theories purport.

If a theory or an idea about your condition carries some course of action or treatment to help you without unacceptable risks, then it may be an idea that merits your careful consideration. You may wish to investigate the efficacy of such a course of treatment along with the risks and costs.

If the theory, on the other hand, carries with it (a) *no course of treatment or action* to be done to help or protect you, or if its treatment carries dangers you are not willing to risk, or (b) it offers some *non-definitive* evidence, and (c) it *only helps to create fear, doubt, and disempowerment* in your life, we suggest you tell yourself, "This is someone's theory. There is no definitive proof for it. It offers nothing to help me or protect me or it carries unacceptable risks. It creates fear and doubt in me. It is okay for me to disregard it as somebody's unproven idea which I will consider if there emerges substantial evidence and/or something to do about it. Therefore I can ignore it as simply someone's unproven idea."

This kind of self-talk is the practice of cognitive therapy. Using cognitive therapy about ideas that tend to promote catastrophic thinking is particularly important because, as we have discussed, anxiety tends to increase symptoms.

Faith

Faith is something that is usually discussed in church about matters that are spiritual. It is rarely discussed in a doctor's office as part of a medical condition. When you have faith, you have confidence that somehow everything is okay. When you have faith, even though you don't know how things will turn out, you feel assured that you don't have to know. You trust that things will simply turn out all right.

Faith is a frame that you hold up and through which you look at your life. It is an attitude that you bring to situations whose outcomes are not immediately clear. Faith is a willingness to believe that even though you don't see the light at the end of the tunnel, there is light there. The great poet Rainer Maria Rilke wrote to a young poet who was upset about his lack of facility and success in poetry. Rilke told the young poet to *have patience with what was not resolved within him and to embrace the very questions and unresolved issues themselves without trying to figure out answers.* It was in living in the questions, in being fully present in the midst of difficulties (without succumbing to catastrophic thinking), Rilke wrote him, that he might *live his way into the answers.*

The 'gift' of pelvic pain and the four horses

While no one would wish pelvic pain on anyone, it can be seen as a gift in that it pushes us beyond what we normally would do to take care of ourselves. It demands that we do whatever it takes to get relief. The following ancient typology of the four horses.

The first horse moves as soon as you jump on its back. No whip or word is required. This horse knows what has to be done and takes off as soon as you mount it. *The second horse* takes off when it sees the shadow of your raised whip. While it is not as eager to move as the first horse, it takes only a hint of the whip to get it going. *The third horse* moves when it feels the light sensation of your whip and the pressure of your heels against the sides of its stomach. It is less anxious to move and requires some physical evidence of your intention to make it move. *The fourth horse* will only move when it feels the sting of your whip in the marrow of its bones.

Most of us are the fourth horse. Most of us only buy an umbrella when it is raining and grease a wheel only when it squeaks loudly. Those who come to us with pelvic pain and dysfunction usually do so after these symptoms scare them, or begin to deeply intrude in their lives.

Even when there is pain and dysfunction, most patients are only willing to do our demanding protocol when they are at their wit's end. Their motivation comes from feeling that they can't go on in the same way that they have been going. When the pain is intermittent or the impact of the symptoms is minimal, patients tend to be less willing to do what we believe it takes to deal with chronic pelvic pain syndromes. When patients are looking for the "quick fix" we encourage them to see if they can find it elsewhere and return to us if they don't. Patients who have not reached a point of some degree of exasperation tend not to be good candidates for our approach because they are not ready to expend the effort and focus necessary for our protocol to have a chance to help them.

Suffering as grace

Ram Dass was one of the spiritual teachers of young people in the 1960's and has remained as a luminary to many since that time. Over the last few decades, Ram Dass proposed the idea that suffering can be seen as grace or a gift. 'Suffering as grace' means that you acknowledge that even though you wouldn't choose to have the suffering you are dealing with, nevertheless it turns out to be something that may have in it the possibility of transforming your life.

Usually the awareness that suffering can be seen as grace is perceived after the suffering has resolved itself. Nevertheless, many people who actively have an interest in their inner life inquire as to how their suffering can help them grow and benefit their life.

Ram Dass also introduced a related idea which we have touched upon that whatever difficulties you may be facing in a particular moment are not distractions from the 'curriculum' of your life, but are the main part of the curriculum itself. Most people believe that their condition has taken their attention away from what they really want to be doing. When you look at your difficulties as your main curriculum, you bring an entirely different attitude to them. This has the power to transform your difficulties because you stop resisting or hating them.

What does this mean for you if you are suffering from pelvic pain? We think that it is useful to view your condition as one of the 'main courses' that you are enrolled in at the 'university' called your life. We are not suggesting in any way that you have deliberately brought this pain into your life, that you want it there, or you shouldn't resolve it as soon as possible. We are suggesting the idea that if you do have pelvic pain and dysfunction that you acknowledge that you have it and ask yourself the questions: What is it asking from me? What lesson does my current predicament contain for me? Am I listening?

Taking a long view: managing your expectations

Unrealistic expectations will make you anxious and increase your pain and suffering. In our view, pelvic pain and dysfunction does not come about out of the blue, even though in some cases it may seem to. It is said that the fruit falls suddenly even though the ripening takes time. It is our view that someone can have a chronically tight pelvis for years without symptoms and then, with age or certain stresses, the symptoms are triggered. Just as the pelvic pain symptoms don't spontaneously appear, neither do they disappear overnight. In our experience, even with our most successful patients, symptoms take a significant amount of time to resolve.

We suggest that patients who begin our protocol give themselves a good year in which to practice it before expecting symptoms to become reliably better. For those who are helped by our protocol, symptoms usually continue to improve as people practice our methodology over time (although flare ups are common with stressful events). Of course, not everyone benefits from our treatment but for those who do, it usually takes a considerable period of time for symptoms to reliably quiet down.

Taking a year does not mean that patients will not experience a benefit quite soon after beginning treatment. Giving yourself a year means understanding that typically a person's condition normally fluctuates, especially at the beginning of treatment.

We suggest that patients resist celebrating when they are feeling better, or despairing when they are feeling worse. Typically during the course of treatment, patients can have twenty or thirty flare-ups, each followed by an improvement of symptoms. Symptom intensity can go up and down often because it is as if we are renovating a building while still living in it.

We have touched on the conflict between resting the pelvic muscles and having the need to use them to function in life. In an ideal world, we would send the pelvic muscles to a tropical island for a long rest. Unfortunately this is not possible. We cannot avoid the stresses and strains that interfere with our healing and trigger symptoms. We tell our patients to give their pelvic floor lots of room to go through its gyrations as they do physical therapy, and the two forms of *Paradoxical Relaxation.*

Why regret and blame are not helpful when thinking about the causes of your pelvic pain

We sometimes hear our patients express regret and remorse about their idea that they brought the condition on themselves. These patients often make themselves miserable with the thought that somehow their current condition of suffering is one they deserve because they were "so stupid" or "thoughtless" in bringing the condition on in the first place. Sometimes they say things like, "I shouldn't have weight lifted. I shouldn't have ridden a bicycle. I shouldn't have put myself in such a position of stress. I shouldn't have experimented sexually," among a host of other regrets that patients have expressed.

These particular thoughts are not helpful. They usually serve only to trigger someone's emotional reactivity, diminish their self-esteem and produce self-loathing. They keep you stuck in the past, binding up your precious energy in negativity and in feelings of helplessness, because the past is over and what was done is done. The truth is that you don't really know what started your symptoms. In fact, nobody can definitively tell you. And most important, if you have muscle related pelvic pain, knowing what triggered your symptoms isn't necessary to get better. All of these ideas and guilt are capable of perpetuating your pain or making it worse.

All of us want to be happy. All of us want to be well. None of us would ever do anything to ourselves if we knew at the time it was going to produce a chronic condition of pain. These thoughts are helpful to tell yourself if you are caught up in a cycle of self-regret or self-recrimination.

It may be helpful to tell yourself, "If I knew back then that what I was doing would bring on what I'm dealing with now, I would never have done it, but I couldn't know then what I know now. I can only do my best given the information I have in the moment." Our usual practice with people who have such remorseful, regretful and self-recriminating thoughts is to help them understand that they were doing the best they could do at the time the condition was in the process of happening. An attitude of self-forgiveness is the only attitude that makes any sense and is helpful for the condition. If you can't seem to get your mind behind this kind of thinking, some limited cognitive therapy can be helpful.

Learning to be unconditional with yourself

One of the major lessons for those dealing with pelvic pain and dysfunction is learning to be unconditional with yourself and do what ever it takes to help yourself. By unconditional, we are referring to an attitude of "I am going to be present with myself while I have this problem. I will be here for myself without limitations or conditions and do whatever it takes, for as long as it takes, to help myself."

We usually treat ourselves the way our parents treated us. Few have had an ideal childhood in which our parents had the time, energy, emotional balance and wisdom to be unconditional with us. Most people want unconditional love, but few have ever experienced it beyond the fleeting moments of infancy. To be unconditional with yourself is to treat yourself the way you always wanted your loved ones to treat you.

Most of us have never completely devoted ourselves to our own care. *The protocol that we use requires time and patience.* We will often tell patients that while we have some general parameters of how long it takes for the symptoms to abate, when the protocol works, it will take as long as it takes. People who come to our treatment with this attitude of unconditionality seem to do the best.

Learning to be a witness to yourself

When you have pelvic pain, it usually becomes a major focus in your life. Earlier, we described how we teach our patients in the relaxation training how to be a witness to the experience of tension and discomfort as a way of reducing it and letting it go. Daniel Goleman in his book *Emotional Intelligence* describes being able to be a witness of yourself as an advanced ability to dealing with your own emotions and those of others. When you can be a witness to yourself, you can step outside and objectively see yourself.

The *Paradoxical Relaxation* taught in our protocol requires that you feel and allow the experience in your body without interfering with it in any way. *As we have discussed, being a witness to your pain and discomfort is usually necessary to relax it.*

The opposite of being a witness to your pain or discomfort is getting lost in it. Goleman refers to being lost in your emotions, rather than witnessing them, as "emotional high-jacking." When you are emotionally high-jacked, your emotions sit in the driver's seat of your life and take you on the ride of their choosing. For instance, when you are 'emotionally high-jacked' by your anger, you can punch someone in the face or do or say something that your rational, ethical self would never do. When you are angry and not high-jacked by your anger, but witnessing it, you feel the anger and contain it and don't "come from it." Your anger does not decide what you do. You do.

In the same way, when you are high-jacked by your discomfort and the fear that often attends a headache in the pelvis, your pain and fear sit in the driver's seat of your life. You get lost in the catastrophic thinking that is associated with such high-jacking. As a reflex, you tense up against the pain even more which causes more pain. You make a difficult situation even worse.

When people are in pain, they tend to forget that they were ever out of pain. And when people are out of pain, they can hardly remember being in pain. We have seen repeatedly that a patient can be out of pain for months. Then circumstances conspire to push them above the symptom threshold and they are back in the old familiar territory of pelvic pain and dysfunction. The tension-anxiety-pain cycle reasserts itself and they lose perspective. They stop witnessing what is happening.

When symptoms go away, most patients find it hard to remember the intensity of their emotions when they were symptomatic. Instead of catastrophic thoughts, they have *anastrophic* thoughts—thoughts that say "my suffering is over forever—it is gone away, never to return."

In both the tendency toward catastrophic thinking when flare-ups occur, or *anastrophic* thinking when symptoms abate, perspective is lost. The ability to witness is lost. The catastrophic thinking that can occur with a flare-up involves suffering. Equally, the *anastrophic* thinking that the pain is gone forever is setting up acute suffering and disappointment when there is a flare-up. Both are unrealistic. Both need to be witnessed and worked with so that you save yourself unnecessary suffering while in treatment.

Desperate patients usually regret desperate decisions

The patients we have seen who have agreed to and later suffered from and regretted heroic measures like pelvic surgeries, for the most part, were seized by their emotions. In agreeing to these kinds of interventions, they were often in a state of near panic and desperation. "Just do something—anything to make my symptoms stop" is the message they brought to the doctor. Unfortunately, they often found a doctor willing to participate in their desperate need to do something by experimenting with interventions and surgeries that often left them worse off.

When you are willing to be a witness to your pain and anxiety you are expressing your faith that somehow it is all right that in the moment, fear and pain exist in you. In our experience, in that moment of allowing them to simply be there, they tend to relax. Not that we are saying that they all immediately go away. Witnessing tension, anxiety, and pain, however, almost always reduces suffering. As we have examined in the section on *Paradoxical Relaxation*, relaxation occurs with an attitude of it is okay for this pain/discomfort/tension to be here as it is in this moment.'

Jean Klein, a physician and meditation teacher, noted that the moment that you observe that you are inside a cage, you have stepped out of it. Being the witness to yourself allows you to face fear instead of simply reacting to it by fighting or fleeing. When Walter Cannon observed that the reflex response to danger is fight, flight, or freeze, he was commenting on the reflex reaction of the human mammal. When we are willing to witness our unhelpful fight, flight, or freeze reaction, we go beyond our automatic animal programming into a higher domain. Here there is a greater possibility of resolving our concern.

How to gauge your progress once you are in treatment

Witnessing and understanding flare-ups help reduce their impact. When our treatment works, within a relatively short time there is usually some decrease in the intensity, frequency or duration of the symptoms interspersed with regular flare-ups. Typically a patient will notice an easing in the discomfort of the pelvic floor during or after the relaxation or physical therapy self-treatment but the discomfort or pain almost always returns sooner rather than later. The 'windows' of being pain free tend to increase, but the course of healing often is three steps forward and two steps backward.

If you are in treatment, don't evaluate your progress in *all-or-nothing* terms. Often patients will feel better for short periods and then return back to the old sense of discomfort and dysfunction. As the therapy continues, and as the person learns to relax more deeply, the periods of being pain-free and dysfunction-free can increase. Notice if there is a decrease in the *overall* intensity, frequency or duration of the symptoms. This is a much kinder and at the same time more realistic way of evaluating how your personal healing is going.

We tell our patients that they have the capacity to feel as good as the best they feel, and our therapy is aimed at lengthening those good moments and even going beyond them. In other words, in the fluctuating symptoms of pelvic pain, you have the capacity to feel what you feel in your best moments.

Psychotherapy can sometimes make dealing with your condition a little easier

It is our experience that psychotherapy alone does not significantly reduce or eliminate the symptoms of chronic pelvic pain syndromes. That said, there is a use for psychotherapy in an adjunctive and supportive role in dealing with chronic pelvic pain syndromes.

Anxiety about the future which plagues people who have pelvic pain tends to fester when it is suppressed and not given a safe place in which to be expressed. When it is painful to sit, to urinate, or to have sex, many thoughts are stimulated about what this all means and what is going to happen in the future. Unexpressed, this kind of thinking tends to cycle around and around in the kinds of catastrophic thinking we described earlier.

It is often hard for most of us to find friends who can hear our fears and anxieties with any degree of understanding and without reactivity. Many people feel baffled, helpless, and afraid to hear of such strange doings and feelings as go on with people who are suffering with pelvic pain. This is one of the important reasons why people with this condition feel isolated and alone. They feel that they have no one to talk to. They are afraid that if they share their real thoughts and feelings with anyone, no matter how close and caring, that the person won't know what to do with such sharing. In large part they are right.

A safe place to regularly share the burden you carry

Psychotherapy can serve the purpose of having a place to express difficult thoughts and feelings. One of the benefits of psychotherapy is that you are paying someone to be present to hear what is going on, someone who has no history with you. The psychotherapist, whom you might see, however, should have both familiarity with and an understanding of your condition and support you in what you are doing about it. Also, the psychotherapist needs to be free from reactivity or fear when hearing what is going on with you and this is not a small thing.

This kind of psychotherapy can lighten your load a little. When choosing a psychotherapist it is a good idea to find someone who is experienced and who comes recommended. We suggest that patients educate the psychotherapist about their condition by giving them this section of the book to read. It is sometimes advisable for the psychotherapist to consult with someone on our team to learn more about our protocol and the best way the psychotherapist can support it. If you are doing our protocol or are contemplating doing it, it is in your interest to make sure everyone you are working with is going in the same direction. In our view, it is not a good idea to be doing simultaneous treatments that are uncoordinated or in any way, at odds with each other.

We recommend that patients tell the therapist that they want a place to share their feelings and are not looking for advice about what to do about their condition. Psychotherapists are people. They are as likely as anyone else to deal with their own fears, inner discomfort or sense of helplessness upon hearing someone's troublesome situation by trying to 'fix' the problem, especially if they have little experience with pelvic pain. This can come in the form of giving advice or making global psychological interpretations about the meaning of the symptoms. Such psychotherapeutic interventions, in our view, are entirely unhelpful and are to be avoided.

A note to family and friends of someone who has pelvic pain

It is not easy for the loved one of someone who has pelvic pain. The caring wife, husband, child, mother, father or friend of someone who has pelvic pain usually goes up and down emotionally with the person dealing with pelvic pain and we have been asked on more than one occasion if we have any advice for them. Here are some thoughts.

The pelvic pain that we describe in this book is not life threatening. It is not a progressive disease that eats away at someone like cancer. People with pelvic pain do not have a shortened life expectancy because of it. While symptoms can be intense, and in some cases make the normal activities of work and other aspects of life very difficult, symptoms tend to wax and wane.

As we have discussed earlier, if the person with pelvic pain knew that they were going to be out of pain in a week, the pain and dysfunction they deal with would usually be more tolerable. He or she would just wait it out with the expectation of it going away. It is the idea that it will never go away, that they will never be able to be free of pain, that is the real suffering of this condition. In other words, it is the catastrophic thought that is the real suffering. Similarly, if the loved one or friend knew that it was going to be over, the physical pain and dysfunction would be more like your loved one having a cold and there would be the clear expectation that the cold would certainly be over. But when the doctors can't help the pain and dysfunction that goes on and on without the hope that it will stop, and the person in pain is depressed and anxious, the experience of pelvic pain can be a real psychological and spiritual crisis for both the patient and their loved ones. When someone suffers, their loved ones suffer along with them.

The dilemma of the person who is close to someone with pelvic pain is that they know that the person they care about is suffering and in pain, but they feel there is nothing they can do. It is this feeling of helplessness that is so difficult for both the patient and the loved one or friend of the patient. Sometimes loved ones or friends feel they have to do something and yet they find that there is nothing to do. They want to reassure the person and yet they really don't understand the problem and don't know what to say. They don't know if everything will be okay. Those who are close to someone with pelvic pain often feel guilty thinking how their loved one's suffering limits their own life and the way it affects them. The suffering of the pelvic pain patient is usually a lonely suffering, with no one who understands the problem and no one to help. The suffering of the loved one of the pelvic pain patient is equally lonely. Often they suffer for years along side the patient with no one to really talk to and with no idea about what to do.

What can the loved one of a pelvic pain patient do? While there is no quick and easy answer to this question, we have a few thoughts. Being close to a pelvic pain patient requires a certain kind of psychological and spiritual development and maturity. If, in some way, you are related to someone with pelvic pain, we think it is helpful to remember that ultimately, the solution to your loved one's difficulty is not in your hands. You are not responsible. It is helpful to remind yourself that someone dealing with pelvic pain must find their own way and you can simply be loving and understanding without having to figure out or solve the problem. In other words, with kindness and love, it is often helpful to let the person with pelvic pain have the problem. Undoubtedly, if you could fix the problem you would. But you can't. In the end, it is not yours to solve. This is not easy to hear or practice. Under the circumstances, however, it will be most helpful to the person you're close to with pelvic pain if you don't burn out with frustration and depression about feeling helpless.

The friend of a pelvic pain patient once reported that he was in the hospital room of his cousin who was hooked up to machines that were monitoring his vital signs. He noticed that he tightened up inside when the numbers on the machine were not the numbers he wanted to see for his cousin. He eased up when the numbers were more to his liking. His tightening up, he realized, was a kind of irrational attempt to control the numbers. In his desire for his cousin to be well, he unconsciously, irrationally thought that if he tightened up and resisted the 'bad' numbers, they might be more likely to change to the good numbers. He realized after a few hours of doing this that he was emotionally and physically exhausted. He became aware of the impossibility and irrationality of trying to control the read out of the machines he was watching and that if he continued this inner game of inwardly resisting the numbers he didn't like, he would wear himself out and not be able to be emotionally there for his cousin. And of course, nothing positive would be accomplished. He decided to abandon this game he was playing and instead *inwardly permit the numbers from the machines to be whatever they were*, accepting them and not trying to fight them. He found this was the most helpful thing he could do to help his cousin.

This story can be instructive to the loved one of someone with pelvic pain. Doing everything that you can do yet also *permitting the situation inwardly, not arguing with reality, in our view is the best way to deal with the difficult situation of pelvic pain.* Practicing the inward acceptance of what is going on in the moment as it is and not projecting that it is necessarily what the future will hold, not feeling guilty for it, not taking responsibility for it, being willing to do whatever can be done but allowing for the fact that the solution for the problem is out of one's hands are all helpful ideas both to the loved one and the patient. If there is nothing you can do about your loved one's condition, feeling guilty, frustrated, depressed, angry that it is going on, or that you can't do anything doesn't help anyone.

In this way being in relationship with someone you love who has discomfort or pain, but whose condition you can't change, is really a practice in accepting what is. You have to deal with your own catastrophic thoughts about your loved one's condition. In fact both you and your loved one don't know what the future holds. But the tendency of many people who are close to those with pelvic pain as well as those with pelvic pain is to go to the catastrophic conclusion that it will never be better. Catastrophic thinking is a challenge to deal with for both the person with pelvic pain and the loved one of such a person. We discuss catastrophic thinking in this chapter. We deal with the issue of having a loved one in pain in the same way as we deal with other matters in our lives. Practicing the art of noticing catastrophic thinking, evaluating its validity and extricating yourself from its grip is an essential practice in being close to someone you love who may have pelvic symptoms.

Most individuals who deal with pelvic pain don't appreciate being asked all the time how they're feeling. A continual, worried question of, 'How are you feeling?' can strain, frustrate and shame someone who is dealing with the symptoms we describe in this book. If you are a loved one of someone with pelvic pain, it is often better to specifically ask that person whether they want you to ask them how they are feeling. If they say, "If I want to share how I'm feeling at any particular moment with you, I will. Otherwise, it's better not to be asking me how I'm doing," in our view, its best to heed this kind of request. Let the pelvic pain patient be responsible to take care of his or her situation and be responsible to share how they are feeling if this is what they wish. This kind of open dialogue is often helpful.

There are other practical things that can be done. If your loved one comes to a clinic of the *Wise-Anderson Protocol* and you and your loved one are willing, you can learn *Trigger Point Release* methods that will probably be of great benefit to your partner. In general, what quiets down someone's nervous system helps them. You can offer to do foot massage or neck and shoulder massage. This is often very much appreciated by the person with pelvic pain. You can listen to the fears and suffering of your loved one and practice permitting your loved one to have these thoughts and feelings without joining your loved one with your own fearful and catastrophic thinking. You can practice, for any particular moment, accepting your loved one's situation as it is without having to project that it will always be that way.

With your loved one's permission and active participation, you can help your loved one practice some of the processes that deal with his or her catastrophic thinking that stir up anxiety and the nervous system in general. This can be done by asking what the thoughts are, that are so difficult in the moment and by asking the questions inquiring into the validity of such catastrophic thoughts that we discuss in this chapter. Dealing with a loved one's pelvic pain is an opportunity to stay open to not knowing what the outcome is and having faith that it is okay to be in the process of what is going on without knowing the outcome. This requires a real interest in managing your own thinking and emotions.

Finally, take care of yourself. In the airplane, we are instructed to put our own oxygen mask on first before even putting the mask on our children. Similarly make sure you are getting 'enough air.' In other words, make sure that you are making space in your life for the rest and nourishment you need. If your life is upset, you become another burden for your loved one with pelvic pain.

We have helped many people with pelvic pain help themselves. We are very optimistic about the possibility of someone with pelvic pain learning how to substantially reduce or resolve their symptoms. Sometimes pelvic pain goes away spontaneously. This condition can get better. It can go away and even when there is a flare-up, when the patient knows how to treat him or herself, it can be a non-event. That is certainly one of the goals of the *Wise-Anderson Protocol*. In summary, as someone close to someone who has pelvic pain, it is best to take care of yourself, be loving and available for your loved one and see the current situation as an opportunity to be present with what is going on in the moment without jumping to some kind of conclusion that you can't know is true.

EMDR

Beyond using cognitive and supportive psychotherapy, there is a role in psychotherapy for more specific purposes. Approaches that can be of assistance include *Eye Movement Desensitization and Reprocessing* (EMDR) for sexual and physical trauma, cathartic therapies in dealing with suppressed emotions, and relationship therapy in working with the interpersonal difficulties that can occur with loved ones.

A small but not insignificant number of patients have tightened their pelvic muscles chronically as a reaction to physical or sexual abuse. Often the tightening up of the pelvic muscles for these patients was part of their way of defending themselves against the trauma reoccurring. "If I open myself up and relax, I will be inviting something bad to happen so I have to remain contracted" or "If I open myself up, I will be overwhelmed by the pain inside me" represent the kind of unconscious thinking of some people who have experienced trauma-related pelvic pain.

We generally refer patients who have had sexual or physical abuse that may be contributing to their pelvic pain to a psychotherapist experienced in EMDR. This method aims to resolve the frozen feelings and memories that occur in a person's life when such feelings and memories were impossible for the person to process at the time the abuse occurred.

Dr. Francine Shapiro discovered that earlier traumatic events seem to loosen their hold on traumatized people when, in a therapeutic environment and guided by a trained therapist, they move their eyes (or attention) rhythmically while talking about the event. EMDR makes use of the fact that parts of the body connected with processing of experience tend to freeze up during a traumatic event and remain frozen.

To understand this, recall what you do when you have had a difficult encounter during the day. Typically you will want to talk about it and share it with someone close to you. You do this as a way of 'processing' the difficult experience in order to be able to let it go so that you can be free in the moment again. Imagine what would happen if you had a fight with your boss, your spouse or your friend that was not resolved, you were very upset and you were not able to talk about it with anyone. The experience would feel like something stuck inside you that needs to come out but does not. Being unable to share your thoughts and feelings would most likely feel extremely physically and emotionally uncomfortable.

When someone has been the victim of incest, sexual trauma, or physical assault, the level of distress they feel is multiplied by many orders of magnitude in comparison to a simple interpersonal upset. Consciousness tends to freeze during this kind of event as if to control or contain it. From the viewpoint of the traumatized person, the trauma is perceived to be too big to handle. In order to protect itself from being overwhelmed, the body/mind tends to freeze up around the trauma.

EMDR often helps unfreeze a person's frozen consciousness around a traumatic event. The methodology of EMDR allows the event to be processed in the same way you would process an upset with your boss by talking to a friend. The processing that occurs in EMDR around traumas such as sexual and physical abuse or physical trauma such as some kind of painful surgery or procedure, however, tends to be much more dramatic than your discussion with your friend about the upset with your boss. Tears, shuddering, grief, and anger can arise in the EMDR processing. Such reactions were suppressed during the traumatic event. As the event continues to be recalled while the eyes, ears or senses focus on rhythmic movement, the trauma can be processed and resolved.

The usefulness of cathartic psychotherapy

Any difficult life situation that does not allow a person to express strong emotions or feelings can result in a person chronically tightening the muscles of the pelvic floor. For instance we have seen patients whose triggering event appears to be the suppression of grief around the death of a loved one or some other life-shaking loss. We speculate that the pelvic floor muscles are tightened because the emotions are not being expressed and the ongoing nervous system arousal chronically flares up pelvic floor related trigger points.

Catharsis-oriented psychotherapies can be of use in helping our troubled patients vent suppressed emotions. In this way, a major obstacle to treatment can be removed.

Reichian Therapy, Bioenergetics, and Holotropic Breath Work

There are several psychotherapeutic methods that are useful in allowing suppressed emotions to be expressed. *Reichian Therapy*, bioenergetics, rebirthing and holotropic breath work are all methods that have grown up on the periphery of standard 'talking' psychotherapy. They are methods that aim specifically at providing an environment and methodology that can assist a person in directly expressing emotions that have been suppressed.

Wilhelm Reich M.D., the inventor of *Reichian Therapy*, was particularly interested in what he called the muscular "armoring" of the pelvis and the effect of stopping the energy and feeling from moving through it. Reich developed a powerful psychotherapy able to unlock suppressed emotions.

Alexander Lowen, M.D., a New York psychiatrist, popularized *Reichian Therapy* in a form called *bioenergetics*. Lowen wrote several popular books from the 1950's through the 1990's. Bioenergetics is also very effective in dealing with suppressed emotions.

Stanislaus Grof, M.D., developed *Holotropic Breath Work* as a way of reconstituting the therapeutic aspects of the psychedelic experience without the use of drugs. Grof was a researcher who studied the effects of psychedelic substances and was deeply moved by the power of these drugs to produce positive therapeutic effects. *Holotropic Breath Work* is often done in groups, lasts a number of hours per session, and encourages patients to let down and allow their deepest feelings to arise and be expressed. This too is a powerful methodology.

A full presentation of the theoretical underpinnings and methods of *Reichian Therapy*, bioenergetics, and *Holotropic Breath Work* is beyond the scope of this book. We believe these modalities can be useful in helping to express and sometimes resolve emotional difficulties that some of our patients may have that interfere with their relaxation of the pelvic muscles.

Sexual shame and guilt

The issues of shame and guilt with regard to sex sometimes may be related to pelvic pain and are appropriate subjects to be dealt with in psychotherapy that is adjunctive to our protocol. Numerous studies have demonstrated that there is a higher incidence of pelvic pain among women who have been sexually traumatized. While studies have not focused so much on men, in our experience, issues around sex are often related to the onset of pelvic pain. Let's explore briefly the likely relationships between sexual anxiety, shame, guilt, and pelvic pain.

The pursuit of sexual pleasure, the frustration humans often experience in achieving it, the turmoil that often attends it in interpersonal relationships and the religious injunctions against it, are all issues that loom large in human life.

It is our speculation that on a psychological level, tension in the pelvic muscles can be an example of a defense, expressed physically, that is related to sex. Here are some examples. We saw a 40 year old woman, who was raped by her father when she was fifteen. Her core belief was that the only way for her to be safe was that she couldn't allow anything to come into her vagina again. Twenty-five years later she came to see us suffering with vaginal pain. Our treatment included teaching her to relax her pelvis. Her traumatic history, however, fought against the goal of our treatment. Without resolving the psychological issues that continued to support her chronic pelvic tension, her situation, and treatment would be like pressing on the gas pedal with one foot and the brake with the other.

There are usually core beliefs that exist unconsciously in individuals who, like this woman, have experienced sexual trauma and related pelvic pain. These beliefs must be addressed before our protocol can be fully effective. A prominent EMDR therapist reported working with a young woman who was raped by her father when she was three, who held the belief that if she relaxed her vagina, her insides would fall out. Others hold the belief that the only way to protect against the heartbreaking violation of rape or sexual assault is to live with a tight and guarded pelvic floor. Again, this psychological dimension must be addressed in order for someone to give themselves permission to relax their pelvic muscles.

There was an 18 year old man who was nervous about sex. Remarkably, he had never masturbated or had any sexual activity in his life. He began having intense sexual dreams, which frightened him and he tightened up his pelvic muscles as a way of trying to control the sensations and emotions that were arising. After several months, he went to his family doctor and reported having urinary frequency and urgency and pain above the pubic bone. This man's core belief was that if he permitted himself to feel his intense sexual feelings, he would lose control of himself, and that belief deeply frightened him. Asking this young man to relax his pelvic muscles without helping him resolve his sexual anxiety would not be a viable therapeutic strategy.

We have also seen a number of men and women who had been involved in extramarital affairs and later reported the onset of pelvic pain. After seeing a physician to rule out sexually transmitted diseases, they came to see us. In our meetings with them, it emerged they suffered from shame and fear about their extramarital experience. The core belief for these individuals has to do with the idea that in order to control themselves and not act out sexually outside their relationship they must tighten up their pelvic muscles and not allow themselves to feel their sexual impulses.

In these and other examples, the sexual thoughts and experiences of some patients have been strongly associated with the onset of their symptoms. These examples represent a small percentage of our patients. Nevertheless, for certain patients these issues are crucial, and resolving them makes it possible for symptoms to abate.

Pleasure anxiety: when feeling safe feels scary

Psychotherapy can be a useful adjunct when addressing what can be called "pleasure anxiety." Pleasure anxiety refers to an aversion toward pleasure because it triggers an unconscious fear that something bad might happen if one is happy and unprepared for danger. Pleasure anxiety is often seen in individuals who have suffered some life-changing trauma like the death of a parent.

Pleasure anxiety can reach the level of terror in some individuals and the relaxation protocol must be modified to help someone through this anxiety. Sometimes, as people with pleasure anxiety follow the relaxation instructions and the nervous system begins to quiet down, their hearts begin to beat faster, their palms begin to sweat and, to their distress, they feel more anxious doing relaxation. This reaction is simply heightened psychological defense against letting down their guard and vigilance.

While this kind of reaction prompts someone having it to stop doing relaxation, on the contrary perseverance through this reaction is vital—but instead of fighting the defense, one must be gentle with it. Sometime it is necessary to reduce the duration of the relaxation session to a period of one or two minutes so that the subconscious can discover that it is safe to quiet down, even for this short period. As one can tolerate more time of reduced arousal, one increases the duration of the relaxation session. It is a delicate dance and the sufferer needs to rely on someone who understands what is going on and can guide them through it.

Here is an example to explain pleasure anxiety. A patient with pelvic pain experienced the suicide of her mother at a time in her life when our patient was happy and carefree. The news of her mother's death occurred suddenly and shocked her. From the time of her mother's death she remained nervous and wary. In her mind, the experience of being happy and carefree was somehow connected to a terrible event happening.

It was for this reason that she complained that she could never relax. With a psychotherapist, while in therapy, she had noticed that as she grew older and explored her life she seemed to be uncomfortable 'feeling good.' She reported that invariably when she felt a sense of contentment, negative thoughts about things that might happen in the future would come to her mind and her good mood evaporated. Moreover, she reported that she felt strangely naked when her pelvic pain would subside. Her treatment involved a focus on tolerating pleasure and accepting the absence of anxiety. This was no small enterprise.

The core of our treatment for pelvic pain is training our patients to profoundly relax their pelvic muscles. *You can't relax the pelvic muscles without relaxing everywhere else in the body. Paradoxical*

Relaxation means that you 'un-defend yourself.' It means that you allow yourself to be at ease, to feel good, and to let go of vigilance.

Our treatment bumps up against psychological patterns that refuse to let go of psychological defenses. When patients are at a plateau in which their symptoms stop improving, it is often helpful to facilitate a dialogue between the part of the patient who wants to improve and the part that seems unable to move ahead. What often emerges from these dialogues is the fear of the unknown that is imagined if there is no more pain or dysfunction.

Sex and prostatitis

In general, most cases of prostatitis affect a man's experience of sex to one degree or another. In bacterial prostatitis, the pain and urinary dysfunction usually have an effect on sexual functioning or pleasure. After this acute episode is over, however, the bacteria are eliminated from the prostate and the infection is resolved. There is commonly no further impact upon sex. In chronic bacterial prostatitis, we have seen sexuality being affected during acute episodes like those in simple bacterial prostatitis. This impact tends to go away when the infection/inflammation is cured as it does with bacterial prostatitis. In other words, in both bacterial and chronic bacterial prostatitis, sexuality tends to be impacted while a man is symptomatic and sexuality is not affected once the symptoms clear up.

In abacterial prostatitis/nonbacterial prostatitis/CPPS, which represents approximately 95% of all of the cases, sexual functioning and pleasure is usually affected. If the symptoms in chronic pelvic pain syndrome are intermittent, generally speaking, sexuality is only affected when other symptoms are present.

When symptoms are experienced either intermittently or chronically, many men have discomfort during or after ejaculation. Typically, a man diagnosed with abacterial prostatitis/nonbacterial prostatitis/CPPS experiences increased aching, discomfort, or pain after intercourse lasting from a few hours to a few days. This experience takes its toll and while most men continue to experience sexual desire, it is dampened by the sense that there will be pain or discomfort afterward.

It is common for some men to complain of a reduction in sexual interest, problems performing sexually, or a diminution in the strength of their erections. We do not believe that there is a physical basis for these complaints. Rather it is our view that the man's attitude and emotions and/or anticipation of pain can have a powerful effect on the reduction of sexual interest, pleasure, and functioning. Furthermore, the responses of the spinal cord reflexes are dampened by pelvic discomfort.

Pelvic pain can be triggered and exacerbated by engaging in compulsive sexual activity to combat anxiety and depression

There are some individuals who deal with their anxiety and depression by engaging in compulsive sexual activity and masturbation. Anxiety and depression momentarily disappear during orgasm. This disappearance of anxiety or depression after orgasm is almost always short-lived. The fact that there has been a great rise in the availability of pornography on the internet may be a factor that has rarely been taken into account in the treatment of pelvic pain of certain individuals. At this time we have no idea of the number of men who fit into this category although anecdotally it appears not to be large number. Nevertheless, it is a subject that deserves discussion.

It is a common experience that repeated orgasms in close proximity yield diminishing levels of pleasure. The diminishment of pleasure with frequent orgasm also yields diminishing relief from anxiety and depression. It is not well known that compulsive sexual activity and pornography will tend to make anxiety and depression worse and not alleviate it.

Someone indulging in compulsive masturbation in an attempt to relieve anxiety or depression is not unlike someone in Las Vegas who wins a big jackpot at a slot machine and then continues to play the slot machine in the hopes of getting another jackpot, even as the payouts become smaller and smaller.

Forcing an already tight and painful pelvic floor to contract during frequent orgasm will tend to make pelvic pain worse

One of the things that happens when you use orgasm and compulsive sexual activity to fight depression and anxiety, is that the pelvic floor is forced continually to strongly contract and relax during the pleasure spasm of orgasm. This often pushes the prostate, seminal vesicles and pelvic floor muscles to overwork. When the frequency and level of intense contraction of these muscles is sustained beyond a certain point, the pelvic pain may be triggered. If the syndrome is already present, compulsive sexual activity will often exacerbate it.

Very frequent orgasm may trigger or exacerbate pelvic pain, anxiety and depression

The way in which very frequent orgasm triggers or may exacerbate feelings of anxiety or depression and pelvic pain is by making the pelvic floor muscles bear the burden of using orgasm as a kind of antidepressant strategy. During orgasm, there is a transient reduction or absence of pelvic pain, depression and anxiety. When symptoms of psychological malaise are soon felt again and the urge to feel better through orgasm arises, and masturbation is engaged in, orgasm can momentarily make anxiety and depression again calm down. One of our patients said that he could reliably eradicate his feelings of anxiety completely during and in the first few minutes after orgasm.

In the book, *Cupid's Poisoned Arrow,* Marnia Robinson discusses the notion that masturbation and orgasm prompt a surge of dopamine. She goes on to describe the theory of how, after the brief dopamine surge, prolactin is released along with other brain changes, which can lower the state of the pleasure of the orgasm and can foster a sort of anhedonia or pleasureless state. Nevertheless the desire to feel better in someone who compulsively masturbates reasserts itself and repeated masturbation both yields less pleasure and creates more physical and psychological malaise.

The implications of stopping addiction to compulsive masturbation, pornography, and sexual activity

If an individual who has been engaging in compulsive masturbation, sexual activity and/or the use of pornography, comes to realize the importance of stopping such compulsive, addictive behavior, it has been recommended in *Cupid's Poisoned Arrow* that someone abstain from ejaculation for a period of 2-4 weeks or longer. She proposes that this period of time helps rebalance the person's 2 week cycle of disturbance after orgasm. From our view, it can help calm down pelvic muscles that are continually caught in the vice of post orgasm hypertonicity. *Cupid's Poisoned Arrow* is an excellent discussion of the effects of compulsive sexual activity and its remedies.

If you give up compulsive sexual activity, how do you calm down and find pleasure and release?

In the absence of compulsive and addictive sexual activity, joy, satisfaction, reward and pleasure must be found elsewhere. Perhaps what is most important is that the individual find another way to calm down anxiety and reduce nervous system arousal. Using our protocol, it is possible to significantly reduce anxiety and nervous system arousal both with the deeply relaxing effect of internal and external trigger point release and with the reduction of an aroused sympathetic nervous system using Paradoxical Relaxation. Social interaction, friendship, creative pursuits, exercise and other activities that bring meaning and quality into one's life are also needed to replace what is sought by the effect of compulsive sexual activity.

A 'middle way' must be sought to replace the intense, supernormal kinds of stimulation of orgasm induced by pornography. The relief and pleasure of Paradoxical Relaxation can be an important substitute and the level of pleasure of Paradoxical Relaxation does not require a disturbance in dopamine at all. Profound relaxation is a deeply felt pleasure when someone finally learns the methodology. It can be what you call on to feel balanced and at peace, what once you sought in vain to feel through intense sexual stimulation. As Robinson describes in *Cupid's Poisoned Arrow*, one often goes through a real withdrawal as reliance on masturbation/pornography driven orgasm is stopped.

The wisdom of reducing (not stopping) the frequency of sexual activity

In general it is better to reduce (but not stop) the frequency of sexual activity when one has muscle related pelvic pain. This is not for forever but simply when the pelvic floor is very sore and prone to flare ups. Because it is important to reduce, but not stop sexual activity in order to quiet down post orgasm related symptoms, there are some suggestions that may be helpful.

It is sometimes helpful to do stretching and Trigger Point Release after sex. Some patients have reported that they gently stretch their anal sphincter, coccygeus, anterior portion of the levator muscle and other pelvic floor muscles after sex, in combination with relaxation, to reduce or stop their post-orgasm symptoms. It is often useful to take a hot bath, do internal Trigger Point Release and relaxation some time after sex. Sometimes our patient's partner will do the internal trigger point release as part of their intimacy together.

Some patients have escaped the flare-up of sexual activity by taking 5 or 10 milligrams of Valium® before or immediately after sex, although Valium® is hardly an aphrodisiac and not an ideal drug for sexual activity. The point of all of these strategies is to quiet down the tightening of the muscles after sexual activity and to restore their ability to relax after the strong workout of orgasm. These strategies become less important as the pelvis returns to a more overall relaxed state.

Why there is increased discomfort hours or the day after sexual activity in men: orgasm as a pleasure spasm

It is very common for men with prostatitis/chronic pelvic pain syndrome and for women with pelvic pain/pelvic floor dysfunction to experience increased discomfort or pain hours or the next day after orgasm. The reason that there is often an increase in discomfort during or after sexual activity in men and women with chronic pelvic pain syndromes is as follows. Orgasm causes strong contractions of the pelvic, prostate and seminal vesicle muscles lasting about once a second during orgasm. Dr. Jeannette Potts observed that *orgasm is a pleasure spasm*. There is a significant increase in nervous system arousal during sexual activity. The pleasure spasm of orgasm in the form of the increased series of contractions during orgasm will tighten the pelvic muscles further. This increased tightening temporarily contracts an already contracted area which doesn't relax well and it tends to throw the patient further above the symptom threshold. After a while, the muscles relax and return to their baseline level, the normal state of the pelvic floor reasserts itself (which is back to some degree of pain or discomfort when a person has chronic pelvic pain syndrome). For this reason we do not recommend increasing sexual activity when a person has a pronounced increase in symptoms after sex.

When someone has pain after sexual activity, it is helpful to do stretching and *Trigger Point Release* after sex. Some patients have reported that they themselves or their partners gently stretch their anal sphincter and other pelvic floor muscles after sex and in combination with relaxation, their post-orgasm symptoms reduce. Sometimes it is useful to do skin rolling, self-massage or insertion of a gloved and lubricated finger inside the pelvic floor in order to gently stretch spastic or trigger pointed tissue to deactivate any reactivated trigger points after sex. It is often useful to do relaxation before sex or relaxation and a hot bath after sex. Some patients have escaped the flare up of sexual activity by taking 5 milligrams of Valium® before or immediately after sex. The point of all of these strategies is to quiet down the tightening of the muscles after sexual activity and to restore their ability to relax after the strong workout of orgasm. These strategies become less important as the pelvis returns to a more overall relaxed state.

Contrary to the common advice some urologists give patients to increase the frequency of ejaculation, we think it more prudent to suggest to patients that they consider reducing the number of times they ejaculate. This is particularly important advice for men who compulsively masturbate. While the experience of ejaculation usually reduces their anxiety and discomfort for a brief while, it often creates more discomfort or pain hours or the day or two afterward. When our treatment is effective, as symptoms quiet down, the frequency of sexual activity can return to normal.

Increasing sensuality in the midst of the pain and dysfunction of pelvic pain syndromes

Men in our culture tend to be uncomfortable in acknowledging either to themselves or others their needs for closeness, connectedness, and non-sexual intimacy. In our culture men often hit each other on the back, punch each other on the shoulder, or call each other names. These are ways men express their affection and connection with each other while maintaining the appearance of appropriate manliness.

Many men get their need for love, affection, closeness, and reassurance through sexual intercourse. Often anxious men who are not in a sexual relationship will frequently masturbate as a way of lowering their anxiety. *In a word, sex is often used by men to address needs that are not sexual.*

When men have some form of chronic pelvic pain syndrome, *there are many burdens that they must bear that are not discussed.* Men we see in our clinic frequently complain of their reduced interest in sex. *What is rarely expressed however is the fact that when a man has pelvic pain and dysfunction, often discomfort related to sexual activity casts a pall on one of the only ways he can be intimate or relax.*

When the cost of sex is particularly difficult or onerous, we recommend to our patients to choose to cuddle with their partner without the aim of being sexual and having orgasm. We will recommend, for instance, that a man exchange non-sexual massages with his wife, or agree to lie on a couch with his partner and exchange a foot massage. These intimate yet non-sexual moments serve to address the often increased anxiety in a man and helps quiet down the often difficult times that are occurring in the marital relationship.

It is okay to be less sexual for a while

Not uncommonly, some of the men with prostatitis have an idea that their masculinity depends on their ability to have intercourse and satisfy their partner. When we suggest that perhaps they have sex less frequently, these patients may express discomfort and worry at how their partner will react.

We will sometimes suggest that our patient be clear with his partner that he can give her sexual pleasure but will refrain from having orgasm himself. This pleasure might be in the form of sexual massage, or bringing his wife to orgasm without having intercourse. In this way the strain on his relationship, which is often a big concern to our patients, can be softened while minimizing a flare-up of symptoms.

None of these measures is ideal

We do not want to give the impression that simply cuddling, or pleasuring one's partner, resolves the sexual issues brought about by pelvic pain syndromes. These measures are attempts to ameliorate the situation under circumstances that are, at best, difficult. We understand that the best solution we can offer to the issue of sex and the problems that arise between both men or women with chronic pelvic pain syndromes and their partners is for them to be able to help themselves reduce or stop their symptoms.

Practice in relaxing the pelvic muscles during sex

We have found that entering into and completing sexual activity while the pelvic muscles are relaxed can help reduce discomfort related to sexual activity. Below we will outline some steps you can take in changing the often unconscious habit of tensing the pelvic muscles before and during orgasm.

Becoming aware of what goes on in your pelvic muscles during sexual activity

Here are some notes on relaxation related to sexual activity.

- Notice if you are anxious in anticipating being sexual.
- Notice if there are any anxieties that occur during sexual activity.
- Notice if there is any sense of urgency in moving toward orgasm or if there is a sense of leisure about it.
- Notice if there is any unnecessary tightening of your pelvic muscles as sexual sensation builds up, as you get close to orgasm or during orgasm.
- Do your best to notice if you add unnecessary tension to the experience of orgasm.
- Notice what happens when you practice the intention of voluntarily reducing your tension during sexual activity.
- Notice if there is any difference in the quality of the orgasm or in your level of discomfort after orgasm by slowing down and relaxing during sexual activity.

Notice without trying to influence what is going on

This practice of noticing what you are actually doing with your pelvic muscles during sex needs to be done *without interfering with it*. First, observe. Then consider the following:

The instructions of *Paradoxical Relaxation* can also be used for changing the habit of overly squeezing the pelvic muscles during sex.

Your practice of Paradoxical Relaxation will be most clearly seen in your ability to accept and relax with the incompleteness of the sexual experience midway through it. Men commonly are captured by the impulse to get to the orgasm. This impulse is usually accompanied by pelvic tension and lack of ease. Our recommendation is: *instead of tightening your pelvic muscles and rushing toward orgasm in the way that you might normally be accustomed to do, slow down and feel the subtlety of the sensations along the way.* Doing this is not easy at first and requires a certain discipline and willingness to postpone immediate gratification. We will address below the subject of not making sex an emergency.

Not making sex an emergency

When a man has a high level of tension in his pelvic muscles, it is common that he tightens up during sex. Anxiety about performance and "rushing" to the climax is not unusual. When a man squeezes his pelvic muscles at a time when the pelvic muscles naturally contract, there is often a reduction in sexual sensation and an increased likelihood of increased discomfort afterward.

It is for this reason that we offer the idea of not making sex an emergency. What this means in practical terms is that a man practices the relaxation method of our protocol throughout his sexual experience. This means that he stays in touch with his often unconscious tendency to tighten his muscles during sex and instead of reflexively tightening, he relaxes. *Relaxing during sexual activity means that you allow the genital experience to come to you rather than you try to control it.* This practice of relaxing during sex is unknown territory to most men. Doing this requires being receptive more than being active. It means that anxiety is not in the driver's seat during the sexual act. Relaxing during sex tends to be accompanied by an increased level of physical and emotional sensitivity.

Being in a sexual embrace, while being profoundly relaxed, is not a new idea. This attitude has been around for thousands of years and exists today in the practice of what is called 'tantric yoga.' As we will describe in our discussion of managing sexual difficulties with vulvar pain, while tantric yoga has spiritual goals, our purpose in discussing this practice is to help restore the health of the pelvic muscles.

It is important that sex is not an emergency situation. Having sex in a relaxed way in conjunction with the rehabilitation and relaxation of the pelvic muscles, helps keep the pelvic muscles from going into the heightened level of tension that we believe is responsible for the increased discomfort after intercourse. To repeat, deeply relaxing and being receptive during sexual activity is not easily learned. The impulse is often to do it quickly. Learning to deeply relax while being sexual takes time, patience, and perseverance. Aside from reducing symptoms, this practice has other rewards of increased presence, interpersonal connectedness, and pleasure.

Vulvar pain and sexuality

Of all of the varieties of pelvic pain syndromes, vulvar pain tends to have the strongest impact upon a woman's sexual life. The initial complaint of most women with vulvar pain relates to pain associated with intercourse. This problem is most vexing and troublesome because it affects young women who for the most part desire to be in a relationship and have a family. Their vulvar pain impacts either finding a relationship or living happily in one.

The four stages of dyspareunia (pain during intercourse)

It is useful to chart a woman's progress in treatment by the extent to which her sexual activity is affected by her condition. In doing this, it is useful to identify four degrees of dyspareunia (pain during intercourse). Women with vulvar pain, depending on their degree of the pain, report experiencing themselves somewhere in the following stages:

- *Stage one:* A woman can tolerate penetration, thrusting, and the completion of intercourse. However, she experiences some degree of tolerable pain, usually at the beginning of intercourse when her partner enters her vagina.

- *Stage two:* A woman can tolerate penetration, thrusting, and the completion of intercourse with pain throughout.

- *Stage three:* A woman can tolerate penetration, but has difficulty tolerating any thrusting. As a rule she cannot complete intercourse. This stage finds a woman generally being avoidant of sex because of the pain.

- *Stage four:* A woman cannot tolerate penetration. A woman who has stage four dyspareunia has simply stopped having intercourse.

Dr. Howard Glazer, associate professor of psychology in obstetrics and gynecology at Cornell Medical College, strongly recommends that women renew non-penetrative sexual practices that lead to orgasm. He encourages couples to engage in sexual activity that does not bring about pain and yet allows for emotional and sexual intimacy leading to orgasm. This includes clitoral stimulation, mutual masturbation, and the use of dildos and vibrators which usually do not irritate the vulva.

Many women with vulvar pain have simply stopped being sexual because of the painful consequences of sexual intercourse. Glazer's advice is aimed at helping a woman 're-sexualize' herself. When women complain that they don't feel interested in sex, Glazer recommends the resumption of non-painful sexual activity aimed at rehabilitating the pelvic muscles and vulvar tissue that have become used to inactivity.

Furthermore, Glazer addresses what would be considered the psychological aspect that might be present in the avoidance of sexual activity. This includes dealing with unresolved interpersonal problems that may exist in a relationship that would incline a woman to pull away sexually from her partner and from sex in general. Glazer addresses issues of shame, sexual abuse, self-esteem and self-image, and other psychological factors that might impact a woman's sexual activity and interest. In this re-sexualizing aspect of Glazer's work, he recommends a book called *Let Me Count the Ways: Discovering Great Sex without Intercourse* by Kline and Robins.

Glazer calls the work he does with the psychological and interpersonal factors involved in vulvar pain "psycho-education," rather than psychotherapy. He is clear that this focus on the psychological is some small part of the picture of vulvar pain, but by no means the whole picture. He says that while the psychological and interpersonal factors are a small part of the picture, they loom large enough in some women to determine whether a woman resumes an active and enjoyable sex life.

The 're-sexualization' prescription is not only meant for the psychological and interpersonal health of the woman. Glazer has taken into consideration the fact that there is evidence of a reduction of blood flow into the vulvar area of most women who have vulvar pain. Sexual activity necessarily involves blood flow into the vulva and other parts of the vagina. Glazer's intention in recommending increased non-penetrative and non-irritating sexual activity is to promote vulvar health and prevent the atrophy of blood vessels and other tissue that can be involved in abstinence from regular sexual activity.

We generally advise women with vulvar pain to explore ways of being sexual that will not throw them into a flare-up, yet can allow them some degree of sexual intimacy even when they are symptomatic. We don't pretend that these measures are an answer to the problem. They simply offer the possibility of having some semblance of sexual intimacy while the patient is proactively dealing with her condition.

Women with vulvar pain generally hurt upon their partner's entrance into the vagina. The discomfort also occurs during the thrusting phase of intercourse. With some women, the pain is immediate. With other women, the pain or discomfort comes after sex.

When there is improvement in the condition of a woman with vulvar pain, we suggest that patients experiment with the practice of *'tantra.'*

Generally speaking, we suggest this to women who are in the first stage of dyspareunia. *Tantra* allows for a couple to have sexual intercourse with a minimum of movement and irritation to a woman's vulva. This ancient practice prescribes that a man slowly enters inside a woman and once inside that he moves very little. His attention is focused on the sexual sensations in his genitals and in the sexual and sensual connection with his partner. His focus is on relaxing with the combination of sexual pleasure and the sense of incompleteness of holding back from moving toward orgasm.

When the man begins to lose his erection, he will move around to stimulate himself until his erection becomes firmer. He then continues relaxing, directing his attention to the connection between himself and his partner. He remains receptive and in an open state in order to feel the sensations and emotions arising out of the contact between himself and his partner. As the man remains in this state with his partner, orgasm can come without the vigorous movement that usually attends sexual intercourse. Most men who practice this report a greatly enhanced sexual experience. Many couples do tantra, who have never heard of pelvic pain.

Practicing tantra at first is not easy. As we have said, tantric practice requires a willingness on the part of the man to tolerate a sense of incompletion mixed with pleasure that comes from not rushing to orgasm. There are men who are not interested in exploring this practice and feel it is an intrusion upon their independence and freedom. Others resent having to practice such a level of impulse control. There are many men, however, who are in relationship with someone with vulvar pain who welcome any means by which to be sexually intimate. To be sure, even with tantra, most women with vulvar pain experience some degree of discomfort. This depends on what stage of dyspareunia they are in. Tantra, while having this limitation, still can help a woman who has vulvar pain enjoy sexual intimacy while minimizing what causes her pain.

Urethral syndrome and sexuality

If there is pain in the urethra upon touch, a woman can be in pain during intercourse as the penis pushes on the tender urethra. We sometimes recommend that women experiment with non-penetrative sexual activity as we have described above in relationship to women with vulvar pain.

Levator ani syndrome and sexuality

There is no known direct physical cause impacting or impairing sexual functioning in *levator ani syndrome,* other than the exacerbation of levator trigger points or associated spasm. As in other conditions where there is no physical cause impacting sexuality, sexuality tends to be affected whenever someone has pelvic pain.

Chronic Prostatitis/Chronic Pelvic Pain Syndrome Associated with Sexual Guilt or Anxiety

There is a small but distinct group of men who complain of pelvic pain consistent with the typical diagnosis of prostatitis or chronic pelvic pain syndrome that arises after they have experienced a sexual encounter that they later regard with shame, guilt or regret. In this discussion, we will refer to *guilty or anxiety sexual pain (GASP)* from such an encounter.

Typically in this scenario, a man will pay a woman for a sexual massage or engage a prostitute for intercourse or will have a casual or long term affair outside of marriage or engage in some variety of sexual activity about which he retrospectively feels anxiety or guilt.

Commonly, after the sexual encounter, the man fears that he has contracted an STD because of adverse symptoms. All appropriate tests are conducted and no STD is found. In the urological and psychological literature, there is little to explain the relationship between prostatitis/ CPPS symptoms, on the one hand, and the sexual behavior that is related to the symptoms.

We suggest here that men who report GASP-induced pelvic pain tend to share a common psychophysical response to their behavior that results in the perplexing symptoms of prostatitis/CPPS.

Psychophysical mechanism in GASP-induced pelvic pain/dysfunction

Contemporary urologic theory has been less than enthusiastic in implicating psychosocial factors in the onset of urologic disease. A mechanistic, body and organ centered explanation of the varieties of urologic pathology pervades the urologic literature. Here we are proposing a psychological theory of how psychosocial factors are intimately involved in the causation of symptoms of prostatitis/CPPS.

We are suggesting that a person's attitude and psychological viewpoint can result in a physical reaction in a man with GASP-induced pelvic pain/dysfunction. This man tends to operate with a rigid moral outlook. *Events in life are black or white, right or wrong, good or bad.* This moral standard is applied both to others and to himself. There is little room in the mind of these men for events, feelings and behaviors to be objectively viewed as they are, without a moral label.

These men tend to disown feelings or behavior that they judge to be bad or wrong and regard themselves with contempt and rejection. Men whose onset of pelvic pain occurs after a guiltily or anxiously perceived sexual encounter, tend to be hard-pressed to forgive feelings or behavior in themselves or others that they judge to be bad or wrong.

Typically a man with GASP-induced pelvic pain views the sexual event retrospectively with remorse, guilt and fear of either having violated a moral code, being discovered by his partner or having contracted some kind of disease. When we questioned the men about the reasons for their behavior, there was little self-understanding about how they possibly allowed this sexual encounter to occur. When in a relationship, there tended to be no forgiveness of the circumstances and context in which such an event occurred (e.g. they were lonely, sexually frustrated, estranged from their partner and in need of some kind of relief, reassurance, self-esteem that was lacking, etc.). Instead, when asked about the behavior, the response of these men was that, "It was wrong and I shouldn't have done it and I feel guilty and afraid because of it." It is also not uncommon for them to say, "I probably deserve what I have."

Men with GASP-induced pelvic pain/dysfunction give themselves little psychological space to have erred. We propose that their pain and dysfunction is the result of a twofold attempt to punish themselves and control themselves into refraining from such behavior in the future. They do this by tightening the muscles of the pelvic floor to stop the sexual feelings there from overwhelming them and causing them to lose control of their behavior.

Elsewhere we have discussed the theory that pelvic pain is the result of chronically pulling the tail between the legs, and is associated with fear, shame, remorse or guilt. It is not uncommon for a dog to pull his tail between his legs when his owner expresses upset over the dog's behavior. GASP-induced pelvic pain may be related to the biological response of shame and guilt to chronically pull the tail between the legs.

In other words we are suggesting that the primary purpose of the response of these men to their own behavior that they reject in themselves is to chronically tighten their pelvic muscles as a way of stopping their sexual sensations in order to control their behavior. As in other men with muscle-related pelvic pain and dysfunction, this chronic tension and guarding creates an inhospitable environment in the pelvic floor that results in pelvic pain and dysfunction. In summary, guilt about sexual encounter leads to fear about self-control. Primitive response of fear and shame is for the man to 'pull his tail between his legs.' This resultant unconscious prolonged tightening, is aimed at controlling sexual impulses and sexual acting out.

We treated an accountant with GASP-induced pelvic pain/dysfunction. He reported that during tax season, within a period of significantly increased stress in his life, and while at odds with his perfectionistic and judgmental wife, he had an affair with the secretary of one of his partners. He expressed great shame over his behavior as he considered himself a morally upright and religious man. He said that his moral values would never permit his infidelity but somehow he did it anyway. His affair went on for a little over a year. His wife discovered his infidelity and he went through a period of anguish with her. They sought counseling and he expressed his remorse repeatedly during their counseling sessions, promised never to do this again and begged his wife's forgiveness.

Things more or less went back to normal in his relationship, however, it was at this time that his pelvic pain began. Initially when asked whether he had experienced any intimacy, stress reduction or beauty in his extramarital relationship, he could not find any value in it. He had difficulty focusing on the question of whether the affair served him in any way. He appeared not to want to appreciate what he got from the affair and instead repeatedly returned to his self-judgment and self-condemnation. Upon reflection, he reluctantly admitted that his extramarital affair brought him comfort, pleasure, self-esteem and stress reduction but quickly reiterated that these benefits could not justify his behavior.

He had great difficulty in conceiving that he could forgive himself for his behavior. When he was asked what he imagined would happen if he forgave himself for his infidelity, he answered that if he forgave himself he just might go back and do it again.

Men with GASP related pelvic pain we have seen tend to have difficulty in differentiating between thought, feelings, and behavior. When we proposed that it was possible to allow the experience of sexual feelings without acting on them, men with GASP related pelvic pain tended to be perplexed. How you allow impulses and emotions to be present while not acting on them was a strange concept to most of these men. And yet this distinction is a critical one in men with GASP induced pelvic pain to give themselves permission to relax their pelvic floor.

The theory we speculate about this patient and others with GASP-induced pelvic pain/dysfunction is that, in his shame and fear about his behavior, he pulled his tail between his legs continually and could not imagine stopping doing this. This chronic tightening of his pelvic muscles, was his way of ceasing to feel his sexual impulses. Not feeling his sexual impulses was his way of controlling them, thereby controlling acting on them.

The *Wise-Anderson Protocol* for GASP-induced pelvic pain/dysfunction: learning to control sexual impulses without chronically tightening the pelvic floor

We are proposing that there is a psychological requirement for a man with GASP-induced pelvic pain/ dysfunction wishing to overcome this pelvic pain and dysfunction. He would do well to forgive his behavior and come to understand that he can have a relaxed pelvis, feel sexual feelings and that he does not have to chronically tighten up his pelvic floor muscles in order to control his sexual impulses. He would probably help himself by coming to understand that a relaxed and uncontracted pelvic floor will necessarily open up the experience of sexual feelings and that these feelings are natural and need not be judged as wrong or bad in order to control acting on them.

Typically men with GASP-induced pelvic pain/dysfunction disown their experience as they consider it bad or wrong. *This psychological disownment occurs simultaneously with the tightening of the muscles of the pelvic floor.* When this disownment is added to an idea that their bad or wrong behavior should be punished as a way of controlling it in the future, they unconsciously tighten their pelvic floor even more.

Once this period of chronic pelvic tightening occurs, as in other men with muscle-related pelvic pain, the condition takes on a life of its own. This condition is fed by the cycle of tension, anxiety, pain, and protective guarding. Added to that cycle, in these particular men, there is protective guarding against sexual feelings that arise in the pelvis. In summary:

- Men with GASP-induced pelvic pain/dysfunction operate in a right-wrong world and judge what they perceive as their own morally wrong behavior with contempt and disownment

- This disownment is both a psychological event of repudiation and judgment of their behavior and a physical event of implementing this disownment and repudiation by physically chronically tightening up the pelvic floor.

Treatment

Psychological treatment requires both the modification of the self-contempt and the thoughts that say, "The only way I can control myself is by tightening up my pelvic muscles as a way of controlling my sexual acting out." The man has to feel that it is okay to have sexual feelings, that it is okay to have a loose pelvis and to experience sexual arousal, at the same time understanding that controlling sexual impulses can be done without killing the experience of the sexual impulses. It goes without saying that the full protocol we offer, including physical therapy and paradoxical relaxation, be an integral part of treatment.

Physical Exercise and Chronic Pelvic Pain Syndromes

The relationship between exercise and pelvic pain is not often addressed. There is little written about this subject even though many of our patients are anxious for advice about whether to initiate, continue, or stop physical exercise.

Some patients with prostatitis, interstitial cystitis and urethral syndrome have reported that certain kinds of exercise worsen their symptoms while other kinds do not. Others report that they feel better after exercise. Still others report that exercise has no effect on their symptoms.

In general, physical exercise lowers levels of anxiety and is beneficial for the body in numerous ways. Our general advice to our patients about physical exercise is to find a form that minimally exacerbates your symptoms.

Sometimes certain physical exercise is contraindicated. Patients who have enjoyed or benefited from these types of exercise ask us whether they should resume these exercises in spite of their increased pain, or whether they will ever be able to go back to them. Our view is that some kinds of physical exercise can aggravate pelvic pain because they put a strong demand on the pelvic muscles to contract—muscles which are already shortened due to chronic tension. These tensed, shortened muscles don't relax very well. When physical exercise tightens them further, they remain in an elevated state of tension for a while. For reasons upon which we can only speculate, some people's symptoms are affected while others are not.

The kinds of physical exercise that are most likely to aggravate symptoms of pelvic pain and dysfunction include weight lifting and body building, sit-ups, crunches, as well as bicycling. We think that bicycling aggravates symptoms in some people because it pushes on the tender, painful trigger points in and near the perineum. These often highly trigger-pointed and tender areas are often not happy being pressed upon by bicycle seats.

Weight lifting and body-building have been associated with the onset of pelvic pain in a number of patients we have seen. A few patients who undertook a crash course in flattening their stomachs reported that their pelvic pain began after their regimen of 500 sit-ups per day got into full swing. While all exercise causes a contraction of the pelvic muscles, sit-ups and weight-lifting demanding the abdominal muscles to strongly contract, put a large burden on the pelvic muscles. It is not surprising that this kind of exercise can initiate or aggravate pelvic pain and dysfunction that arise from chronically contracted muscles.

There are doctors who insist that when the pudendal nerve is compressed, one must protect it by avoiding exercise like bicycling or rowing which tend to aggravate it. While pudendal nerve entrapment remains a controversial and speculative general explanation of chronic pelvic pain, if one is symptomatic, avoiding exercise like bicycling or rowing is a harmless precaution.

Hatha yoga and stretching

Part of our protocol in the physical therapy component of our treatment involves doing stretches to loosen the muscles in the pelvic floor that have been shortened. These are specific kinds of stretches aimed at assisting with the rehabilitation of the pelvic muscles and we include these exercises as part of our homework for the patient.

The muscles of the pelvic floor can be stretched to some limited degree. We believe the stretching that we describe in Chapter 6 is the best way to use external stretches to lengthen and loosen contracted pelvic muscles. It is a kind of yoga.

Hatha yoga is an ancient practice of physical stretches that are called 'asanas' or postures, aimed at relaxing the body and preparing it for meditation. The popularity of yoga has grown in the west and in many places yoga studios are as common as copy shops or video rental stores. Hatha yoga receives our support as we see it helping the muscles to stretch and lengthen as well as helping the body to quiet. If there is a limitation of time, we encourage our patients to do the stretches described in this book that are specifically aimed at the lengthening and relaxation of the pelvic muscles.

The only caveat we offer with regard to yoga is that it be done with plenty of time to relax in between poses. Furthermore, we do not recommend yoga that requires prolonged awkward poses that tighten the pelvic floor up.

Massage and body work

Whatever calms you and soothes you is good for pelvic pain. Full body massage, while sometimes costly and time consuming, is a very good activity for someone who has pelvic pain. Swedish massage, Shiatsu, Rolfing, Esalen massage, Jin Shin Jitsu, Reiki, Rosen Bodywork, Feldenkrais, Trager, Craniosacral Therapy, Tui Na, and reflexology, are all types of bodywork that usually have the effect of relaxation and quieting. A number of our patients have unsuccessfully sought out these approaches as a primary treatment. In our view, none of them has any lasting benefit for pelvic pain. Nevertheless, we consider them useful in quieting down anxiety and nervous system arousal.

Other Relevant Issues

Medications for pelvic pain and dysfunction

We know of no curative medications for the kinds of pelvic pain and dysfunction described in this book. While there are generally no effective pain medications, there are some medications that can 'take the edge off' the pain on a temporary basis for some patients.

In general there are no really effective medications to deal with chronic pelvic pain. Alpha blockers like Flomax®, Hytrin®, Cardura® and Uroxatrol® can offer modest relief to some patients with pelvic pain, but there can be considerable side-effects for some patients including nasal stuffiness, elevated heart rate, dry mouth, and fatigue. Elavil®, originally used as an antidepressant, is sometimes prescribed in non-antidepressant doses for pelvic pain.

Perhaps of all the medications that have a limited efficacy for discomfort in the pelvis, the benzodiazepines like Valium® can help give the sufferer a 'break' from the discomfort. Sometimes patients will take 2 to 2½ milligrams of Valium® every four hours for a day or two or 5 or 10 milligrams of Valium® every third day to help sleep, and in order to reduce the constant discomfort or pain. Patients should exercise caution about addiction and sedation with these medications and consult with their physicians about their use.

Narcotic medications

While narcotic medications can reduce pelvic pain, there are complications to these drugs which include addiction, lowered pain threshold, a need to increase medication over time, constipation, and general mental dullness. Some of our patients have a harder time getting off of the narcotics than they do in releasing their pain. In general, when possible, we would discourage the use of narcotic medication. We can however work with people who are on narcotic medications, even though these medications tend to complicate treatment to some degree.

Bladder retraining

As we've discussed previously, it is sometimes helpful to modify the tendency toward frequent urination when one is symptomatic with a pelvic pain syndrome. The bladder receives about 1cc of urine per minute. If the bladder has gotten into the habit of urinating frequently and this persists even though symptoms have clearly improved, it is sometimes useful to change this habit by gradually postponing urination for up to an hour or two. This is done in small increments so long as such postponement is comfortable. In this kind of retraining, bladder capacity may be increased. This retraining should be done under the supervision of a physician.

If I am in pain, do I continue working or do I take time off?

There are advantages and disadvantages in holding down a full time job and functioning in every aspect of life while you are dealing with pelvic pain and dysfunction. The advantages are that you usually keep up your self-esteem by functioning fully in your life while you have symptoms. The obvious other advantages have to do with maintaining your reputation and financial stability and keeping up with your obligations. Members of your family who rely on you are probably going to feel better knowing that you are continuing to function in a way that allows them to feel secure. The disadvantage of continuing to work exists when your work exacerbates your symptoms.

It is useful to consider the following questions with regard to working or taking time off. What best serves my recovery from my condition? What best serves my long-range goals in life? What best serves my self-esteem? What is the best course of action that I can take that allows me to be an inspiration to myself? If I were ninety-five-years-old and peacefully lying on my deathbed looking back at my life, what would I advise myself about what I should do now? There are few universal answers to these kinds of questions.

Why pelvic floor biofeedback is not a reliable indicator of the usefulness of our protocol

The following article was written by David Wise, Ph.D., edited for the 5th edition, as a response to a question on the Internet about the usefulness of pelvic floor biofeedback.

… I am responding to a request for a comment about the usefulness of intrapelvic biofeedback measurements in determining if pelvic pain is a tension disorder and appropriate for the *Wise-Anderson Protocol*. My short answer is that electromyographic measurement of the anal sphincter and/or muscles near the opening of the vagina with a biofeedback sensor, used alone, is generally an unreliable measure of what is going on inside the pelvic floor. Unremarkable readings of the anal sphincter and/or vaginal opening should not be used to rule out tension related pelvic pain or to dismiss the appropriateness of the *Wise-Anderson Protocol*.

Here is the longer answer. Let me say first that I have been a biofeedback supporter and practitioner for over 25 years. I had the best of training over many years from one of the luminaries of the field and have worked with many patients over the years with multimodal biofeedback for anxiety, functional cardiac disorders, and urinary incontinence among other problems. I continue to do neural feedback training with Steve Wall, one of the geniuses in the field of biofeedback and the designer of the remarkable biointegrator system. In addition, I did biofeedback assessment and training in intrapelvic biofeedback at Stanford for a number of years with many patients.

I think biofeedback that measures skin temperature, galvanic skin response, muscle tension, brain wave activity, and respiratory sinus arrhythmia for problems other than pelvic pain is remarkable and enormously helpful. What I am saying below refers to pelvic floor biofeedback for chronic pelvic pain syndromes that we discuss in our book in which a sensor is inserted rectally and/or vaginally where readings are measured on an electromyography in microvolts. It does not refer to intrapelvic biofeedback for urinary incontinence which I happen to think is the best and safest treatment that exists for incontinence.

In my own case, when I was symptomatic, I did an hour or two of pelvic floor biofeedback on a daily basis for a year. After many months of diligent practice, my resting anal sphincter tone was a remarkable zero after about 15 minutes of relaxation. And I was very dismayed, like the person whose comment you sent to me, to find that I was still in pain at the moment that the anal sensor registered zero. I was also disappointed as a clinician experienced in the successful use of biofeedback for other problems to find that the biofeedback measurement seemed to indicate (erroneously) that tension was not a central problem in my pelvic pain.

I didn't understand then what I understand now, which is that the electrical activity in the anal sphincter and/or vaginal opening is, for the most part, the only area that the biofeedback sensor measures, and often says very little about what is going on with the other 20-some odd muscles within the pelvic floor and external muscles related to pelvic pain. Furthermore, the biofeedback sensor measures dynamic muscle tension, but not chronically shortened tissue without elevated tone. It is possible to have a relaxed anal sphincter and/or vaginal opening and have pain referring pelvic floor trigger points deep inside that can make one very miserable. In this case, elevated tone and active trigger points inside the pelvic floor are not reflected in the anal sphincter and/or vaginal opening measurements.

Shortened, contracted tissue inside the pelvic floor, symptom-recreating trigger points inside and outside the pelvic floor when palpated, the habitual tendency to tighten the pelvic floor under stress or to reflexively guard against pelvic discomfort and a tension-anxiety-pain cycle are the culprits in most people with pelvic pain that we successfully treat. This can sometimes but not necessarily include a chronically tight anal sphincter and/or vaginal opening. All of these factors are diagnostically significant. For example, in my experience at Stanford, people with levator ani syndrome almost always have an entirely normal resting anal sphincter tone while palpating the painful trigger points on the levator and other internal muscles. Resolving those trigger points and relaxing the inside of the pelvic floor can resolve this pain without much change in the measurement of the tone of the anal sphincter before or after treatment.

On our website, www.pelvicpainhelp.com, we have video clips of an important study, replicated many times, demonstrating that at rest, the electrical activity inside a trigger point in the trapezius, monitored by a needle electromyographic electrode is quite high while the electrical activity of the tissue less than an inch away from the elevated electrical activity is essentially electrically silent. If you used a regular biofeedback sensor to measure the general tone of the trapezius, you may well find nothing remarkable and yet to rely on this information is entirely misleading and would incline you to miss the treatment that could substantially reduce or abate the pain and dysfunction coming from the active trigger point.

The bottom line here is that in my experience, electrical measurement of the anal sphincter and/or the opening of the vagina, used alone, is often a poor measure of what is going on inside the pelvic floor. While I believe biofeedback is remarkably successful for many other disorders and is one of the treatments of choice for urinary incontinence and vulvar pain, I am unimpressed with the usefulness of biofeedback in treating most pelvic pain.

The best gauge of the usefulness of our protocol that treats pelvic pain of neuromuscular origin is a thorough examination of the pelvic floor for trigger points that recreate symptoms and palpating for tightened and restricted muscles inside the pelvic floor. This must be done by someone with a significant amount of experience in working with pelvic pain and with the kind of myofascial *Trigger Point Release* and relaxation methods that we use. An inexperienced person will miss all this and I have seen many times that even practitioners who specialize in treating pelvic pain miss trigger points referring the symptoms to and inside the pelvis.

We sometimes find pelvic floor electromyography useful when there is a high pelvic floor resting tone, because it provides an objective marker that we can compare readings to after the patient has used our protocol. The idea that pelvic floor biofeedback measurements are a reliable test of whether pelvic pain is a tension disorder represents a misunderstanding of the problem and should not be relied on, especially when the readings are normal. Pelvic floor electromyographic measurement monitoring the anal sphincter and/or vaginal opening is one of those medical tests where a positive finding may mean something and point toward the proper therapy and a negative result doesn't necessarily prove anything.

How to think about the 1½ hours of self treatment we ask our patients to do

Ultimately those with pelvic pain do a grand experiment with regard to what works and what doesn't. Almost everyone we see for treatment has consulted multiple doctors, done a variety of conventional treatments, and has not been helped by these treatments.

Our program requires about 1½ hours of self-treatment per day for many, many months and when self-treatment is successful in significantly reducing or stopping symptoms, some level of self treatment is required on a maintenance basis. Such a time commitment is usually not easy with the normal demands of work and family and having a life.

One woman came to see us from overseas who had 5 children whom she was schooling at home. Aside from that daunting task, she held down a part time job. Her husband offered her no assistance at home. The entire burden of raising and educating her children along with running the household fell on her shoulders. When she got away from her family and had time to do our protocol, her symptoms improved. In the normal course of her life, with no real time for herself, she floundered and her baseline level of symptoms remained.

She was very conflicted about taking any time for herself. Her idea was that she was selfish to take time for herself. Selfishness was to be shunned and so any time she took for herself felt almost like a sin. In these circumstances, her condition did not improve. This kind of attitude and lifestyle gives our protocol little chance of working. Daily self treatment is the heart of our protocol. There is no way of short changing the time necessary for self treatment if you want to benefit from what we have to offer.

There are some individuals, often used to the privilege of wealth, who do not take well to the idea of self-treatment. These individuals resist doing the treatment themselves. They will often go back home after seeing us and hire a physical therapist for the physical therapy component of the protocol. And often they do the relaxation protocol minimally. To the extent that these individuals persist in refusing to take on direct responsibility of self treatment, their ability to get better remains limited.

The majority of individuals with pelvic pain have tightened their pelvic muscles for a long time before the symptoms ever manifested themselves. This inner tightening is a default mode of dealing with difficulties in life. It is a way in which someone unconsciously protects themselves in the various situations in life where anxiety or stress arise.

Reversing the consequences of this inner posture is a huge undertaking. Releasing pelvic floor muscles that have been tightened for many years is a very ambitious aspiration. Changing the habit of tightening the pelvic floor under stress, and the psycho physical pathways that make the pelvic floor take the brunt of stress and anxiety is a major event in someone's life. It is an inside job. No one else can do it for you.

We have said that no drug or surgery can accomplish this change. Only a concerted, dedicated effort can begin to bring this about. This is why drugs and surgery have failed to help muscle related pelvic pain. This is why we advocate 1½ hours of self-treatment per day.

Understanding that the treatment falls on your shoulders requires a shift in understanding about how healing occurs. Once we have instructed you in self-treatment, the responsibility for the treatment falls into your hands. Like Home Depot, *you can do it and we can help.* The emphasis is on you can do it and are most likely to get the best results from our program when you take on that responsibility.

Monitored Kegel exercises

At the time of the writing of the 5th edition of this book, many patients who speak to us report that they have done pelvic floor biofeedback as a treatment for pelvic pain. Pelvic floor biofeedback usually involves doing Kegel exercises, (tightening of the pelvic muscles as if stopping urination and then alternatively relaxing the pelvic muscles). This alternation of tightening and relaxing typically is done for 5-12 seconds of tightening and then 5-12 seconds of relaxation.

We generally do not believe Kegel exercises are useful with pelvic pain and, in fact, they can exacerbate symptoms. Kegel exercises were developed to help women restore their continence after childbirth. They are exercises to strengthen and tighten muscles, not to relax them. Kegel exercises usually add tension to an already tense area in someone who has pelvic pain. While Kegel exercises can be very useful for women who have vulvar pain or incontinence, we generally think it is contraindicated for pelvic pain.

Using the *Wise-Anderson Protocol* for other manifestations of a headache in the pelvis: constipation, anal fissures, hemorrhoids, irritable bowel syndrome, and post bowel movement pain

The consequences of chronically holding tension in the body are not limited to pelvic floor pain and dysfunction. A modified *Wise-Anderson Protocol* may be useful in other conditions that arise from chronically holding tension in the body. The conditions we discuss include constipation, anal fissures, hemorrhoids, irritable bowel syndrome, and post bowel movement pain.

One of the larger conclusions of our book extends an idea that we have quoted earlier, namely that the development of a solution to any difficult problem is often not found within the confines of the field designated to study it. The basic tools of conventional medicine in general and the specialty of urology in particular confine themselves to pharmaceuticals and surgery. Certainly pharmaceuticals and surgery have revolutionized modern civilization, and have extended the lifespan and health of human kind. In the case of pelvic pain however, the diagnostic tools of urology that rule out structural pathology are essential, but the therapeutic tools of drugs or surgery have not helped, and sometimes have actually complicated or hurt the problem. In a word, pelvic pain of the kind we treat has not been adequately diagnosed or treated by the tools and conceptual framework of conventional urologic evaluation and treatment. The protocol that we have developed is cross disciplinary and is outside of the box of the conventional urologic world view. In the same way, we propose that other conditions might well benefit from our cross disciplinary methodology that reaches beyond the conventional diagnostic and treatment tools.

Constipation

The colon and rectum are structures that operate together in the activity of the evacuation of stool. Normal bowel elimination involves a complex mechanism which includes the reflex relaxation of the internal anal sphincter when the rectum is full. This sensory muscle, which is autonomically controlled, can differentiate between gas or stool and signal the pelvic floor muscles to relax if it is appropriate to eliminate (along with appropriate peristalsis in the colon). However, if it is not socially appropriate or convenient, an individual can voluntarily tighten up the pelvic floor and help quiet down the sense of urgency that is felt.

Heightened anxiety can lead to increased tension in the pelvic floor. This interferes with the ability of the muscles to release at the appropriate time, at the same time disturbing normal peristalsis in the bowel. There are also individuals who have learned to do the opposite of what needs to be done in order to eliminate. Instead of relaxing their pelvic floor muscles, especially the pubo-rectalis muscle, they contract it while attempting to eliminate, causing a frustrating condition called paradoxical puborectalis contraction. Fortunately this condition is relatively easily diagnosed, and reversible with neuro-muscular re-education. It is important to stop the habit of this paradoxical contraction, as prolonged bearing down can result in prolapsing pelvic or abdominal organs.

Anal fissures

The anal fissure is like a paper cut in the mucosal lining of the anal sphincter. It is understood by many researchers that the anal fissure is called an 'ischemic ulcer.' Ischemia is a condition in which there is a significant reduction in blood flow to an area. The current understanding about anal fissures is that because there is elevated tension, the blood flow in the anal sphincter is reduced, thereby impairing the tissue which then becomes fragile and vulnerable to injury from a hard bowel movement or from the pressure of bearing down during defecation.

It is generally agreed that the source of the anal fissure in large part involves a chronically tightened internal anal sphincter. Both surgery, the procedure of stretching or dilating the anal sphincter under anesthesia, and the application of topical agents to the internal anal sphincter are aimed at relaxing the anal sphincter. The surgical concept for anal fissures is based on the peculiar idea that cutting the sphincter is the best way to reduce the tone, tension and spasm in the anal sphincter. While surgery can be successful, there is a risk of short-term and sometimes long-term fecal incontinence.

Hemorrhoids

At some time or another, many people find a little blood in their stool, usually after a particularly hard bowel movement. One can become confused and upset at such an event. At other times, alarmed individuals go to the doctor complaining of rectal pain after a bowel movement with no apparent blood in the stool. Often the doctor gives the diagnosis of anal fissure or hemorrhoids to these complaints. Hemorrhoids constitute another condition that is painful and sometimes the source of blood in the stool. A hemorrhoid is a kind of varicose vein, which tends to balloon out when straining on the toilet.

One French study showed that one-third of women had hemorrhoids or anal fissures after childbirth. This is probably because of the great pressure exerted by bearing down during childbirth in addition to the prevalence of constipation during pregnancy. Millions of people in North America suffer from hemorrhoids. Anal fissures and hemorrhoids are common in both men and women. These conditions are often related to constipation and diarrhea. Constipation has been related to chronic tension in the pelvic muscles in adults and recently to refractory constipation in children in a study done at the Mayo clinic.

While most anal fissures and hemorrhoids resolve themselves after they flare up, some colorectal surgeons lean toward an aggressive procedure or surgery to treat hemorrhoids and anal fissures. We have seen patients who are anxious about their rectal discomfort talked into treatment of the fissure or hemorrhoid involving surgery.

Conventional treatment of constipation, anal fissures and hemorrhoids tends to ignore the relationship between body and mind

Like the conventional treatment of pelvic pain, the relationship of a person's mindset, level of relaxation during bowel movements, and management of stress is almost entirely ignored in the literature on the treatment of these conditions. Instead, there is a narrow focus on immediately reducing symptoms of these conditions. Procedures, surgery, laxatives and medications are the usual options.

Most of the patients we have seen who have had surgery for anal fissures or hemorrhoids have reported that the physicians they saw offered few options related to quieting down the anxiety and habitual straining and tightening related to these conditions. Instead of seeing an anal fissure, for example, as an expression of anxiety and chronic pelvic tension, conventional treatment sees its symptoms, including chronic anal tension, as something that needs to be mechanically or pharmaceutically stopped. Little regard is shown for the big picture of a person's life and how one's symptoms are a response to this big picture. It is our view that the symptom is the way our bodies are trying to communicate. If we refuse to understand the message because we don't understand the body's language, we needlessly suffer and don't deal with the root problem prompting the symptom.

In the large majority of cases, it is the chronic tension in the pelvic floor, including the anal sphincter, usually combined with diet, anxiety and time urgency around bowel habits that strongly contributes to constipation, anal fissures and hemorrhoids. The chronic pelvic tension, diet, and bowel habits associated with most constipation, anal fissures and hemorrhoids do not come out of the blue. In a word, a person's mind, body, and lifestyle are involved in the creation and perpetuation of these conditions.

We propose that a modified *Wise-Anderson Protocol* might be of significant benefit for the treatment of constipation, anal fissures and hemorrhoids. The overriding principle is that all of these conditions tend to occur as the result of someone expressing anxiety by tightening the pelvic floor, and in the case of constipation, inhibiting normal peristaltic movement in the colon. *Where sphincterotomy, or the partial cutting of the internal anal sphincter, to reduce anal sphincter tension is often used for anal fissures, we believe that it is perfectly possible to learn to relax the anal sphincter with no surgery whatsoever.* This can be accomplished by teaching patients the *Trigger Point Release* and *Paradoxical Relaxation* protocols we use for pelvic pain syndromes. A devoted effort of self-treatment in the *Wise-Anderson Protocol* that we teach in our 6-day clinics, we believe, would be more than sufficient training for someone suffering from constipation, anal fissures and hemorrhoids. Of course, the modification of the *Wise-Anderson Protocol* would have to include diet and bathroom habit reeducation, teaching the patient not to strain unduly and not to resist the feeling of urgency to go to the bathroom.

Irritable Bowel Syndrome (IBS)

IBS is common in the general population and is reputed to account for up to 50% of visits to gastroenterologists. The symptoms of IBS typically include: abdominal pain, abdominal bloating or fullness, diarrhea or constipation, sometimes heartburn, early feelings of fullness and incomplete bowel emptying. Typically it is treated with certain medications, avoiding colon irritating food and drink, increasing intake of water and fiber, exercise, etc. It is a distressing disorder and it often comes and goes with periods of stress.

A modified *Wise-Anderson Protocol* and the treatment of IBS

In our 6-day pelvic pain clinics, a few patients who also suffer from irritable bowel syndrome have reported improvement in their IBS symptoms. These patients have reported that this improvement occurred after doing a specific kind of abdominal self-treatment to be discussed below, in combination with *Paradoxical Relaxation*. This brief essay discusses the treatment and a proposed mechanism to explain the possible efficacy of this modified *Wise-Anderson Protocol* for IBS. We do not advise someone do this method for these conditions without physician instruction and supervision. The reason for this is that if one does not understand abdominal anatomy and the appropriate pressure to be used, blood vessels and structures in the abdomen can be damaged.

IBS is common in both male and female patients whom we have treated for pelvic pain. The purpose of the *Wise-Anderson Protocol* is to teach patients targeted self-treatment methods. One of the methods we show patients is the use of a self-treatment pressure release device that allows them to easily do abdominal *Trigger Point Release*. Some of our patients with IBS, had dramatic improvement of their symptoms of abdominal or esophageal discomfort when they exerted *Trigger Point Release* pressure to areas of tenderness or pain throughout their abdomen. This was done in conjunction with the regular practice of *Paradoxical Relaxation*.

Proposed mechanism of the modified *Wise-Anderson Protocol* on IBS

In their classic book *The Colon*, Wolf and Wolff observed in patients with abdominal fistulas (open holes in the abdomen) that permitted direct visual examination of the colon in different emotional states, the colons of subjects studied tended to become slowed down and contracted (hypodynamic), stopping their rhythmic movement, during periods of fear, dejection, futility or defeat, dissatisfaction, boredom, tension, and mild depression. The subjects' colons became hyperactive (hyperdynamic) in moments of anger, resentment, guilt, humiliation, anxiety and conflict. When the emotional states of these individuals became quiet and calm, the colonic behavior normalized and the rhythmic peristaltic movement and color resumed. Wolf and Wolff stated:

"In the patients described, it was common to find a disturbance of colonic function characterized either by a hyperdynamic response with diarrhea, or a hypodynamic response with constipation. Hyperfunction was characterized by hyperemia, a contraction of longitudinal muscles together with shortening of the colon and increase in rhythmic contractile activity of circular muscles in the caecum, ascending, and transverse loops while the descending and sigmoid colon showed no rhythmic circular contractions but assumed a rigid tubular shape due to longitudinal muscle activity, with pallor of the mucosa. In colonic hypofunction with constipation, rectal, anal and perianal muscles were usually contracted so as to further impede emptying.

...The hypodynamic reaction was encountered when individuals reacted...with feelings of fear, dejection, futility, or defeat, dissatisfaction, boredom, tension and mild depression... sustained or recurrent colonic hypofunction in patients was found to be associated with constipation... may be looked upon as a part of a general reaction of 'grimly holding fast' under circumstances that threatened the individual.

The hyperdynamic reaction of the colon, on the other hand... (was related to) symbolic assaults which included anger, resentment, guilt, humiliation, anxiety, and conflict. Catastrophic or shocking situations or those arousing feelings of being overwhelmed also evoked hyperfunction of the large bowel... (this can be called) the ejection-riddance pattern of colonic hyperfunction."

Early in the 20th century Walter Cannon, originator of the terms '*fight, flight, freeze*' and '*homeostasis*' noted a similar reaction in the colon of a cat that rhythmically moved when undisturbed but stopped its movement when a dog was brought into the room. IBS symptoms including abdominal discomfort or pain, bloating and fullness, burning, constipation and diarrhea have long been known to be associated with hyper- or hypo-arousal of the autonomic nervous system.

The premise of this book is that there is a self-feeding tension-anxiety-pain cycle that occurs in pelvic pain. We suggest here that this cycle may also be at work in IBS. Furthermore, the intervention we are suggesting, a modified form of the *Wise-Anderson Protocol*, may help break this tension-anxiety-pain cycle in IBS.

Here is a thumbnail sketch of our proposal for using the *Wise-Anderson Protocol* in modified form for this condition. The patient diagnosed with IBS is taught to do *Trigger Point Release* performed gently but firmly, with increasing pressure over a number of weeks, throughout the abdomen where trigger points have been established. This is done for a period not exceeding 90 seconds for each place where pressure release is performed. The focus of pressure follows the ascending, transverse, and descending colon. This is done while the patient relaxes during the pressure release and then practices *Paradoxical Relaxation.*

The simplicity and cost effectiveness of this methodology is obvious. No drugs are used. Patients are empowered to help themselves. The risks are minimal. We are not proposing the reader of this book use these proposed methods for constipation, anal fissures, hemorrhoids, or irritable bowel syndrome without medical supervision. We continue to endorse an experimental evaluation of this method for the symptoms of IBS.

Post bowel movement pain

One distressing symptom of pelvic pain occurs when a bowel movement flares it up. Little is written about this symptom when it occurs in the absence of hemorrhoids or anal fissures, but in our experience it is common.

In this section, we wish to propose an explanation of the mechanism responsible for this symptom and an intervention for it. The mechanism of defecation typically involves the filling up of the rectum with stool, which then sends a signal for the internal anal sphincter and puborectalis muscle to relax and triggers the experience of urgency to have a bowel movement. Once the stool passes through the relaxed anal sphincter and out of the body, the internal anal sphincter reflexively closes.

When someone has pelvic pain and exacerbation of symptoms after a bowel movement, we propose that the internal anal sphincter tends to 'over close.' That is, it tightens up more than it was tight before the bowel movement and sometimes appears to go into a kind of painful spasm. This is the reason why we suggest that some people have increased pain after a bowel movement.

Our patients with post bowel movement pain often insert a gloved, lubricated finger into the anal sphincter after a bowel movement to help release the over-tightened sphincter. This maneuver can reduce post bowel movement pain and sometimes can reduce or eliminate its appearance over time.

Post bowel movement pain appears to occur less frequently when someone is relaxed and not hurried, and whatever contributes to a more relaxed state during a visit to the bathroom may reduce this symptom. The toilet manufacturer Toto makes a warm toilet seat called a Washlet® that sends a warm stream of water, then air, to clean the anal opening after a bowel movement. This kind of post bowel movement care may also be helpful for this symptom.

Squatting vs. sitting during defecation as a way of helping the relaxation of the pelvic floor

Most people throughout history have squatted when they have evacuated their bowels. The modern toilet is relatively new in the history of mankind and has been adopted as the standard of a civilized bathroom appliance. The perennial hole in the ground over which one squatted to defecate is considered primitive in modern western society. A website, www.naturesplatform. com, devoted to promoting the advantages of squatting during defecation writes about the history of the modern toilet:

"Human beings have always used the squatting position for elimination. Infants of every culture instinctively adopt this posture to relieve themselves. Although it may seem strange to someone who has spent his entire life deprived of the experience, this is the way the body was designed to function.

The modern chair-like toilet, on the other hand, is a relatively recent innovation. It first became popular in Western Europe less than two centuries ago, largely by coincidence. Invented in England by a cabinet maker and a plumber, neither of whom had any knowledge of physiology, it was installed in the first dwellings to use indoor plumbing. The "porcelain throne" was quickly imitated, as the sitting posture seemed more "dignified"—more suited to aristocrats than the method used by the natives in the colonies.

Two other influences also favored the adoption of this new water closet. One was the headlong rush to modernize all existing sanitation facilities (which were in fact non-existent). The public assumed that all the benefits of modern plumbing required the use of the seat-like toilet, since it was the only one having the proper fittings to connect to the pipes. This assumption was incorrect, since toilets with all the same flushing capabilities could be (and have since been) designed to be used in the squatting position.

Secondly, in nineteenth-century Britain, any open discussion of this subject was considered most improper. Those who felt uncomfortable using a posture for evacuation that had nothing to do with human anatomy were forced to keep silent. How could they denounce the toilet used by Queen Victoria herself? (Hers was gold-plated!).

So, like the *Emperor's New Clothes*, the water closet was tacitly accepted. The general discomfort felt by the population was indicated by the popularity of "squatting stools" sold in the famous Harrods of London. These footstools elevated one's feet while in the sitting position to bring the knees closer to the chest—a crude attempt to imitate squatting.

The rest of Western Europe, as well as Australia and North America, did not want to appear less civilized than Great Britain, whose vast empire at the time made it the most powerful country on Earth. So, within a few decades, most of the industrialized world had adopted "The Emperor's New Throne."

A hundred and fifty years ago, no one could have predicted the effect of this change on the health of the population. But today, many physicians blame the modern commode for the high incidence of a number of serious diseases. Compared to the rest of the world, people in westernized countries have much higher rates of appendicitis, hemorrhoids, colon cancer, prostate cancer, and inflammatory bowel disease."

There is compelling evidence that sitting on the toilet to evacuate the bowels is inferior to squatting in a number of ways. Squatting tends to relax the puborectalis muscle, which is essential in defecation. A long study examining the effect of squatting during defecation and hemorrhoids showed improvement or elimination of hemorrhoids as the result of squatting during defecation. Doing the Valsalva maneuver in which one bears down to initiate defecation while holding one's breath has been sometimes associated with heart attack or episodes of atrial fibrillation because such a maneuver increases pressure in the thorax and interferes with venous blood returning to the heart. The heart rate can significantly drop during this activity. Defecating while squatting can reduce the need to bear down during defecation.

The modern toilet makes squatting during defecation problematic. Nevertheless, with a little innovation, it is possible to squat on a toilet. On www.naturesplatform.com, a device is sold that allows one to easily squat during defecation. When pelvic pain also involves constipation, anal fissures, or hemorrhoids the issue of integrating squatting during defecation might well be considered.

We would like to see research on a non-invasive and self-administered treatment of anal fissures and other headaches in the pelvis following a modified version of our protocol for pelvic pain. This may involve the rehabilitation of a tight pelvic floor using *Trigger Point Release*, modifying the habit of tightening the pelvic muscles habitually under stress using *Paradoxical Relaxation,* and relaxing the pelvic floor while squatting on the toilet. While there is little research done on the treatment of these kinds of conditions using this perspective, we strongly support an independent study evaluating the efficacy of a modified *Wise-Anderson Protocol* including squatting on the toilet, for the treatment of constipation, reduced urinary flow, bashful bladder syndrome, slow transit time, irritable bowel syndrome, anal fissures, hemorrhoids, and other manifestations of headaches in the pelvis.

CHAPTER 9

STORIES OF PATIENTS IN THEIR OWN WORDS

We have begun to collect stories from patients who have been trained in our protocol. We hope these accounts, in the patient's own words, can offer a flavor of what our treatment feels like as the patient and what is possible in terms of results from our program. Each patient below is writing after a certain amount of time of doing our protocol. We believe the results can continue to improve as their skills at relaxation deepen.

Stories of recent patients undergoing the protocol

Story of 52-year-old physician

I am a 52-year-old internist (family doctor for adults) with a busy practice in Los Angeles and the married father of 2 small children (ages 4 and 9). In addition to all the responsibilities of my practice, my colleagues and myself were in the early stages of organizing a move of our medical practice a few miles away (we actually started our planning in January, 2005). This process began to take up an extraordinary amount of my time. I should add that I also have been very involved caring for my children. I was, to say the least, quite busy. I always felt that I had previously handled stress quite effectively. I always had a plan of action and somehow got through the task at hand methodically. At no time prior to June of 2005 did I ever have any physical symptoms that I could recall related to stress other then the occasional sleepless night. As a result, I was completely caught off guard by the symptoms that I was to develop.

I was awakened one morning in June of 2005, at about 6:00 AM quite abruptly (I usually get up at about 6:30AM). A pain deep in my pelvis somewhere between my rectum and testicles had developed. I got up to void and was relieved that the pain had resolved promptly. Prior to this particular morning I had on occasion had an episode of what I presumed to be *prostatitis*. From time to time I would have some mild dysuria (pain on urination) and would take 7-10 days of an antibiotic-usually "Cipro" (also known by its generic name of ciprofloxacin). This episode was different in that I had no dysuria-just pelvic pain. I started the Cipro again for 10 days but noticed that I was getting these intermittent episodes of pelvic pain in spite of the antibiotics. The episodes were intermittent over the next month but no other symptoms had developed. I sometimes went a week or so without the pain and was just hoping whatever "inflammation" was there would go away by itself. I flew back East in July of 2005 to spend a few days with my brother and a friend from medical school at the New Jersey shore. The pain was becoming more frequent and starting to wake me up at night. I was becoming quite concerned that I had developed something a bit more serious than "prostatitis." I didn't want to tell my friend from medical school as he would have instructed me (rightly so) to get further (appropriate) evaluation and I feared I would find out I had cancer right in the middle of my life!

Back in Los Angeles after this vacation the pain became more frequent and it was beginning to wake me almost every night. I began taking anti-inflammatory medication (ibuprofen is the generic but is also sold as Advil, Motrin, as well as under other names) but this didn't seem to do much for the pain. I then began to develop low and mid-back pain which raised my panic level. I was trying to think of a patient with this constellation of symptoms and couldn't quite think of anybody.

Over the years I had seen multiple patients with what I thought was "prostatitis" and treated them with antibiotics-sometimes for months but didn't appreciate that they might have had pain this severe. I would occasionally refer them to urologists who would continue the antibiotics and recommend that they take hot baths and have frequent sex. But when this back pain developed I felt that I indeed had something more ominous then *prostatitis*. I had back films taken which were entirely within normal limits but due to the severity of the pain I then had an MRI scan performed of my spine and pelvis.

I assumed at this point that I had metastatic cancer and the scan would basically be my death sentence. I reviewed the scan with several radiologists who all felt it was unremarkable. In spite of these normal studies I was still convinced that I probably had some, as of yet, undetected malignancy because of the severity of the symptoms. The pain was becoming continuous and now it was becoming very difficult to sit. I had to continually shift my weight back and forth or the pain would be triggered or exacerbated if I sat incorrectly. My mood was becoming somber as I knew I had an undetected fatal disease.

I began to take sleeping pills (Ambien, etc.) which seemed to allow me to sleep for some of the night free of pain but I would always wake up abruptly with pain. Unfortunately, after taking these pills for more then 2 or 3 consecutive nights they became ineffective and I couldn't think straight during the day. I never took any time off from work but I stopped my in-line skating (usually skated about 30 miles per week) as I felt that this might have somehow been the trigger. One day I noticed my urine was dark and tested it for blood and it was positive. I now knew that I had a cancer of the urological tract (kidneys, bladder, prostate, etc.) and became completely depressed.

I had no choice but to seek out the opinion of one of my urological colleagues who would do the appropriate studies and tell me that I had a cancer. The only problem with all of these thoughts is that I couldn't think of one of my patients in my career of now over a quarter of a century who had pelvic pain like I was having and found a cancer. In fact, prostate cancer almost never causes pain at it's origin in the pelvis (although one of the urologists that I consulted told me he knew of one case!). It does cause back pain after it has spread but by that time your x-rays are very abnormal-which mine were not. With much trepidation I consulted one of my urological colleagues who was quite kind and caring. I finally had a belated digital prostate examination (using a gloved finger) by the urologist who assured my prostate felt normal (except that the actual examination was quite painful). In fact, my prostate was of normal size which is actually a bit unusual by the time you reach your fifties. Most men by then have some non-cancerous enlargement of the prostate gland known as benign prostatic hypertrophy (BPH). My PSA (prostatic specific antigen) and other laboratory studies were normal.

The PSA test is a test used to help diagnose prostate cancer. He was still concerned however by the blood I found in my urine (rightfully so) but also told me he has seen that in others taking large amounts of anti-inflammatory medication (ibuprofen). I was panicked but now underwent a CAT (computerized axial tomography) scan of my kidneys, bladder and the rest of the urogenital tract. Unfortunately, the CT scan showed some abnormality at the base of the bladder. The urologist assured me that this was probably a variant of normal but in light of the blood in my urine and my pain he recommended a cystoscopy. This is a procedure I have had performed on many of my patients and seldom heard that it was particularly uncomfortable. It is frequently used to evaluate blood in the urine. A very long thin tube with fiberoptics in it is inserted through the tip of the penis and is passed until the bladder can be visualized. It is something I never want to go through again! It is extraordinarily painful and my symptoms for the next few days were even worse then before. I was now in complete agony.

I was getting increasingly depressed. I had near constant pelvic and low back pain and slept poorly. I began to fear going to sleep at all and was exhausted all day long. The urologist had reassured me that there was no evidence of cancer as evidenced by a normal physical examination, normal laboratory and x-ray studies, and a normal cystoscopy. He concluded that I had *chronic prostatitis* but was puzzled because "most of those guys were really uptight." He said my prostate was congested and needed to be de-compressed. He suggested frequent hot baths, frequent ejaculations, and a trial of medications. The medications recommended were either "alpha blockers" such as Flomax, Hytrin, Cardura, or Uroxatral or drugs that shrink the prostate such as Proscar or Avodart. The alpha blockers are usually used to help alleviate the urinary frequency and decreased force of stream caused by BPH.

I have prescribed these drugs many times over the years to many of my patients. I tried 2 of these drugs, exactly one time each to see if they would help with my symptoms. I promptly developed a rapid heart beat and dizziness with each of these drugs and had to discontinue them. Of course, they had no effect whatsoever on the pain. I then began Proscar (also used for BPH symptoms), being warned that this drug may take many months to be effective for prostatitis. I was also concerned about the the potential side effects of this drug which includes erectile dysfunction as well as gynecomastia (breast enlargement in males)! While I was concerned about these side effects my symptoms were increasingly taking over my life and I felt I had to do something as I was starting to feel that I don't want to live if this continued.

I thus began taking the Proscar. I had by now stopped taking the ibuprofen due to stomach upset and it seemed to have no impact on the pain anyway. I would take the sleeping pills every 3rd night or so. It was a kind of "treat" so I could sleep more then 2 hours and not be awakened with pain. Unfortunately, the pain continued and I was now crying intermittently. This was making life difficult at home and at work. The summer was over and the kids were back to school and I was miserable. I then began to experience urinary frequency. It began gradually but over the next several months I developed the need to urinate almost every hour. At its worst I would be going every 15 minutes and it made it difficult to see patients. My staff knew something was wrong since I seemed to always be using the bathroom. To make matters worse, I couldn't quite get all of the urine out and it would wet my underwear and trousers occasionally making this very embarrassing. I was beginning to see why some people might contemplate suicide with severe medical problems. I was also losing weight as my mood worsened and I didn't want to eat.

I consulted several other urologists during this period. These were doctors in my community that I knew and respected. They felt that I had chronic prostatitis and warned me the symptoms could go on for some time. This I didn't like to hear. One had suggested that he felt drinking a large volume of liquid was important and he thought beer was particularly well suited to this. I dutifully increased my fluid intake (not beer though-it made medical practice a bit difficult) which unfortunately just exacerbated my urinary frequency. Another urologist recommended a supplement called "Quercetin" which I dutifully began taking. The increased sex which was highly recommended by all (sounds like a great idea in general) did not seem to help and in fact, was becoming uncomfortable. I experienced no difficulty having an erection but it was painful and orgasm uncomfortable. I was feeling as despondent as could be. I now was developing constipation which required stool softeners, fiber supplements, and frequent suppositories.

It all came to a head in November. I had tickets for a rock band that I had seen several times since the seventies. They were performing in LA for only one night at the Kodak theatre (where the Academy Awards have been held in recent years). I was becoming nervous because my seat was not an aisle seat and I feared having to go to the bathroom frequently and bothering people. I also wasn't sure that I could make the trip in Los Angeles traffic without having to stop to go to the bathroom! In any event, as soon as the first number was being played I had to urinate. The rows were so close together that everybody had to stand to let me out. By the time I reached the aisle I was crying uncontrollably. I stayed ultimately to half-time but only in the lobby. I couldn't bear going back to my seat and went home very depressed. I was truly at my wit's end.

My wife started to check out Internet web sites to see if there was something else new to treat "chronic prostatitis." I must admit I didn't encourage my wife in this regard. I assumed (wrongfully in retrospect) that it was unlikely to yield any help for me. As a physician with twenty-five years experience and after having consulted several urologists I thought it unlikely that I would find any help there. I also remember how many patients brought me useless Internet information with regards to their health problems. My wife printed out a few pages from Dr. Wise's web site (www.pelvicpainhelp.com) and put them on my desk at home. She pointed out that my constellation of symptoms were almost exactly what Dr. Wise discussed. She read about the *Stanford Protocol* and correctly concluded that my symptoms were stress-related and he might be able to help me.

I still was not quite ready to accept having a stress-related disorder. I reluctantly purchased the book (I have never bought a self-help book in my life). When the book finally arrived I started to read it but had to put it down when I noticed that some people had these symptoms for decades. I didn't know this and this made me feel more discouraged and didn't feel I could even keep reading! Meanwhile, there was no let up at all in my symptoms. My life revolved around pain, urinary frequency, constipation, and increasing depression. I found no joy in anything, including my children.

It was now November of 2005 and I didn't know where to turn. My wife finally coaxed me into calling Dr. Wise to see if he could offer any help. I was pretty skeptical. I assumed that if he had the answer— everybody would know it. Effective treatments for diseases are not secret and if they are successful everybody realizes it sooner or later. The urologists I had consulted would have the same information-right? When I spoke with Dr. Wise in November he seemed to know about my symptoms in some detail and also that my only relief (however temporary) was from the sleeping pills. This relief from sleeping pills comes, in part, from their effect as muscle relaxants. Other drugs in this general category include benzodiazepams such as Valium (diazepam), Ativan (lorazepam), and Xanax (aprazolam). I never did take any of these medications as they are generally used in anxiety type disorders.

I still didn't think my symptoms were related to something like that. In any event, Dr. Wise felt that he would be able to help and urged me to come up to Sebastopol for the *Stanford Protocol* clinic. I signed up for the December, 2005 session. I felt some brief alleviation in my symptoms after this conversation-likely related to some relaxation due to feeling there maybe some help for me after all and I was going to do something about it. I picked up *A Headache in the Pelvis* again and read on before my trip North. My brief and slight improvement in symptoms was extremely short-lived as the time got nearer to going for the *Stanford Protocol*. It just seemed to me that this was going to be a waste of my time and money and I was utterly despondent, although I had some faint hope that maybe this treatment would help.

The time had come. I flew to the Bay Area and rented a car to see a urologist who confirmed the diagnosis of the "chronic pelvic pain" syndrome. While waiting to see him I remember going out to eat (although I no longer had any appetite) to get some strength and feeling that I should just turn around and go home because I really felt that nothing could be done. I drove up to Bodega Bay and spent the night absolutely despondent in a very beautiful and serene location. I could not even enjoy these beautiful surroundings and felt that if I can't get help here there is no solution at all. When I arrived in Sebastopol, I was taking Proscar, Quercetin, Cipro (in case there really was an infection!), mineral oil, psyllium (fiber supplements), suppositories (in case the oil and psyllium didn't work), and of course, sleeping medication.

I drove out the first morning to Dr. Wise's compound expecting nothing and feeling ridiculous having come all this way. I met the other dozen or so patients who also made the journey with symptoms more or less similar to what I was experiencing—many of them had had symptoms for years! The surrounding was peaceful and the environment created by Dr. Wise and his staff quite nurturing. We spent long days together doing group relaxation, learning stretches, and having *Trigger Point Release* by Tim Sawyer. By the end of the first day I noticed that somehow the need to urinate had improved slightly and that I didn't have to always get up during these sessions. I also noted that the pain itself would diminish (although at first just temporarily) after the *Trigger Point Release* sessions.

I was still symptomatic that first evening but had a glimmer of hope that there may be something to these interventions. I certainly wasn't ready to abandon any of my pills yet! There were four additional days of relaxation sessions, stretching, *Trigger Point Release* (this entails direct pressure with a gloved lubricated finger on tender areas in the rectum which in effect transmits pressure to the underlying muscles which are in spasm) and discussion. I woke up on the third morning (after 2 days of therapy) and had my first normal bowel movement in months. This is not normally reason for celebration but I was feeling increasingly hopeful. I experienced progressive improvement over the ensuing days of the program with diminution of all of the symptoms I had been experiencing. The symptoms did wax and wane and I was hopeful when they improved but still depressed when they returned. I completely stopped the Proscar, Quercetin, and Cipro on the last night. I concluded that these drugs play absolutely no role in this disorder. (The other possible explanation which I consider highly unlikely is that suddenly all of these drugs "cured me"—I finally had taken them long enough!).

My pain, constipation, urinary frequency, and most importantly, mood, had dramatically improved. I distinctly remember sitting in the airplane terminal in Oakland going back to Los Angeles and feeling completely euphoric! I was totally asymptomatic! I have never enjoyed being in an airport so much in my entire life. I did not have to use the bathroom even one time from my arrival at the airport until I touched down in Los Angeles (probably a total of 3 hours overall). That was the longest voiding interval I had in probably 3-4 months.

Alas, much as Dr. Wise predicted, my euphoria and lack of symptoms were not to last. When I arrived back in Los Angeles and went back to the stress of my career and life the symptoms came back over about a weeks time, although not to the extent they were before the *Stanford Protocol* clinic. I continued to listen to his tapes as much as possible and do the stretches I was taught 3-4 times per day. It was time-consuming and I was trying to do everything I was taught including reducing work and personal stress which is probably the hardest thing to control. The symptoms again improved over the next several months using the tapes and stretching and I was feeling hopeful although there were continued exacerbations and remission of my symptoms. I did not initially have the *Trigger Point Release* done when I came back to Los Angeles as I was trying to see if I could get by without it. I had improved significantly but now hoped for complete resolution of my symptoms. I asked my physical therapist (who I had known and used for years for a variety of minor musculoskeletal conditions) if he would be willing to learn the technique. I gave him a copy of *A Headache in the Pelvis* which he read. After several sessions he was able to perform the *Trigger Point Release* effectively. Luckily for me he previously used *Trigger Point Release* techniques extensively in a variety of musculo-skeletal conditions and he was quite sensitive to the obvious delicate nature of this particular type of intervention. I began the *Trigger Point Release* therapy weekly in Los Angeles in March of 2006 (approximately three months after leaving Sebastopol). With the addition of this to my daily stretching and 2-3 times weekly relaxation tapes I have had minimal symptoms since about the beginning of May, 2006. I attribute all of the success to the method that Dr. Wise and his colleagues have worked out. I take no medication whatsoever right now and have no constipation, urinary frequency, and virtually no pain. I also can sit in any chair I want without a cushion (which I failed to mention that I had to take to restaurants when my symptoms were at their worst).

It might be nice if there were a "simpler approach" that was successful. Who wouldn't want resolution of something like this with a couple pills for a week or two. Unfortunately, I do not believe that exists. I actually find it remarkable that the therapy (at first blush somewhat complex) could be figured out at all. It requires a multiple modality approach over time. It is not a simple therapy which a 15 minute office visit is going to solve. As I discovered when trying to eliminate the *Trigger Point Release*, it is clear that all of the recommendations by Dr. Wise appear necessary (at least they were for me). I also strongly feel that the intensive initial approach to this disorder (such as the *Stanford Protocol*) is necessary. I think that had I tried all of the components piecemeal I might have still improved but I think it would have taken much longer… maybe never.

As a physician I am almost shocked about the lack of knowledge and ridiculous suggestions about this disorder by the urologists I had consulted. I mentioned earlier the recommendation to drink beer. Some of the other sexual recommendations are almost comical such as "not holding back" during sex and having sex exactly 3 times per week. To their credit, they didn't seem offended when I offered to give them a copy of Dr. Wise's book. As Dr. Wise pointed out in his book there are a multitude of reasons that urologists are not enlightened about this disorder which is indeed unfortunate as it is one of the most common disorders for which urologists are consulted. It certainly has changed the way I treat patients with this disorder. As a primary care physician I see many patients with this disorder first. After appropriate evaluation and a clear diagnosis I recommend Dr. Wise's book. I would only have them see a urologist if there is something unusual which requires intervention that only a urologist can offer. Hopefully there will be further research on this disorder but there is no doubt in my mind that the approach of Dr. Wise is the correct one for those afflicted with this disorder.

A day has not gone by since I returned from Sebastopol when I have not thought of my experience there and how grateful I am to Dr. Wise that I have been able to return to my life.

Story of a 39 year old woman

I struggled with pain during intercourse since I lost my virginity at age 17. It was extremely painful that first time and continued to be so for nearly 20 years. For many years, I had no idea that it wasn't supposed to hurt. I was in major denial not wanting to face this very personal and sensitive subject. While I always heard others (personally and in the media) talk about the joys of sex, I absolutely could not relate. Sex for me was filled with anxiety, fear and literal physical pain. I suffered from embarassment and shame when hearing others talk about sex (as well as during my own sexual encounters since I could never be honest with my partners).

After meeting my husband at the age of 34, I finally faced this situation. I considered surgery but then got pregnant shortly thereafter (through painful intercourse). Since the doctors thought a vaginal birth might help with my pain, they advised to wait until I gave birth. Unfortunately, I had a c-section. A few months later, my husband and I visited Dr. Wise's clinic in Sebastopol. After learning and doing the physical therapy and breathing exercises for just a few weeks, we had nearly pain free sex and I got pregnant again! I continued with the breathing exercises and physical therapy daily for the following 9 months. I credit the relaxation I achieved from these exercises with helping me have a vaginal birth with no drugs whatsoever (this was only 12 months after a drug-filled c-section!). The vaginal birth has made a tremendous difference for me. I oftentimes now have no pain or discomfort during intercourse. I hope that continuing with Dr. Wise's protocol will make me 100% pain-free in the near future.

Dr. Wise's protocol is not an easy fix. It takes time, patience and perseverance. But I do believe it helps shift the anxiety response that my body has been conditioned into after nearly 20 years of dealing with painful intercourse. It has helped me be more comfortable with my own body and in relating sexually to my husband with more comfort, pleasure and therefore, intimacy.

Story of 27-year-old businessman

"My pelvic pain started at the left tip of my penis. I went to over twenty doctors, checked myself into the hospital emergency room, did a CT scan, ultrasounds, and many other schemes to find the cause of this pain. Gradually my pain spread and sitting, sleeping, walking and every part of living was painful. Through my research on the Internet I believed I may have pudendal nerve entrapment. I had a pudendal nerve latency test. It came back positive, showing irregular reactions from my pudendal nerve. PNE was a term that horrified me. The information on the Internet indicated that given my test results I would never be able to have pain-free sex, sitting would always be painful, and as time went on I would get worse. I read online that some people were trying new physical therapy techniques to improve their condition. I found a local therapist and started to work with her. I started to feel slightly better with internal trigger point releases. However, despite the temporary relief, I always found the pain returning. She gave me a bunch of books to read. One of them being *A Headache in the Pelvis*. I was overwhelmed that there was a book out there that described my condition in full detail. The approach to healing also made sense to me. I attended the clinic and learned the complete guide to self-healing.

I was finally empowered to take control of my condition. I completely dedicated my life to healing. I would spend anywhere from four to eight hours per day doing *Paradoxical Relaxation*, stretches, skin rolling, jogging and hot tub. I actually invested in a hot tub and a treadmill. That's how dedicated I was. Within four months I was completely pain free. Through my process, I had many realizations. The most important was, in order to fully recover in the minimum amount of time, the protocol had to be followed religiously. If I did three out of the four steps, I would have relief, but not full recovery. I evaluated my therapy, and tried to improve it. I realized that I couldn't do skin rolling on my back side as effectively on myself as a therapist could. So, I went to a PT just for skin rolling. Sure enough, that was the missing piece in my puzzle. Once I complied with the protocol 100%, I felt 100% better. I just want to thank Dr. Wise again, you have saved my life, without the protocol, I probably would have been in physical and mental pain forever, THANK YOU!"

Story of a 44 year old male hedge fund manager

I have been meaning to write you a note for some time. I have benefitted greatly from your program and my symptoms have decreased to the level of being insignificant. I continue with the protocol and have taken up yoga on a regular basis to improve my stretching. I have used your relaxation techniques repeatedly to help deal with the stress I have experienced with my work. While this has probably been the single worst year of my career and I have lost significant amounts of money in my business (I manage a hedge fund), my pelvic pain has disappeared using your protocol. I used to experience discomfort while sitting and I have not experienced this since October. Additionally, my urination has returned to normal. I continue to stretch and relax and while I have reduced the frequency, I continue to do the internal trigger point release. Most of all, I have the confidence that I have the tools to deal with the symptoms should they reoccur. My life was hell for a few months during the first half of 2008 due to pelvic pain. My working life has been hell since September due to the stock market crash, but I am so thankful that I have my health and wellbeing and am amazed that I have been able to get better while experiencing the severe stress caused by the lousy stock market.

Once again, Thank You and Happy New Year

Story of a 47 year old woman

I picked up the second edition of this book and couldn't put it down. For once someone understood, it got straight to the heart of the matter After 30 years of mild pain followed by 7 years of chronic and severely debilitating pain I knew I was on the right path. It had felt for years that I was in emotional solitary confinement, unable to share the extent of the pain with anyone who could really know what I was talking about.

I had read articles that depicted pelvic pain sufferers as the lepers of the medical world. Consultants had made me feel psychotic, untreatable, and an "interesting and perplexing" case. Complementary and physical therapists had been supportive and really helped. However many years on and £30,000 later I had some of the jig saw pieces and had started to make some progress towards full health but it wasn't until I read this book that the full picture emerged.

It was time to bear the cost and take my pelvic pain thousands of miles away to Dr Wises' seminar. A decision I didn't regret. I arrived in California and met fourteen men and women with the one common denominator of pelvic pain and its debilitating effects on life. However we didn't wallow in mutual pity as each one of us had the positive intent to return to full health. Some had feared that a mixed group of pelvic pain sufferers would be embarrassing but we quickly got to know each other and respect each other's privacy. We would talk candidly and even have moments of humour about our pain.

Our discretion was assured through the protocol being called a "seminar" rather than clinic. If anyone had peered into the room of neatly layed out mats with pillows and blankets they may have wondered what was going on. This was our paradoxical relaxation room where Dr Wise in his unflappable manner talked us through his immense knowledge of the subject. It was also where he taught us the art of paradoxical relaxation. We shuffled, scratched, snored and fidgeted but eventually, one by one, found moments of peace where we could truly sink into the feeling of letting go, accepting how our bodies felt and giving up the fight to control the pain. Throughout our lives many of us realised we had strived; for perfection, to excel, to achieve and … to get better. We had worked hard at getting better, very hard, and now we were learning that the secret was exactly the opposite; NOT to work hard at it! Here in Santa Rosa was the dawning realisation that to get better we needed to let go of doing anything, accept our pain and learn how to relax; profoundly.

Every day of the protocol we each had a session with Tim Sawyer, the protocol's chief Physical Therapist. I wondered if Tim had ever dreamed as a child of becoming a therapist. One who excelled at teaching patients to self massage pelvic muscles which lay deep inside their "private parts." Possibly not. And yet what a gift he gave all of us. He taught us to find trigger points, those knotty sore areas of muscle that triggered pain elsewhere. There was no embarrassment thanks to his professionalism and I now feel quite adept at this strange but wonderfully relieving skill.

Five days later I left Santa Rosa feeling renewed in spirit and knowing that I was on a journey that would lead to a full recovery. Eleven months after my visit I am 90% better. I have learnt to recognise tension and to relax, not just when I'm listening to the tapes, but as I climb stairs, walk the streets, work, lie in bed, watch TV and do every day chores. My levels of awareness are heightened and I am able to recognise what may cause a "flare up" and how to avoid it. Together with Claire, my physical therapist in the UK, I am learning to exercise again, breathe properly and to build up the other muscles that remained weak as my overly-strong pelvic muscles took the strain. I am learning new habits to replace those that have exasperated the pelvic pain and to sink into Dr Wises' protocol and work with it rather than "try hard" at it.

You can't beat this pain by trying, striving or driving for a cure. You have to be with it, allow it, almost befriend it and then slowly it subsides; that's the amazing paradox.

Story of 25-year-old attorney

In 2001, when I was twenty-three years-old, I was walking to class and started to feel a pain at the tip of my penis. It was a mixture of stinging and burning, and it would hurt terribly as it rubbed against my clothes. I figured I had a urinary tract infection, and went to the school infirmary to see a general practitioner. The doctor found no infection, and referred me to a urologist. The urologist also found no infection, and said that there was nothing wrong with me. In a way, I believed him wholeheartedly, and even wanted to. Of course, the pain was still there. For over a year, I simply put up with the pain, not wearing blue jeans or other rough clothing. Sometimes the pain wasn't that bad, sometimes it was terribly annoying. I developed other symptoms: pain in the urethra during ejaculation and afterwards, frequency and urgency related to urination. Although not relating it to my pain then, another symptom that I had dealt with since a teenager was nervous stomach, that is, always seeming to have a bowel movement before any significant event of pressure. However, the severity of my symptoms always stayed manageable, and I carried on without telling a soul about my symptoms.

I had always been a popular and successful young man. I did very well in school and always had a plethora of friends and girlfriends. I never had any social anxiety, and was extremely gregarious and outgoing. Looking back, however, it is clear that I dealt with extreme anxiety. I am an intense, type A personality, always having to do more and more and more, and no amount of work or pressure or activity ever seemed enough. I lived almost manically in my professional and personal life, and I could never seem to get enough of any aspect of life. I was searching for something, but had no idea what it was. Again, looking back, I can see that my pain and symptoms, combined with my manic and unpeaceful personality, was causing deep emotional and psychological problems in my life. I lost relationships with people that I loved very much. I began to withdraw from social circles, and spent more and more time alone.

As I graduated from professional school and started my working life, my pain started to get worse. I was in a high-stress job, and my pain began to spread into my legs, perineum, hips and back. From 2001 until 2004 (when I discovered the *Stanford Protocol*), I went to several different urologists, and basically I got the same treatment as most other men diagnosed with prostatitis: antibiotics, anti-inflammatories, and even anti-depressants for "psychosomatic" pain. Nothing helped. The drugs actually made things worse because they masked my natural intuition about what was going on with me. Finally, my pain exploded, and I could no longer carry on my routine I was in so much distress. I hurt 24/7, and I fell into severe depression. I truly believed my life was over. I had a dark night of the soul.

Then, I found *A Headache in the Pelvis* on the Internet. I read it and it described perfectly what I was experiencing. In fact, I never had a doubt from the beginning regarding the muscular basis of the *Stanford Protocol*, as I had been abusing myself through the old, high-school athletic modes of weightlifting and contraction. My entire body, and especially my pelvis, was riddled with trigger points. Immediately I went to California and attended one of the clinics. I learned *Paradoxical Relaxation* from Dr. Wise and the basics of trigger point therapy from Tim Sawyer, both internally and externally. I immediately felt better, but knew that I had a very long way to go before I could consistently reduce my symptoms.

During these past two years that I have been practicing the *Stanford Protocol*, there have been many ups and downs. However, I never doubted the efficacy of the program and knew that such steps forward and back were what had to occur for true healing to happen. Drugs are easy and mask the problem; true healing takes faith, commitment, and compassion for oneself. I have always continued to improve. In fact, the setbacks for me were not that I physically felt any worse, but rather I had to work through my anger about no one ever teaching these wonderful truths about my muscles to me, and how it related to the central nervous system arousal in my life. I was mad that I had not been raised on the teachings in a Headache in the Pelvis. Of course, the *Paradoxical Relaxation* helps tremendously when these suppressed emotional responses begin to surface.

My pelvic musculature is, I would say, about 97% healed, and I know over the course of the next year it will slowly dissolve.

Story of an 82 year old woman

You may very well forgotten me since we have not communicated by phone since the spring of 2004. It is about time that I reported to you on my progress.

With the recommendation of Dr. Jeanette Potts, Cleveland Clinic, you agreed to give me instruction by phone detailing your wonderful program on pelvic pain. At that time in my life I could not possibly have flown to California since my pain was so constant and intense. I regret that, of course, and know that I would have benefitted greatly.

However, I want you to know that since 2004 I literally immersed myself in the tapes, exercises and your book. I did a tape and exercises every day and a therapeutic massage nearly every week until the end of 2007.

My whole mindset has changed. The more knowledge I gained the more my body calmed down. My lifelong pattern of trying to be perfect has eased considerably. Looking back over the years I can see the tension I created for myself. And I finally admitted that I was the one who had to change and take the time to retrain myself. And it has taken time. I have been free of pain for over five months. This is totally wonderful since I began this situation in 1988.

I continue to do the tapes and exercises several times a week and from time to time read a few pages of your book. These things seem to be necessary to maintain my good health, etc. now that I am approaching 81 (!) there will hopefully be a few more good years!

My sincere thanks to you and Dr. Potts, as well as Betsy O'D. and my massage therapist. You all have contributed to my well-being so greatly. I appreciate all of you and pray that your good work will continue to help others.

I neglected to mention how supportive my wonderful husband is. He has gone through a lot with me.

Story of a 22 year old male

I attended the clinic you held this past December and I wanted to take the time to update you on how I'm doing.

When I came to you I was in dire straits. I had seen probably 20 doctors, spent months in physical therapy, and had a 'pelvic floor repair' operation, all without any positive results and increasing frustration and depression. I had played football my whole life and had always been a physically active person. I was unable to do anything involving exercise for about two and a half years since the symptoms got to their worst point. I had to stop playing football and eventually left college altogether. Attending your clinic was truly going to be my last attempt at getting better before I planned on resigning to a life of inactivity and unbearable depression.

I'm still somewhat astounded at my own focus in staying with the protocol even when after a month or two I wasn't feeling better. I actually don't even want to give a summary of my recovery because I don't feel far enough away from it to revisit it. But a couple months ago I started to notice improvement and now I feel almost back to normal. As I've told the friend from the clinic I've stayed in touch with, if I was about 50% when I arrived in California, I'd say I'm about 90-95% now, and still getting better. I've rekindled most of the relationships that I cut off during my time with the symptoms and it seems like there's only good things ahead. I'm going back to college this fall and plan on playing football for the school.

There's no way to express how thankful I am for you and your staff. I really don't know what to say other than I honestly believe this protocol saved me from going to a bad place emotionally, to say the least.

I know saying thank you doesn't even begin to cover it, but thank you,

Patient report after 2 years of practicing protocol

In the summer of 1998 at the age of twenty-one, I started to experience urinary frequency. It started out mild. In the mornings I would wake up to urinate and then lie back down in bed and not feel that I had completely emptied my bladder. I ignored it at first but after it persisted for a couple of weeks I decided something must be wrong and went to see a urologist. He was unable to culture anything from my prostatic fluid, the extraction of which was the first of many uncomfortable and unnecessary procedures. He decided anyway that I must have a low-level infection of the prostate. I started taking antibiotics and it seemed to help initially--the first of a myriad of expensive and unnecessary medications which seemed to help at the outset. Before I finished the medication the symptoms returned and after it was finished they remained.

The urologist was unable to provide any further recommendations. The next urologist I saw in December of 1998 had me pee into a uroflow device to measure my flow rate. He printed out a nice little graph to show me how my flow rate was lower than average and informed me that I had a urethral stricture which would require a dilation under general anesthesia and a prescription to Hytrin®. Anxious to be rid of my symptoms, I eagerly underwent the procedure. Improvement lasted only about 2 weeks.

When I called the urologist several weeks later to ask about my returning symptoms he instructed me to keep taking the Hytrin®, which I did for several months to no avail. My symptoms gradually worsened, but I did not experience any pain––only frequency.

I moved to San Francisco in August of 1999 and made an appointment to see a doctor at a prominent university whose specialties included chronic pelvic pain syndromes. He suggested that I might have interstitial cystitis and recommended I undergo a hydrodistention under general anesthesia to verify this. In February of 2000 I underwent the procedure and the results were uncertain. It was a "soft call" as to whether I had IC. I definitely lacked classic IC symptoms (no pain, no prominent food sensitivities) but the doctor could think of nothing else it was likely to be.

Soon I began a cycle of trying out new medications, becoming excited that they were working at first and then quickly becoming disappointed as my symptoms returned and remained. The frequency gradually became worse than it had ever been before, but still it was only frequency and not pain. There was some extremely uncomfortable frequency at times (bathroom visits 15-20 times a day and 4-6 times a night) but nothing I would describe as pain ever manifested. Also at this time I was beginning a new job which was significantly stressful. In retrospect I think this was a major factor in the worsening of my symptoms, along with a spiral of hopelessness as each new medicine I tried failed to help. I tried the usual battery of meds that is prescribed for IC and after 6 months when it seemed they were not working at all I began to try other things such as numerous over-the-counter herbs, additional prescription antibiotics of different types, the hypertension drug Amlodipine®, etc. etc.

I estimate I tried 20-25 different medicines or products over the life of my symptoms, none of which helped me to any significant degree. I tried transcutaneous electrical nerve stimulation. I underwent two urodynamic evaluations at two universities (both requiring catheterization while awake) and there were no remarkable insights gleaned from either study. I spent countless hours combing the

Internet and the university medical library for some additional scrap of information that might prove useful.

Eventually I stumbled onto an article written by David Wise on www. prostatitis.org called "The New Theory of Prostatitis as a Tension Disorder." I contacted David and since he was in my area I went to see him in November of 2000. I made some half-hearted attempts to start the relaxation therapy at home but didn't really begin it in earnest until early January, 2001. It was very difficult to sit through an entire tape at first and I squirmed and fidgeted throughout most of the tape. The therapy certainly teaches you patience. At this time I also began seeing a physical therapist recommended by David who specializes in CPPS.

With the combination of relaxation twice a day and physical therapy once a week I slowly began to see some steady improvement in my frequency over many weeks' time. It was always the case that I felt better for a day or two and then felt worse again for a stretch of days, but over time the good days began to outweigh the bad. The good days that I did have were the best days that I'd experienced in over a year. These days were extremely encouraging and the memory of them is what carried me through the bad stretches, although after many bad days in a row it was often easy to think that I had been fooling myself.

When a good stretch occurred, though, it seemed unmistakable that my symptoms were improving. I had many good stretches that occurred with increasing frequency throughout March, April, and May, and by June '01 for the first time since they had begun I felt that I had a solid handle on my symptoms—that I was on the sure path to healing myself completely. I would definitely become cocky at times and stop doing the relaxation or stretches. My symptoms would not immediately return but if I persisted in a chronic state of stress for some time without paying attention to what was going on in my pelvis then they would creep back and suddenly demand my attention. In fact I can still say that this is the case—that I experience low-level symptoms from time to time but they are not something I fear anymore because I understand the factors that lead to their appearance and the factors that lead to their abatement. In addition, the intensity is very, very minor compared to what it was at the height of my misery. When symptoms do occur they are so subtle that they hardly enter my consciousness and I experience myself as having completely normal bladder behavior.

I practice the formal relaxation less frequently now (2-5 times a week depending on how things are going) and my pelvis seems to be perfectly happy with that. I live my life in a more relaxed state overall and that makes all the difference.

I consider myself lucky when I read other peoples' accounts of their experiences with CPPS. However I would not hesitate at all to describe my own experience as a waking nightmare. I remember in the midst of it coming home from work exhausted and collapsing onto my couch in tears, not sure if I could hold down my job, if I would have to move back home with my mother, etc. My social life was severely impacted. I skipped countless activities on account of how uncomfortable I felt and because I dreaded having to go to the bathroom every 30 minutes in public. I didn't date for 3 years. I sunk further and further into misery and desperation and I believe my symptoms would have continued to worsen had I not found David's article online.

The relaxation techniques were a godsend for me. They have helped me in more ways than in just the abatement of my symptoms. I feel more centered now, more at peace in general. In one way of looking at it I can consider my symptoms to have been a gift, because they are the only thing that could have led me to devote so much of my time to the relaxation, which in retrospect I desperately needed though I have never thought of myself as an uptight person. I have never battled with depression except as a result of my symptoms. I have only experienced mild anxiety from time to time and always as a result of outside circumstances. However I believe now that I am genetically predisposed to holding the tension that I do feel in my pelvic muscles. I say it's a genetic predisposition because of the fact of my maternal grandfather's identical symptoms and the existence of bladder problems in general on my mom's side of the family.

A metaphor I have found useful is that one's pain can be like a compass –it's trying to lead you to where you need to be. The story of my own struggle has in a sense been the story of learning to read my personal compass and to trust it and check in with it every now and then, with the goal of not having to check in with it at all because I am following it all the time without effort. When I was physically suffering it's like the compass was shoved in my face and I would get really gung-ho about the relaxation. When the symptoms abated I started to wander off the path, but like I said this was necessary for learning. Now the compass is much clearer to me even when I'm not suffering and I can detect the path intuitively.

In sum, I suffered from prostatitis/CPPS for three years and my life became absolutely miserable. I received four different diagnoses from four urologists, tried over 20 prescription medications, vitamins, and herbs, and underwent several very uncomfortable and expensive procedures, all of which did hardly anything to help my symptoms which had slowly been increasing in intensity over time. Using the protocol described in *A Headache in the Pelvis*, I slowly I began to heal myself, without any medication. Six months later my symptoms were diminished significantly and nine months later I felt I was healed. It is now 2-1/2 years after I first started to practice these methods and I feel that I have been freed of this horrific condition.

There are many schools of thought regarding this syndrome and I studied all of them obsessively at one time. I feel very strongly however that over the coming years the ideas in this book will eclipse the other models of this disease and come to be recognized as the most powerful methods for dealing with it as more and more people are seen to have solid and long-lasting benefits. Mine is not the last testimonial you will see. I should say however that it is not a simple or quick solution and it requires a lot of devotion, but chances are the end-result will be your freedom. My advice to those who are still suffering is "best of luck; do not abandon hope until you have given these methods your most sincere effort."

Patient report after practicing protocol for 8 months

I am a 35-year-old male who, until recently, suffered from chronic prostatitis for over fifteen years. I am writing to share my experience in hope that someone else currently suffering from my predicament can heal as I have.

Starting at about age eighteen, I began to notice symptoms of high urinary frequency and a great sense of urgency when I felt the need to urinate. By the time I was twenty-four, the symptoms reached the point where I was uncomfortable much of the day. I went to see multiple doctors, including several urologists who did several invasive procedures. I had diagnoses that ranged from chronic prostatitis to a narrow bladder neck. Other than taking alpha-blockers, doctors told me they could not do much to help me.

I somehow learned to get by with my symptoms. I always sat on the aisle row of a movie theater or airplane to facilitate my many visits to the restroom. I would map out the restrooms first upon entering a new mall or other unfamiliar place. I tried to avoid any event where I would not be assured access to a restroom hourly. I typically felt the urge to urinate every hour during the day. Multiple visits to the restroom at night were not uncommon. I budgeted more time to sleep because the quality of my sleep was so poor.

In October of 2002, the inconvenient and annoying symptoms of my condition turned into a persistent pain. Urinating no longer relieved, even temporarily, the pain and sense of urgency to urinate. I felt pain in and around my urethra, my bladder, and my prostate. Multiple visits to several urologists resulted in a diagnosis of "chronic prostatitis." I started taking any pharmaceutical that the doctors suggested, including antibiotics, alpha-blockers, Ambien® to sleep at night, muscle relaxants, and anti-inflammatory drugs. None of these helped. By Thanksgiving, I wasn't able to sleep more than a few hours per night. I began missing work. I spent entire days in tears. I suffered from panic attacks. I went to the emergency room. I started to avoid people as much as possible. My increasing anxiety made the pain even worse.

I can remember thinking in December 2002 that everything I had spent my whole life trying to achieve was coming to an end. I had an MBA from Harvard Business School. I had a great job. I had a loving wife and two children. I had a strong relationship with God. Yet, I couldn't see how I was going to survive. I didn't see how I could possibly maintain my job with this pain. I didn't even think I would be able to enjoy watching my children grow older. Sex was out of the question because it just exacerbated the symptoms. I would have gladly given up all my money and material possessions to be cured of the acute pain that plagued my every moment.

In desperation, I turned to the Internet. Fortunately, I learned about the work of Drs. Wise and Anderson. Contrary to many other approaches I read about on the Internet, their approach appealed to me because:

1. It had a fundamental basis. In other words, it made sense that the pain I was feeling was the result of constriction of the pelvic region.

2. It did not entail pharmaceuticals or surgery. Surgery is permanent. Pharmaceuticals were not working and had bad side-effects. I was intent on not resorting to narcotics of any kind.

3. Their approach allowed me to be proactive about my pain. Some Internet sites claim that chronic prostatitis is caused by an as-yet unidentified and untreatable infection. What good would it have done me to convince myself that I had an untreatable infection?

4. The symptoms I felt and the way I felt them matched those described in *A Headache in the Pelvis*.

5. My symptoms historically have been linked to stress. Having increased tension in the pelvis during times of stress seemed to fit my profile as well.

My wife drove me to San Francisco to start therapy. I first saw a urologist who ruled out other possibilities and confirmed that I might benefit from this course of therapy. I attended daily physical therapy with a therapist trained in the techniques. In addition to internal stretching performed by the therapist, I was put on a program to stretch various muscles and fascia daily. I began learning "moment-to-moment" relaxation. I also began learning and practicing the *Paradoxical Relaxation* technique. Within a week, I was much better. My wife drove me home to Los Angeles, where I continued physical therapy twice a week and later once a week for about three months. I became better and better at "moment-to-moment" relaxation of the pelvic muscles, to the point that I didn't need to think about relaxing those muscles any more. I continue daily *Paradoxical Relaxation* using tapes provided by Dr. Wise. Amazingly, the pain has diminished with each week that has passed. While there are occasional flare-ups the general trend was and continues to be in one direction–better.

It has now been eight months since I started this program. I have had to dedicate significant time to this effort. However, I feel like a miracle has been granted to me. My urinary frequency has dropped to only once per night and once per two hours, at most, during the day. I feel little, if any, pain. I feel almost no pain following sex. I am better than I have been in over 15 years!

Patient recovery with no physical therapy or formal relaxation training

While most patients require both *Paradoxical Relaxation* training and intrapelvic *Trigger Point Release*, we have received numerous emails from people reporting that their symptoms improved after the reading of our book and of hearing of a possible solution to their difficulty. Here is the story of a patient like this.

I first experienced prostatitis when I was around 23 years of age. Basically, I developed a rather noticeable pain in my left groin that simply irked the heck out of me and would not go away. Numerous urologists diagnosed it as epididymitis, but the funny thing was that it wasn't particularly responsive to the antibiotics that were prescribed. Moreover, it had this rather strange tendency to occasionally migrate to the right side, in which case the strong pain I had felt on the left would totally vanish. For about a year, it manifested primarily on the right side. Then, it switched back to the left. The discomfort generally didn't go away, though over time, what initially felt like a pretty distinct pain in my scrotum generally became a more generalized feeling of discomfort. It stuck with me throughout my graduate studies. Even during my first professional job in an office, it was there, without any sign of relief. Basically, it not only irritated me but also worried me tremendously.

After about eight years, I had pretty much resigned myself to living with that condition indefinitely, which was not a rosy picture at all. Luckily, by that time, the Internet had taken off as a vital source of medical information. After reviewing numerous websites, I came across the findings of Dr. Wise. I was struck by two things. The first was the startlingly accurate description of my condition in his writings. It seemed he had a handle on what was going on, which was namely that this "condition" seemed to be in a category all its own. The second thing was the real breakthrough: the possibility that the ultimate source of this discomfort was not any infection, not any structural abnormality, but simply TENSION, muscular tightness that restricted the entire area that was affected.

To make a long story short, this basic insight was nothing less than a breakthrough for me. I eagerly contacted Dr. Wise, to learn as much as I could about his "theories." I was always pleased to see that his model of prostatitis seemed to accurately reflect all the rather subtle qualities of this strange condition with which I had been living. For example, I noticed that my discomfort would increase dramatically whenever I had caffeine, or whenever I became stressed over anything. Perhaps the most important discovery offered by Dr. Wise was the knowledge that this condition had its origin ultimately in my own state of mind, or mental state of disease. As such, I knew I, myself, could fix it, simply by "unwinding," so to speak.

Within about a six month period after simply learning about what was really going on, I basically found the symptoms disappearing. In other words, simply realizing that my own thoughts and beliefs were at the root of this proved to be the best medicine. Simply by refusing to worry and, even simply by just understanding my condition, miraculously, the pain went away! Now of course, this does not mean there was no effort involved, or that it happened overnight. But the one thing that is clear is this: the less helpless I felt towards my situation, the more it improved.

Basically, the first step was just plain knowing that "nothing was wrong," and the second step was making a concerted effort to relax and work through and accept the pain, even when it was still there. By learning to see the pain as acceptable, so to speak, I managed to put it out of mind. Once I had gotten into a pattern of really being able to stop thinking about it (which is much easier once you know it has no real "physical" basis, at least not in the form of a virus), it just plain vanished! Basically, I am now free of prostatitis.

Patient report after practicing protocol for 2 years

In October of 2000 I had a vasectomy performed by a urologist in Toronto. Before the operation I inquired about its safety and the possibility of side effects. I was told the operation was routine and there was no possibility of any problems. In June of 2001, I began to experience severe pains in my testicles. These pains were severe enough to force me to give up employment. For several months I was unable to do much more than stay in bed. In addition to the pain I was unable to ejaculate. I saw a urologist at Mt. Sinai Hospital in Toronto who recommended a vasectomy reversal. It was scheduled, but as the pain spread from the testicles to the perineum and the entire pelvic area, my urologist felt that the reversal might do more harm than good.

He instead put me under the care of the pain clinic at the hospital. I was given large doses of opiates, 36 mg of hydromorphine contin per day, which lessened the pain but did nothing for the underlying condition. In November 2001, I came upon your article, "The New Theory That Prostatitis is a Tension Disorder." I spoke to Dr. Wise a number of times on the phone and in December 2001 went to California. I was seen by Dr. Rodney Anderson, urologist and Tim Sawyer, physiotherapist. My wife accompanied me on the visit and learned the technique of myofascial release inside the pelvic floor from Tim Sawyer.

At first my wife was unable to perform the internal massage because it was too painful, but after a month of external massaging, she was gradually able to do the internal work. She did this twice a week for about two months. It gradually became easier to do and eventually the frequency of the massages was much reduced. At the same time, I began daily relaxation exercises, using a course on tape. I also did various stretches recommended by Tim Sawyer.

The pain grew gradually less severe during 2002 and I gradually reduced the number of grams of painkiller I was taking. By the late months of 2002, I was taking only one mg. per day. Since January 2003 I have taken no painkillers on a regular basis. I visited Dr. Wise and Tim Sawyer again in March 2003. Tim was able to confirm a significant loosening inside the pelvic floor. I continue to feel some pain every day but rarely is the pain severe enough to take any opiate. The degree of pain from day-to-day varies a great deal.

Some days are entirely pain-free except for occasional discomfort in the pelvic area; some days involve pain for longer periods and more intensely. There is usually some pain during and after sexual intercourse, but ejaculations are normal. Occasionally I use aspirin or ibuprofen.

In general I would say I'm pain-free about three-quarters to seven-eighths of the time. For the other quarter or eighth the pain is present but bearable.

For a long while I was taking a drug called Imovane to help me sleep at night. I discontinued the Imovane about a month ago, but I am now frequently awakened by the need to urinate during the night, which is a disturbing problem. I have been advised to try Flomax, which I used at the height of the problem but discontinued about a year ago.

The relaxation exercises, myofascial release, and stretches seem to have helped me reduce my pain very significantly. Although I am not back at a full-time job I have been able to work part-time as a consultant and university lecturer. The alleviation of the pain has of course made life much more worth living for me. I am grateful for your patient and understanding help.

Patient report after 4 years of practicing protocol

Beginning in about 1992 (age 27), I experienced occasional pelvic pain, primarily the right side in an area stretching from my groin and extending upward. It was a dull ache. I am a military lawyer. I saw a civilian urologist who conducted a thorough pelvic and prostate exam and concluded there was nothing wrong with me (except a small, benign, and unremarkable spermatocele resting on the top of the right testicle). He examined my prostate fluid under a microscope with negative results. The pelvic pain was worse just above and to the right of the pubic bone and in the lower abdominal area.

When I was stationed overseas from 1994-1996, the pain became progressively worse. I tended to usually have a dull ache in the pelvis just above the pubic bone and to the right. The pain was worse if I had to stand for a long time (e.g. in a courtroom or on a subway). I got to where I would want to sit down and "rest" to relieve the ache, even though I was physically fit and not tired. I didn't want to walk anywhere. In concert with the pelvic pain, I experienced pain that would radiate down my right inner leg and back thigh and rear, sometimes as far down my leg as the calf.

Another symptom was that my urine flow was typically very, very slow. It would sometimes slow to an intermittent trickle, and I learned that if I took a deep breathe and exhaled while standing at the urinal, the flow rate would accelerate a bit. Usually, it took me a long time to urinate, and after going, my bladder still felt full. I remember during some of my first court trials in 1995, I had an intense urge to urinate, even after I just went, and it would feel as though I had to urinate virtually the entire day. During this time I started feeling an occasional, sudden, sharp pain somewhere inside the rectum. This pain would last for up to 10 seconds and would slowly release on its own. It was sometimes so intense and sharp that I was seized with pain and couldn't move until it subsided. (Imagine a severe toe cramp in your rectum). The pelvic pain level would fluctuate from between 0 to 4 or 5 on a scale of 10, and it was usually between a 1 to 3.

In addition to the pelvic pain, the pain in the inside thigh, and slow urination, I usually also felt a tight feeling in the area between the testicles and rectum for about an hour after sex, as though the path for the sperm had been tightened or blocked. In 1996, I moved to the West Coast, and these symptoms continued.

I went to several military urologists, both overseas and in California, who diagnosed me with chronic prostatitis. In 1997 I experienced these symptoms on and off. In 1998, the symptoms became worse. I was prescribed Ciprofloxin® 500 for about 75 days for chronic prostatitis. The doctors never found any evidence of a microbe infection in my prostate fluid. One doctor also inserted a lighted camera into my urethra and examined the path leading up to my kidneys and bladder—all tissue was healthy. After the antibiotics and tests, I still had an aching pelvis, and was still "double eliminating" (on the advice of one of the doctors, urinating 10 minutes after I urinated in order to try to make the bladder fully empty). My side ached nearly all the time and no one knew why.

Fortunately, the military urologist had heard a paper delivered by Dr. Rodney Anderson at a conference on prostate massage. The urologist thought Dr. Anderson might be able to help me, so he referred me to Stanford Medical Center. Dr. Anderson did a complete physical examination. That exam found the unremarkable spermatocele, but more importantly, some "pressure points" of pain. Dr. Anderson sent me immediately to see Dr. David Wise.

When I first began the treatment I was skeptical; I could not believe that my pain was unwittingly a self-inflicted wound. After I learned to be conscious of my body, and to reflect on the holding and tightness in my pelvis and the pain I felt, I became convinced. It took some time—months, and I cannot recall when I crossed the line, but I became absolutely certain that my symptoms were relieved by the protocol.

Over the course of my year of training in progressive (paradoxical) relaxation, I learned to totally relax my mind and body. When I received myofascial release therapy from a physical therapist prescribed by Dr. Wise, I could actually feel when the tension inside was released by stretching the tissue; it was instant and soothing relief when a "tight" spot was stretched. It got to where I could feel where the pressure point was and could direct the therapist to it quickly. My wife has also been trained in the myofascial release therapy, and she occasionally treated me in 1999 and early 2000, but stopped after the pain subsided. She stands willing to continue that protocol if the pain flares-up.

In the last four years, I have integrated this relaxation method into my life. Each day, I practice momentary relaxation and the deep relaxation, stretching (taught by the physical therapist), and breathing in concert with relaxation. I try to make time for one complete session of progressive (paradoxical) relaxation session each day, but in my current position I cannot always do so.

At the present time, I do a complete session of 45-55 minutes 2-3 times per week, and a shorter session of 15-25 minutes on all other days. I also practice conscious effortlessness throughout the day by relaxing the pelvis, and practice contractions, and stretches, which were taught by the physical therapist. I also do a continuous, almost subconscious series of checks throughout the day to search for and release any tightness and holding in my body, particularly in my pelvis and the sides of my face. When I practice relaxing my body, my head and neck become so relaxed that my head bobs gently and unconsciously with the flow of the blood to the head. As a result of this relaxation, the blood vessels in my body relax and widen, and after a few minutes, my hands and feet become flush with blood.

Because of my military job and lack of privacy in Washington, D.C., I have adapted and learned to practice a full session of progressive (paradoxical) relaxation while lying with my head on a towel in the building gym—with a loud game of basketball taking place on the court next to me, or while laying on the sidewalk or grass as planes landing at National Airport roar overhead. These conditions are not ideal for relaxation, but it does work well. Because I have been taught to effectively abandon effort, I can focus on my breathe and heartbeat rather than the noise. I don't fight or stress about the noise around me, but just let it be there as I drift away. I have done the same thing on a ship—with bells clanging and announcements being made over the loudspeaker. I have learned to be profoundly relaxed.

Usually I have no pelvic pain. It is usually nonexistent, but will fairly rarely be present at a low level if I become very stressed or busy at work. This stands in stark contrast to before I began the protocol when the pain was there all the time and occasionally severe.

One of the most important benefits is that I am certain of the source of the pain, conscious of the feeling and aware of the tendency to subconsciously tighten or hold the pelvis. I now feel how I tighten (and can focus on releasing) the tension. I am also aware of how the level of pain is linked to the pace of stress in my life. One more thing: until I wrote this, I had forgotten the emotional and mental worry, and fear that I had over what was mysterious pain and symptoms. Now I feel I am in control, the worry and fear have vanished. I know the recipe for getting well—discipline for exercising daily relaxation.

Until I wrote this I had also forgotten the slow urine flow that I used to have—standing at a urinal taking as long as four or five other men to urinate. My urine flow is now strong. I had also forgotten how I always had the feeling that I had to urinate soon after I already went. Now, I have a feeling of a totally empty and comfortable bladder. The discomfort after sex has now abated except for rare instances—it now occurs about twice a year. This treatment and protocol has changed my life.

Patient report after 5 years of practicing protocol

In late September of 1997, two years after retiring, I started having problems with urination. Some brownish colored "sediment" started showing up at the end of urination and then pelvic pain started. My pain was in the rectum and prostate areas. When I woke up in the morning there was generally no pain, but it built up during the day and was worst in the evenings. My internist prescribed an antibiotic and referred me to a urologist. The urologist prescribed traditional treatment for prostate infection including antibiotic and ibuprofen. After six weeks of treatment virtually no progress was made. I observed during this period that pain killers provided no relief but muscle relaxants did help. Naps on the floor were the only other thing that seemed to help.

The symptoms were ruining my life and at times I was depressed. I was losing weight and there didn't seem to be any light at the end of the tunnel.

A close friend got me an appointment in mid-December 1997 with Dr. Tom Stamey, the pioneer of urology who was still at Stanford. Dr. Stamey determined in one hour that I had no evidence of infection in the prostate gland and referred me to Dr. Anderson and Dr. Wise. I had no idea what form of treatment they would provide.

Dr. Anderson had me see a physical therapist that specialized in myofascial pelvic floor muscle pain relief. He relieved "trigger points" in various pelvic floor muscles and even taught the procedure to my wife who happens to also be a PT. I bought medical textbooks on myofascial pain and read extensively about the subject.

Dr. Wise started to teach me *Paradoxical Relaxation*. Gradually I started to make progress. One of the difficulties is that progress is an up and down process. I remember several times getting discouraged and phoning Dr. Wise. His calm, steady, reassurance was very helpful. One day, a few months after starting his therapy I asked him how long it would take to perfect his technique. He hesitated for a while but finally said "about two years."

After two months I had made enough progress to know that things were on the right track. Oddly, knowing it might take two years was encouraging as I knew what to expect and not to think that I would be all cured in a month. My progress steadily got better and after a year I was 80% better. After two years I felt like I had reduced my symptoms by 90%.

It is now about five years since I first started treatment with Drs. Anderson and Wise. I feel that my symptoms are 99% gone but more important I know how to deal with symptoms if they occur. Happily, I seldom think about the problem any more.

Story of 44-year-old physician

I first met Dr. Wise at age 44 with a fifteen-year history of constant urinary urgency and suprapubic discomfort. My symptoms were exacerbated by any exercise requiring sitting in a squatted position such as rowing and biking including a recumbent bike. Also, constipation and sex could worsen my symptoms in addition to ill-fitting seats, including car seats. I had been on multiple antibiotics, Hytrin, Elavil and Flomax without improvement. I did have a cystoscopy with hydrodistension and was told that I had mild interstitial cystitis. The Cysto gave me temporary severe urethritis, but it did improve my symptoms about 75% for two months.

After meeting Dr. Wise I began to see a massage therapist every two weeks for external pelvic deep tissue work which helped somewhat. I also got some internal work from a therapist in weekly blocks for a month at a time - total of about ten sessions over a year with continued mild improvement. I was slow to take to the tapes but did manage to listen. Approximately one year ago I had two back-to-back sessions with Marilyn Freedman and had marked improvement. She also added some stretches and core strength exercises. I fell somewhat back, yet did see Marilyn again in December 2005 for two additional sessions which again helped a lot. I do some sort of cardio workout every day and also light weight training four days a week. I have added squats (not heavy weights) –-to my regimen and I believe strengthening my quads takes weight bearing pressure off my pelvis as I spend most of my day standing at work. I am religious about stretching out my pelvis and have combined it with relaxation techniques each night before bed. I do four or five deep stretches including a child's pose, gluteal stretches, and sitting in a deep squat. This process is combined with quiet breathing and takes approximately twenty minutes. Overall I believe there is a 90+% improvement for me and after 15+ years of pelvic pain I am very grateful.

CHAPTER 10

MORE THAN YOU EVER WANTED TO KNOW ABOUT THE MEDICAL SCIENCE OF CHRONIC PELVIC PAIN

Chronic pelvic pain syndrome

This chapter offers insight into what physicians and scientists have learned from scientific investigations of chronic pelvic pain syndromes (CPPS), focusing more on male pelvic pain. Many individual physicians and medical centers take a special interest in this problem and the plight of those suffering from it. The National Institutes of Health (NIH) received a directive from the Congress a few years ago to pursue effective treatment modalities for CPPS and, through a consortium of national awarded medical centers, is dedicating significant efforts to new scientific studies in this endeavor. In 2008, NIH invited proposals to study in greater basic biologic detail what underlies the cause and behavior of these maladies.

CPPS exists as a non-malignant pain emanating from structures around and inside the pelvis. There are no gold-standard objective tests that define CPPS. No one can verify and quantify the amount and intensity of pain. Only a few stalwart physicians and scientists have endeavored to uncover the possible biological basis for its existence and attempt to find any kind of rational medical treatment.

Although there are *more than two million office visits a year in the United States for complaints about prostatitis,* and variations of this disorder make up almost 10% of a typical urologist's practice, they are sadly not the most welcomed of patients because there are no definitive therapies to help these individuals. Physicians want to help patients and when they have treatments that are ineffective not only they but the patients are frustrated and dismayed. In this chapter we review the current knowledge gained from many scientific studies devoted to characterizing and managing chronic pelvic pain syndromes. We also present some of the forward thinking that may advance our knowledge about CPPS and lead to development of new therapeutic approaches.

If one looks at the history of medicine, the pelvic malady of *prostatitis was only first described in the middle of the 19th century.* Imagine all those men suffering for centuries without a clue as to what might have been going on. In the first part of the 20th century someone introduced the theory of a possible role of bacteria and examined prostatic fluid microscopically. The secretion was cultured for the first time in 1913.

It was not until 1968, however, that Dr. Thomas Stamey and Dr. Edwin Meares at Stanford University established an appropriate, detailed patient examination that allowed the urologist to document scientifically when bacteria were truly originating from the prostate gland and not the urethra or the urinary bladder, or if there were no bacteria at all.

Prostatitis is an incorrect label for most cases of men with pelvic pain and encourages the ineffective use of antibiotics

We soon learned that bacteria were rarely the cause of CPPS, but when it was, treatment of true bacterial prostatitis was relatively easy. Chronic prostatitis is an incorrect label; we are dealing with a variable set of pain conditions with no objective markers and multivariate symptoms.

The disorder typically does not exhibit prostatocentric symptomatology and pain sites exist between the belly button to above the mid thigh. The European community has promoted the term prostate pain syndrome (PPS) as a more generic term over the USA category label of chronic prostatitis/chronic pelvic pain syndrome (CP/CPPS). Still, they both smack of a prostatocentric approach, which is probably to be avoided for lack of evidence, and *the diagnosis encourages physicians to use antibiotics as standard therapy that clearly lacks efficacy.*

By definition, prostate pain syndrome is persistent discomfort or pain in the pelvic region with sterile specimen cultures and either significant or insignificant white blood cell counts in prostate specimens--semen, expressed prostatic secretion or urine collected after prostate massage.

Evidence of inflammation by itself in the prostate offers little help in guiding any effective therapy for symptoms of pelvic pain and dysfunction in men

There does not appear to be any diagnostic or therapeutic advantage to differentiating between those patients with significant or insignificant white blood cells from the prostate. Remarkably, in the authors' experience, men with *no prostate inflammation* appear to suffer greater degrees and longer duration of pelvic pain on average.

We believe that chronic testicular pain and so-called pudendal nerve entrapment should be included in the general term of chronic pelvic pain syndrome or CPPS. Women with pelvic pain, particularly interstitial cystitis type pain, fall under a general diagnostic designation termed bladder pain syndrome (BPS). In this chapter we use prostate pain syndrome or CPPS as a model to discuss scientific investigations and treatments.

The anatomy: organs, muscles and nerves

Our viewpoint about prostatitis/CPPS centers differs from the conventional practice of routinely identifying and treating pelvic pain in men as a prostate infection. We do not see the prostate as the source of the problem of most male pelvic pain. What we have proposed for many years has to do with our view of the anatomical areas of the pelvis that actually cause the pain and how that pain is created.

Discovering the culprit of pelvic pain

Of course all pain messages transmit through *sensory nerve receptors, then coalesce into fine webs of nerves ending in the spinal cord and, ultimately, forwarded to the brain* where it is perceived subjectively in different ways and interpreted by each patient. Physicians traditionally assign *blame for pain to the various organs of the pelvis.* Reproductive organs such as the uterus, the vagina, the testicles, the penis, the prostate gland, and excretory organs such as the rectum and urinary bladder, receive this blame. We attribute pain to these organs rather than suspecting the supportive structures of these organs—connective tissue such as ligaments and tendons, muscles, blood vessels and nerves serving these structures.

It can be difficult to understand the dull and diffuse nature of pelvic pain unless you understand how nerves work and that there can be communication between nerves (cross-talk) as well as intermingling of signals from various nerves that can confuse someone about where the pain really originates.

There is also the phenomenon known as "referral" whereby pain coming from an organ may not be felt in the organ itself but can be felt in remote areas including the skin. Because of the intimate relationship between the nerves, a strong signal from one area may stimulate a neighboring nerve, even though that neighbor nerve was not being irritated by the stimulus. This represents the method whereby muscles become tense although not related to the source of irritation.

There are 20-plus different muscles and an exhaustive distribution of nerves in and around the pelvis associated with the bony structures and organs. These muscles obviously play an indispensable role in association with the organs they support.

Understanding the muscles of the pelvic floor

As the myriad of nerves interlace throughout the pelvis, the stimulating nerves responsible for smooth muscle contraction and organ function, as well as motor nerves that control supporting muscles, balance and complement each other. We divide muscles into *smooth* muscle and *striated* muscle. Smooth muscles exist in the walls of the intestines and provide the motility of our intestinal function; similarly the urinary bladder, the uterus, the ejaculatory ducts, the prostate and even the heart function with various types of smooth muscle.

Our skeletal or striated muscles are responsible for voluntary movements and offer support and balance to the pelvic structures. Adrenaline, in the form of a biochemical called norepinephrine, stimulates smooth muscle through the adrenaline receptors embedded in the muscles. These receptors *are extremely sensitive to small amounts of norepinephrine.* We designate these smooth muscle receptors as alpha- and beta-receptors. The heart is full of beta receptors, for example, and when one is excited, even mentally, adrenaline causes the heart to go into a racing configuration. *The smooth muscles in the pelvis,* while confined primarily to the organs, *respond in the same way to mental signals that release adrenaline* and cause a reaction in the pelvic muscles. *There are also adrenaline receptors in the contracting or striated muscles* of the pelvis that can be excited by release of excitatory biochemical substances like adrenaline—these are responsible for the "fight and flight" response that gives us extra energy. This is why people can sometimes perform heroic maneuvers in stressful situations.

Dr. Steven Kaplan and colleagues at Columbia University reported that the inappropriate contraction of the external urinary sphincter during voiding can be misdiagnosed as chronic prostatitis. An interesting observation in their review included the fact that 91% of the subjects in this study were firstborn sons. Dr. Kaplan's group felt that behavioral modification and biofeedback to teach the appropriate relaxation approach to urinating was a good therapeutic option.

The misnomer of chronic prostatitis as the model of pelvic pain in men

Chronic prostatitis means different things to patients and doctors. It is a common diagnosis, but clearly a misnomer. There are three cardinal symptoms associated with the diagnosis of chronic prostatitis—pelvic pain and discomfort, disturbances in urination, and abnormal sexual function. *The primary symptomatic complaint that becomes chronic is pain or discomfort.* Patients may or may not have accompanying urinary and sexual problems as well. It is frequently the pain during urination or pain during or after ejaculation that is associated with the urinary or sexual problems. The physician and patient need to understand the circumstances at the time of onset, how long and cyclic the discomfort has been occurring, what degree of intensity is involved, and where the pain is located. We also evaluate the patient's attitude towards his pain, whether the pain is variable or constant, and if he or she is having pain-free intervals.

The second set of common symptoms includes *disturbance of urination*; typically a sense of urinary urgency and frequency, inhibition of the ability to release the urine, a burning sensation or "dysuria" with voiding, and depressed flow—lower urinary tract symptoms. There may be dribbling of urine at the end of emptying the bladder because of poor balance between the sphincter muscles and the contraction of the bladder, often resulting in "trapping" of urine within the urethra as it runs through the prostate.

The third set of symptoms is *disturbance in sexual function* that may include loss of libido or sex drive, inability to attain erection, or to maintain erection for satisfying sexual intercourse and, most importantly, discomfort with ejaculation. Sometimes there can be a spasm-like discomfort immediately after ejaculation or a discomfort that lasts as a nagging annoyance for several hours or days. There may be changes in the spermatic fluid such as decrease in volume, blood staining on occasion, and watery or clumpy, discolored semen.

Medical History

The typical patient is a young to middle-age man with variable symptoms of chronic, irritative and obstructive voiding accompanied by moderate to severe pain in the pelvis, low back, perineum and genitalia. To qualify as chronic pelvic pain the condition should occur longer than 6 months, and for research purposes, continuous within the previous 3 months. *It is one of the most common genitourinary diagnoses in men under the age of fifty years.*

The urologist's first order of business when referred such a patient is to accept the challenge seriously and treat the man suffering with this condition with respect, interest, and compassion. The patient is understandably tense, wary and defensive having encountered frustration and rejection previously. The physician should listen to the patient's complaints and accurately document the circumstances surrounding the onset of the disorder—sensory descriptions, various treatment modalities and outcomes, noting particularly the time course of events and associated triggers that may have caused a flare in his symptoms. The United States national cohort study by the NIH reported a typical duration of patient complaints averaging 4 years.

The urologist evaluating pelvic pain in a male must rule out associated urinary bladder or prostate diseases. Errors in diagnosis and inappropriate therapeutic pathways may ensue if less than a systematic evaluation is undertaken. Both prostate and bladder cancer as well as urinary stone disease have been missed because of an inappropriate diagnosis of "chronic prostatitis". It is crucial to have empathy for the suffering patient, documenting his description of the physical characteristics of the pain complex: what makes it worse, what helps, where is the pain referred, and what associations exist with sexual function? The psychosexual behavior and influence of sexual partner relationships play a significant role. How has the chronic pain affected libido, the ability to attain adequate penile erections, accomplish intercourse, reach orgasm and have pleasurable ejaculation?

Associated alimentary tract complaints such as irritable bowel disorder, constipation, dietary exacerbations, and bowel function may point to further clarifying aspects of the disorder. Further, the psychosocial medical history should probe for genetic or acquired personality types: tense, anxious, chronic tension-holding patterns, possible childhood issues of sexual or physical abuse, traumatic toilet training, abnormal bowel patterns, teen sexual problems, excessive masturbation, suppressed homosexuality, excessive weight lifting, gymnastic maneuvers and activities such as dance training. Identifying such issues helps to create a specific phenotype of the pain condition and may ultimately suggest appropriate multi-modal therapy.

In our research we utilize symptom questionnaires and validated instruments to detail patient psychological issues. These tools help quantify the baseline, eventual progress and outcome of our management techniques. The most widely used research tool is the National Institutes of Health Chronic Prostatitis symptom Index (NIH-CPSI). This widely used symptom scoring analyzes pain, urinary symptoms and quality of life as three separate domains. Almost every meaningful clinical trial of treatment has used this scoring system to evaluate efficacy outcome. We state the percent improvement in the CPSI score when available in the treatment studies described below. The CPSI has also been modified by Dr. Clemens from Michigan to allow symptom scoring for women. An alternate type of CPPS symptom questionnaire—the Stanford Pelvic Pain Symptom Score (PPSS)—has also been useful in our hands, although not usually reported in scientific studies. The PPSS expands the description of named painful anatomical locations and grades the severity of pain at each site (0 to 4+); it includes urinary symptoms that mimic the International Prostate Symptom Score

(IPSS), and scores sexual dysfunction aspects of the patient condition as a separate domain.   Our group utilizes both symptom scoring questionnaires in the treatment outcome analysis of CPPS therapy.

The physician's examination

When physicians examine a patient *they typically focus on the organs* of the pelvis; they perform a rectal or vaginal examination and attempt to palpate the uterus, the ovaries, the rectum, the prostate, the bladder, and testicles, but usually *ignore the important integration of the muscles and the fascia or ligaments holding these organs.*

It is our considered view that when evaluating a patient with chronic pelvic pain *it is imperative to do a thorough evaluation of the muscles and ligaments surrounding these organs.* It is our duty to elicit with the examination what the patient experiences and attempt to correlate what we find with any possible abnormality that may be occurring either in the organs or in the pelvic muscles. This is not a simple task. The majority of patients suffering with chronic pelvic pain have no classic standard findings that can be easily detected. There are, however, certain basic urologic evaluations that should be done including a careful lower body neurologic examination, urinalysis, and serum PSA in men over fifty.

In our *evaluation at Stanford*, as do most urologists, we *examine the prostate for microorganisms and inflammatory white blood cells.* This requires the patient to urinate a small amount prior to examination, to compare this sample microscopically to what may be found in voided urine after massage of the prostate. We palpate the pelvic muscles looking for actual trigger points or specific discomfort zones, especially surrounding the prostate. We then feel the prostate gland itself; we determine its consistency, whether it is soft or "boggy," whether there are areas of induration or hardness—this may represent fibrosis or scarring from previous inflammation—but we must remain ever vigilant for cancer.

We methodically massage the prostate gland, beginning at the base and milking it toward the center on each side to express prostatic fluid into the urethra. The prostate gland is composed of 20-30 small microscopic tunnels (acini) emanating from the periphery of the prostate. Each glandular unit is connected to the outside world by a pinpoint duct that opens into the urethra on each side of the main seminal vesicles' ejaculatory duct located in the center of the prostate. These tiny ducts expel the enzyme-rich prostatic secretion with smooth muscle prostate contractions at the time of sexual ejaculation.

The easiest way to perform this pelvic examination is with the patient lying supine with the legs spread in stirrups (the female position). This allows the examiner to have leverage and direct visualization of the penis and the urethral opening to collect prostatic fluid. We have found it convenient to collect the fluid with a tiny sterile glass pipette, the prostatic secretion drops accumulating with capillary action as they appear at the penis opening or meatus, particularly when there are only one or two drops that are quite precious to be able to examine and culture.

Once the prostatic fluid has been collected, the patient will urinate a small volume to provide a washout of prostatic fluid that can be separated, analyzed and submitted for bacterial culture. This is particularly important when no prostatic fluid is expressed out. We advise patients to refrain from any sexual ejaculation for seven days prior to coming in for the examination to afford a better opportunity to maximize collection of prostatic fluid. Older men typically have more prostatic fluid because the gland is larger. Younger men find it a challenge to refrain from sex for a week.

We take the patient's prostatic fluid to our office laboratory where a simple examination under the microscope (after staining the fluid with a dye) helps identify white cells and improves the analysis. We count the number of white cells in the prostatic fluid to compare with counts from normal, asymptomatic men and to track changes as a treatment program is instituted. Unfortunately this detail of performing careful analysis of the prostatic fluid is usually conducted only in academic or university medical centers where an intellectual curiosity prevails.

How common is infectious prostatitis?

Acute bacterial prostatitis, as described earlier, is a *fairly easy diagnosis to make*. It is associated with pain in the prostate, difficulty urinating, high fever, chills and weakness. It is serious because bacteria can spread into the blood stream causing sepsis or blood poisoning. Acute bacterial prostatitis requires aggressive antimicrobial therapy and sometimes needs catheter drainage of the urinary tract. Inadequately treated acute bacterial prostatitis may potentially become dormant and develop into *recurrent* chronic bacterial prostatitis. We typically treat acute prostatitis for a total of 28 days using potent antibiotics. We administer antibiotics for about 6 weeks when true chronic bacterial infection is established through a microbiology laboratory.

Chronic prostatitis is caused by bacteria in only 5% of cases of pelvic pain

There has been great debate about whether chronic pelvic pain represents an infectious disease. *The consensus of expert opinion today is that chronic prostatitis, as a medical disorder, is probably caused directly by microbial agents in only about 5% of the cases.* Most of these episodes of bacterial prostatitis are without symptoms between infection flare-ups. *Men who complain of chronic pelvic pain and who have been diagnosed with prostatitis may possess increased bacterial counts found in the prostatic fluid. But the bacteria are normal flora, or normal types of bacteria in the urethra, and they colonize the prostate ducts in low numbers just as we find normal resident bacteria in the vagina, the mouth, the rectum, and other parts of the body.* Uropathogens, however, are bacteria not normally found in the genitourinary (GU) tract and are known to be invasive and cause inflammation of both the prostate and bladder. These bacteria are organisms from the intestinal tract. When a physician identifies significant numbers of these bacteria in the genitourinary system, either in the urethra, the bladder, or coming from the prostate gland itself, he or she considers this to be bacterial cause of the symptoms. Are we not trying hard enough to find poorly detected microorganisms that may be responsible for inciting this condition? Some have suggested we should culture the body fluids for a longer time to detect the slow-growing bacteria that may also be hiding out under biofilms. Dr Cohen, a pathologist from Australia, has just produced evidence that acne organisms can be found in the prostate if carefully cultured. There is evidence that the bacteria were there as sleuthed out using DNA tracking. It appears that those individuals who suffer from CPPS do indeed have a higher incidence of the positive DNA fingerprints when you take biopsies from their prostates compared to men who never had CPPS *but as we discuss below, this appears to be irrelevant to their symptoms*

Serious investigators have looked at multiple microorganisms that might be the cause of chronic prostatitis, including microbial forms such as *Chlamydia, Ureaplasma,* and even parasites or protozoans such as *Trichomonas. While very small percentages (3-10%) of patients have been found to carry these unusual organisms, there have never been convincing studies to prove that these organisms are specific causative agents.* Dr. Andrew Doble and associates from England performed an exhaustive search for infectious agents in chronic prostatitis syndromes using ultrasound-guided tissue biopsies of the prostate. They found that 88% of their patients had chronic inflammation in the tissue, but only 15% of patients had any organisms that were cultured or grew from the tissue, and actually *these were considered to be contaminants from the skin. This information again reinforces the concept that we are dealing with a painful disorder and no proven microorganism as a cause. Unfortunately, most physicians and patients believe chronic prostatitis to be an infectious entity and are searching for the Holy Grail of antimicrobial treatment that will once and for all eradicate these pesky organisms from their system. We believe this is a fruitless quest.*

Another controversy that continues to be debated among urologists and microbiologists is whether *gram positive organisms* (a laboratory stain classification) such as *Staphylococcus* and *beta strep*, commonly found as normal flora in the urethra, may indeed act as pathogenic bacteria or organisms that would invade and cause inflammation. These gram-positive microbes are usually found on the skin and in the mouth, as opposed to gram- negative microbes that come from the large intestine. While some patients may have large numbers of these organisms in the urethra and colonizing the prostate, use of antimicrobials to eradicate the organisms does not *seem to provide improvement in symptoms and there is very little association with the cause and effect of symptoms.*

Dr. Wolfgang Weidner from the University of Giessen in Germany is an important contributor to evaluating the occurrence of microorganisms and inflammation in CPPS. He published a paper in 1991 demonstrating a thorough search for microorganisms in hundreds of consecutive patients. He found high numbers of bacteria and several sub-bacterial species of *Ureaplasma* in a typical prostatitis pattern associated with increased numbers of white cells in the prostatic secretion. At that time he felt there was an important difference in the classification between patients with and without inflammation in the prostatic fluid, and that there were differences in the symptoms from those patients that had no white cells and pain in the prostate (the NIH classification difference between IIIA and IIIB).

Our own anecdotal experience suggests a difference between the two categories in symptoms and in response to therapy. *We believe that patients who have no inflammation seem to have more neuromuscular dysfunction, more myofascial trigger points, more pain and respond more rapidly to the Trigger Point Release* therapy and *Paradoxical Relaxation.* However, a careful NIH-sponsored study concluded that there is no correlation between evidence of infection or inflammation in the prostate and the symptoms of prostatitis/chronic pelvic pain. The precise relationship of prostate inflammation and chronic pelvic pain remains to be elucidated.

The inflammation debate

In the first place we have only small shreds of evidence that inflammation may be involved in causing the pain of CPPS. Even less well understood is what biologic or physical entity may be inciting the inflammation. In a few instances, some tissue has been available for sampling—bladder, prostate, rectum, vagina—and no obvious microbiologic substance appears to be an initiator. Furthermore, the presence and degree of inflammation does not correlate quantitatively with the degree of pain.

As stated previously, the NIH study found no relationship exists between infection/inflammation and severity of pain and dysfunction in prostatitis. The occurrence of infection/inflammation in chronic prostatitis/CPPS fails to be consistent and not helpful in diagnostic terms. Dr. John McNeal, a devoted research pathologist at Stanford University, has worked on prostate disease, particularly prostate cancer, his whole professional life; he found many years ago that between *5-15% of men over the age of 60 have inflammation in their prostate tissue on microscopic examination but absolutely no complaint of pelvic pain.*

Doctors can determine that there is inflammation in the prostate ducts when they look at expressed prostatic secretion under the microscope at 400 times magnification. However, it is not always possible to massage prostatic fluid from a patient. We then must rely on a post-massage voided urine specimen and separate prostatic fluid by centrifugation from the urine for analysis. Again, our male patients with prostatitis who have high numbers of inflammatory white cells in their expressed prostatic secretion actually seem to have less pain on average than those with few or no white blood cells coming from the ducts of the prostate. There is no current scientific information to explain why this is so.

As we do not have proof of infectious agents causing chronic pelvic pain syndrome, the unanswered question remains; what is causing the inflammation? Many investigators believe that it has to do with *dysfunction of the voiding mechanism*, an imbalance in the urinary muscle control causes reflux or pressure of urine and hence toxic substances of urine backing up into the prostate gland ducts and creates an inflammatory and irritated condition. In simple language, tension in the pelvic muscles may be inhibiting the free flow of urine, causing it to reflux or back up into the prostate. This "backed-up urine" may then cause the mild inflammation that is found in approximately 1/3 of patients with a diagnosis of prostatitis.

Dr. Linda Shortliffe, a urologist at Stanford, performed an analysis of the prostatic fluid proteins in an attempt to look at differences between men with bacterial and nonbacterial prostatitis. She reported that even patients without bacterial prostatitis could have elevated levels of prostatic immunoglobulins, the body's response to infection or inflammation. In 1995, Dr. Robert Nadler reported the effect of inflammation on prostate specific antibody (PSA) levels--the enzyme blood test used to test for the possible presence of prostate cancer. The presence of inflammation was quite common, and nearly all of the men with high PSA levels had a least one biopsy specimen positive for chronic inflammation. Confusing the issue, however, 77% of those with normal PSA levels also had small areas of inflammation on biopsy. In many cases, acute and chronic inflammation were more prevalent in the high PSA group (63%, versus 27% in the normal PSA group). *They concluded that a quantitative demonstration of acute and chronic inflammation in the tissue was not necessarily associated with clinical bacterial prostatitis, or even symptoms, but may be an important contributor to elevated PSA levels in the blood.*

Possible immune response may occur with nerve growth factors and associated inflammatory agents known as cytokines and this raises some intriguing possibilities. Firstly, it may reveal biological markers that could be analyzed to show an abnormal presence and provide potential therapeutic blocking agents for the inflammatory condition. Very small amounts of nerve growth factor, perhaps released because of primary prostate nerve damage, can increase sensitivity to both thermal and mechanical stimulation. These chemical changes relate to altered sensitivity to pain and could be responsible for the dynamics of fluctuation in this chronic pain syndrome.

Not finding an elusive inflammatory inciting agent or evidence of obvious inflammation does not detract from our belief and supporting evidence that the central nervous system—the brain and spinal cord—in conjunction with powerful immune regulating mechanisms known as the hypothalamus-pituitary-adrenal (HPA) axis may be intimately involved in altering inflammatory events in the body related to CPPS.
Neurogenic inflammation (inflammation resulting from the local release

of biochemical substances from nerves) is a phenomenon that has been demonstrated in many experimental models. It is clear that the autonomic nervous system, particularly the adrenergic or sympathetic system, plays a very important role. Sensory nerve endings are activated and they then release cytokines and many other inflammatory mediators, which in turn affect the surrounding tissue. Small micro vessels dilate and become permeable, increased blood flow (causing redness) and exuding blood plasma allows white blood cells to accumulate. This is acute inflammation. This inflammatory process may, in turn, excite or activate the stress system, causing anxiety and recycling the neurogenic inflammation. The hallmark of chronic inflammation is infiltration of tissue with mononuclear inflammatory cells ("mononuclear cells," "round cells," i.e., monocytes, lymphocytes, and/or plasma cells). Generally, good tissue has been (and is being) destroyed, and there will be some evidence of healing (scarring, fibroblast proliferation, new blood vessel proliferation).

We believe that distress related immune dysregulation may be one core mechanism behind a large and diverse set of health risks associated with negative emotions. We label this field as *Psychoneuroimmunology* and *Psychoneuroendocrinology.* This book cannot serve as the forum to expound on the multiple scientific studies that show these relationships and pathophysiological phenomena. We must, however, always hold our beliefs in abeyance and remain open minded about the possibilities in our quest to understand this CPPS malady.

Imaging of the prostate in chronic prostatitis

The best way to look at the prostate gland tissue is to use transrectal ultrasound (TRUS). This method of evaluation can often be quite valuable in demonstrating inflamed tissue, the presence of stones in the ducts (representing urinary mineral deposits), swelling and thickening of seminal vesicles (semen storage organs behind the prostate) and accurate measurement of the size of the gland. Japanese investigators

have used computerized x-ray images and angiography or dye in blood vessels to evaluate chronic pelvic pain. They demonstrated excellent three dimensional graphic images of veins around the prostate and found considerable congestion in these veins behind the bladder and along the sides of the prostate in patients suffering with pain. The veins on the surface of the prostate were much thicker in diameter than in subjects with no pain. This basically represents varicose veins of the prostate. This is suggestive of heightened tension in the muscles of the pelvic floor and is supportive of our view that chronic pelvic pain syndromes are associated with muscle tension.

It is quite common for urologists to look inside the urethra, prostate and bladder in patients suffering from this disorder with a technique called *cystoscopy*. This consists of passing a pencil-sized flexible probe with magnifying optical lenses, high intensity fiber optic light, and associated video camera up the penile urethra. *However, cystoscopy may be the least productive procedure that can be done.* Some urologists will say to the patient "Oh, yes, I see some inflammation in the prostate." This is anatomically impossible because they are only looking at the surface of the urethra and not at the prostatic tissue itself. There is rarely, if ever, any obvious inflammation on the surface of the prostatic urethra in the condition of prostatitis.

Urodynamics

One investigative tool to evaluate urinary and prostate function consists of physiological measurements with a procedure called *urodynamics*. Such testing should be suggested only if it would benefit the physician to understand and treat specific abnormalities. This testing procedure evaluates physiologic function of smooth and striated muscle function in the bladder, prostate, and urinary sphincters. We place a small pressure-sensing catheter in the bladder to detect changes in bladder pressure; the catheter simultaneously monitors the urethral voluntary sphincter pressure activity and associated pelvic floor function. An important component of this testing includes a catheter balloon in the rectum to monitor abdominal pressure. We utilize electrical sensors patched to the skin around the anal muscles to detect electrical activity within the pelvic floor, both with relaxation and voluntary contraction, but primarily to determine how much relaxation is achieved when attempting to urinate. Comparison of symptoms, morphological, microbiological and urodynamic findings in patients with CPPS have existed for decades. A common theme emerges suggesting *functional* obstruction at the level of the bladder neck and external sphincter, high sensitivity during filling, and poor or interrupted urinary flow. Abnormally low urinary flow rates is found in 65% of patients. Some patients respond to alpha-nerve blocking agents as therapy for CPPS while most do not.

Muscle tension and chronic pelvic pain syndrome

Because we have so little to document a cause of chronic pelvic pain, theories and partial bits of evidence are discussed interminably. Clearly, we need evidence for specific treatment, but multimodal shotgun therapy still prevails. Many investigators publish articles reviewing the evidence for abnormalities and potential treatment approaches but progress requires strong scientific studies. Fortunately the NIH, through the NIDDK branch, is providing funding for cooperative basic science and translational investigation and we hope this gathering of the minds will bear fruit.

Comparison of symptoms, morphological, microbiological and urodynamic findings in patients with CPPS have existed for decades. Neuromuscular imbalance, or dysfunction in voiding, continues to be a prominent suspect of causation in chronic prostatitis/CPPS. This certainly fits our model of tension myalgia and chronic pelvic pain syndromes leading to imbalance in urinary function causing inflammation in the prostate. A study published in 1987 by Dr. Wayne Hellstrom and colleagues from the University of California, San Francisco, promoted this concept with case reports. Their physiologic studies revealed elevated urethral pressures where the urinary channel runs through the middle of the prostate, causing reflux of urine minerals and toxic metabolites into the peripheral or outer zone of the prostate, the location of most of the inflammation. The peripheral zone ducts are perpendicular to the course of the urethra and are susceptible to high pressure in the prostate. Specific measurements of intra-prostatic pressure have been undertaken in patients suffering from chronic prostate pain and one series of 42 patients showed significant elevation of prostate hydrostatic pressures.

Dr. George Barbalias from Greece proposes this mechanistic cause of chronic prostatitis. He advocated long ago the use of potent alpha-receptor blockade as a method of treatment. He actually used needle electrodes to measure electrical signals from the external urethral sphincter. While he found normal motor unit potentials in the majority of the patients and discovered that there was a coordinated function of the bladder and the external sphincter during the voiding with no difference between inflammatory and non-inflammatory patients, both groups had decreased urinary flow rate. He said this was a *functional* urethral obstruction but not an actual physical obstruction. This *functional* urethral obstruction represents chronic pelvic muscle tension.

Some key pioneer clinician-investigators attempted to evaluate the neurophysiology of the pelvic floor and its relationship to chronic pelvic pain. Dr. Dirk H. Zermann, and colleagues at the University of Colorado in Denver, showed that in men with chronic pelvic pain there was a strong association with neuromuscular and myofascial (muscles and ligaments) dysfunction. In a clinical evaluation of 103 patients seen at their clinic, 91 men (88.3%) had abnormal tenderness of the striated or voluntary muscle of the pelvis, and this myofascial tenderness was virtually always associated with inability to relax the pelvic floor efficiently. Diane Hetrick, a physiotherapist, and the team with Dr. Richard Berger at the University of Washington in Seattle have recently confirmed the opinion that musculoskeletal dysfunction occurs in men with chronic pelvic pain syndrome.

A higher percent of increased pelvic floor muscle tone, pain with internal palpation, increased tension with external palpation, and pain with external palpation were found in patients with CPPS as compared to healthy controls. Furthermore, these investigators at Washington showed that there exists hypersensitivity in the pelvic (perineal area) sensory nerves of patients. They used a flash heat technique to create a painful heat stimulus in the perineum. When compared to healthy volunteers there was definitely more sensitivity to the heat pain in those patients suffering from chronic pelvic pain syndrome.

Many physician specialists (rheumatologists/immunologists) working with arthritis believe that the primary abnormality leading to expression of symptoms in fibromyalgia and related conditions consists of errant central nervous system function. This concept promotes the idea that there may be skeletal muscle abnormalities in patients having pain. It appears that a generalized disturbance in the pain perception threshold and the tension phenomenon from the central nervous system underlie these disorders.

Central Nervous System Stress and CPPS

Throughout the years, many physicians noted the features of stress and/ or anxiety contributing to pelvic pain syndromes. In 1986 a group from Sweden (Lars Gatenbeck) studied rats that were stimulated and stressed with or without hormone additives. They investigated the microscopic changes of the prostate under these conditions. Inflammation of the gland was thought to occur because of stress reactions increasing output of adrenaline and other biochemical neurotransmitters.

In their experiments, rats were submitted to stress stimuli for ten days. Examination of the prostate tissue after this kind of activity demonstrated moderate infiltration of inflammatory cells—there was a significant difference in those rats that received stimulation and those that did not, the latter having little or no inflammation. At the same time, they found a reduced serum testosterone level, but it was not clear what the influence or importance of this hormonal change could be. The other feature that was noted was that the lobes of the rat prostate having the least advanced drainage system had a greater involvement in inflammatory manifestation. This is an example of one of the very few experimental attempts to document the behavioral effects on both physiologic and microscopic changes. *It is not a difficult leap of imagination to transfer this to the human condition and understand the effects of stressors and anxiety that contribute to the chronic pelvic pain syndrome.*

In 1988 Dr. Harry C. Miller studied 218 men who had complaints typical of CPPS. Sixty percent or 134 of these patients were followed carefully and managed only with stress control. *This psychological approach alone improved 86% of the patients who reported that they were better, much better, or cured. Most importantly, repeat cultures, prostatic massages, instrumentation, and medications were not utilized at all in this group of patients as he relied solely on stress management.*

Study at Stanford of cortisol and CPPS

We recently studied a group of 45 men with CPPS and 20 normal age-matched men and found the patients to have significantly more perceived stress and anxiety. *These men were also found to produce a more rapid rise in morning awakening levels of cortisol in their saliva.* We then followed up on this phenomenon and invited these patients to come in for acute stress testing in the laboratory. Compared with the normal control men, our patients showed a *depressed* afternoon ability of the brain to produce the precursor (ACTH) for cortisol production from the adrenal glands compared to normal control men. Perhaps the blunting or cortisol of men with CPPS in the afternoon represents the fatigue of the cortisol production machinery of the brain.

Treatments and clinical research trials

The National Institutes of Health (NIH) promote clinical research regarding the pervasive disorder of chronic prostatitis and chronic pelvic pain syndrome. They want to find a satisfactory treatment. Progress in treatment requires documentation of results with strong levels of evidence that something works. The best level of evidence occurs when patients are treated with an active drug or treatment method and a similar group is randomized to treated with a sham procedure or placebo drug and do not know it. We call this a blinded control clinical research trial. These are very expensive and difficult to perform. Sometimes it is impossible to blind the patient from knowing that they are not receiving the real thing.

Cipro®, Flomax®, Lyrica® and Uroxatrol® shown to be no better than placebo for CPPS

A good example in a recent nationwide study evaluated the two most common medication treatments for the disorder: oral Ciprofloxin (Cipro®), a potent fluoroquinolone antibiotic, and/or oral tamsulosin (Flomax®), a potent alpha nerve receptor blocking agent for the smooth muscle of the prostate and urethra. These two pharmacologic agents were tested in a blinded fashion against a placebo or sugar pill as a treatment of these syndromes. This was an important study because no one had ever systematically evaluated the effect of antibiotics for these "nonbacterial" disorders, although many doctors and patients claimed improvement.

The outcome of this study showed that the symptom scores improved slightly regardless of whether the patients took the antibiotic, the alpha blocker, or the placebo. The contribution of an alpha-blocking smooth muscle relaxant continues to be debated with regard to its efficacy. *In our own practice, virtually every patient who comes to see us has been previously treated either with potent antibiotics and/or alpha blocking agents, but they continue to have recurrent complaints.* Further testing patients with shorter term CPPS with an additional randomized clinical trial of another alpha blocker-- alfuzosin (Uroxatrol®) demonstrated no difference over a placebo. And finally, a recent study of pregabalin (Lyrica®) as an oral treatment for CPPS was not found to be any better than a sugar placebo when taken over several weeks. Our oral medication clinical trials continue to disappoint.

Dr. Daniel Shoskes investigated the use of an herbal dietary supplement known as a bioflavonoid. Quercetin was given to patients with chronic prostatitis/CPPS in a blinded fashion for one month. Patients taking the substance had their symptom scores decrease from 21 to 13 (67% improvement). This therapy seems to be well tolerated and offers significant symptomatic improvement in many men with chronic pelvic pain syndrome. Larger national studies need to be performed for a high level of scientific evidence. Another herbal approach from Europe suggests that a formulation of rye grass pollen (Cernilton®) has some anti-inflammatory effects and has been popular as treatment for nonbacterial prostatitis. A well-done study from Germany evaluated the primary outcome of treatment (change in pelvic pain) over a 12-week period. In a group of 139 patients, half on pollen and half on placebo, the pollen group dropped their pain scores an average of 45% and the placebo group an average of 29%.

What about acupuncture and electrical stimulation therapy? Drs Chen and Nickel reported in 2003 that acupuncture treatments given twice weekly for 6 weeks improved total CPSI and pain scores by 70% on average. This was a small study in 12 men with no placebo control. A more recent trial was reported from Turkey in 2010. Ninety-seven patients received 6 weekly acupuncture treatments and at 24 weeks follow-up the total CPSI score improved by 57% and the pelvic pain score by 45%. Another percutaneous needle study, also from Turkey, tested the efficiency of posterior tibial nerve (at the ankle) stimulation in CPPS. They had 89 patients randomized to needle electrical stimulation or sham 30 minutes once weekly for 12 weeks. Success was defined as a 50% decrease in pain scores and 66% of the patients achieved this level of relief at the end of 12 weeks. Of course electrical stimulation therapy like this cannot be done easily on a long-term basis. The same holds true for internal pelvic high frequency local electrical stimulation that was tried on 88 patients in Switzerland. Electrode catheters were placed into the prostatic urethra as well as the anal canal. Stimulation was performed for 30 minutes twice weekly for 5 weeks. The CPSI total score and pain improved 52% by the end of therapy but symptoms recurred by 3 months later.

Obviously the most convenient way to apply electrical stimulation would be surface or transcutaneous electrical nerve stimulation (TENS). In 24 patients treated with this technique, applying the electrode pads to the pubic and perineal area and treating for 20 minutes daily, 5 times a week for 4 weeks, the CPSI scores improved 45%. Patients receiving antibiotics improved their scores by 22%. This trial requires sham treatments and longer follow-up.

What about electrical stimulation using permanently implanted electrodes? Dr. Siegel from Minnesota implanted small electrodes (Medtronics Interstim ®) through the posterior skin and sacral bone openings to stimulate the sacral nerves in 9 women and 1 man. He documented an average 53% decrease in pain on a simple pain scale, but there were 27 minor complications associated with the implantation procedure.

Heat therapy of the prostate

While heat therapy (hyperthermia) is not an approach we advocate, some studies have reported favorable results. Thermal therapy consists of various forms of heat induction—microwave, radiofrequency, laser, and ultrasound energy—where in place of 'cutting' tissue as in surgery, the prostate tissue is heated to a temperature that may cause tissue destruction. A publication in 1993 described 54 patients who had significant prostatitis symptoms for a period of over two years despite several courses of antimicrobial or anti-inflammatory therapy with no significant clinical benefit. The method of treatment utilized transrectal hyperthermia and the target temperature was only 42.5°C, therefore not creating any significant damage of tissue. Transrectal ultrasound could not detect changes in the prostate volume or shape after the procedure. Overall, 50% of the patients reported an improvement in the quality of life; 47% reported no change. *This would be consistent with a strong placebo effect.* In 1994 Dr. Curtis Nickel reported using transurethral microwave thermal therapy at higher temperatures ranging from 45-60°C that do cause death of prostatic tissue. Patients with nonbacterial prostatitis showed significant reductions in their symptom severity indices; 47% had a marked improvement at three months. A similar study utilized cooled transurethral thermal therapy on 35 men in 2004 in the United Kingdom. These investigators found 51% improvement in the CPSI total score and 60% improvement at 12 months of follow-up. However, this *again is not far from what one would expect from a simple placebo effect* but has the attendant risks associated with inserting a microwave device in the prostatic urethra and destroying prostate tissue.

Other reports from various investigators from 2002 to 2004 initially showed no improvement in CPPS using transurethral prostate needle radiofrequency heat ablation vs. a sham procedure. One Taiwanese report on treatment of 32 patients using this technique in 2004 suggested a 68% improvement in a non-standardized pain score.

Prostate and pelvic massage

Prostatic massage has been utilized by several generations of urologists, particularly prior to the advent of antibiotics. In a report from a Philippine study, repeated prostatic massages revealed occult organisms. This study received attention and popularity as a therapeutic benefit from massage expression of ductal contents that were not being emptied. This treatment may diminish prostatic pressure. The frequency of prostatic massage seems best when done twice weekly.

Dr. Daniel Shoskes proposed massage plus antibiotic treatment. His patients underwent prostatic massage plus antibiotics for 2 to 8 weeks and 40% had complete resolution of symptoms, 20% had significant improvements, and 40% had no improvement. There was no correlation between inflammatory content and bacterial cultures. Our opinion gained from research at Stanford as expressed in a review article from *Techniques in Urology*, favors repetitive massage of the prostate, not for emptying the gland, but rather to relieve pelvic tension and release myofascial trigger points. *We continue to be extremely skeptical of the concept of occult bacteria that needs to be "massaged out." A simple analysis of repeated prostate massage is a "blind approach" to treating the disorder, wherein occasionally the right trigger point or myofascial source is appropriately touched.*

While we do not advocate biofeedback, there is emerging interest in utilizing behavioral pelvic floor rehabilitation techniques in treating male CPPS. A group from Northwestern University Medical School in Chicago promotes the use of biofeedback in pelvic floor re-education as well as bladder training for this disorder. They recognize that pelvic floor tension myalgia contributes to the symptoms. They looked at a small group of 19 men, average age of 36 years, and treated them with this non-interventional process. The men showed improvement, particularly in their urinary scores, but also had a significant decrease in their median pain scores, from 5 to 1 on a scale of 0 (no symptoms) to 10 (worse symptoms). This was a preliminary study, but it confirms that a formalized neuromuscular re-education of the pelvic floor muscles benefits some patients.

We are not the first doctors to have considered the kind of treatment we are describing in this book. As early as 1934 there were a few physicians who understood that pelvic pain is related to tension or spasm of the pelvic muscles. George Thiele, MD was a proctologist (now referred to as a colorectal surgeon), who developed a physical treatment for pelvic pain that he generally included under the name coccygynia (pain of the coccyx or tail bone). Thiele's findings were later confirmed by Shapiro in 1937 who referred to pain around the coccyx as the Thiele Syndrome. In an article in 1963, Thiele reported on 324 patients who had pelvic pain in and around the rectum and anus. He, along with several other researchers, recognized that coccygectomy (surgical removal of the tail bone) failed to help anyone with pelvic pain other than those who had severe trauma to the tailbone. Furthermore, he acknowledged that there was no evidence of any disease of the coccyx or adjacent areas.

Thiele's contribution of applied massage to the levator ani and coccygeus muscles yielded remarkably good results. In some papers in the colorectal studies that followed, his treatment was referred to as Thiele Massage. He reported that over 90% of people that he treated improved after such treatment. He was a pioneer in this area, and while he published his results for doctors in his field to consider, somehow his work disappeared and is rarely referred to in the literature on pelvic pain. The reason for this may be both economic and ideological. There is little economic incentive for colorectal surgeons to do Thiele Massage. Furthermore, colorectal surgery indicated by its very name, tends to be surgical, and massage of the pelvic muscles may not be seen as a good use of the surgeon's time. Alternatively, other specialists or physical therapists would be more likely to utilize this form of therapy for patients with CPPS.

Mehrsheed Sinaki, M.D. was a physician at the Mayo Clinic in the department of physical medicine and rehabilitation throughout most of the 1970's. Doctor Sinaki reviewed the medical records of patients who had a diagnosis of pelvic pain in general, but at that time more often referred to by the terms piriformis syndrome, coccygodynia, levator ani spasm syndrome, proctalgia fugax, or simply rectal pain. Absent were reports of urinary symptoms or of diagnoses including prostatitis, interstitial cystitis, or some of the other conditions we include in this book. Sinaki's important article documented that the treatment that yielded the best results in these patients was as discussed earlier, the Thiele Massage. He acknowledged that the conditions he examined were obscured by many vague and chronic complaints. Furthermore, he found, as we find today, that a general medical exam and routine laboratory and x-ray exam are unremarkable. Sinaki believed that the definitive test for the conditions he was reviewing was the digital-rectal examination in which the doctor inserts a gloved lubricated finger into the rectum to feel the state of the muscles. He observed, however, that the normal digital-rectal examination was inadequate to assess the tenderness of the muscles.

Segura and other colleagues of Sinaki at Mayo Clinic reiterated Sinaki ideas in the Journal of Urology in 1979. They wrote, *"Patients with symptoms suggestive of prostatitis or prostatosis who do not have pathogenic bacteria in the prostatic secretions may in fact not have prostatic problems. The possibility of pelvic floor tension myalgia should be considered."*

Trigger points and pelvic pain

Drs. Hubbard and Berkoff, Department of Neurosciences at the University of California, San Diego, discovered that trigger points, which we usually find inside the pelvic floor of our patients, show abnormal spontaneous electrical activity. Drs. Travell and Simons, who introduced the concept of muscular trigger points and myofascial release, defined the standard by which trigger points could be identified.

Those standards were as follows:

1. Palpable and firm areas of muscle, usually referred to as the taut band

2. In the taut band, a little spot of great tenderness and sensitivity, especially upon the use of manual pressure

3. A pattern of sensation involving pain, sometimes in combination with tingling or numbness when this area is palpated digitally

4. What has been called a "local twitch" of this spot of tautness when the trigger point is pressed

Until the time of this study, trigger points could only be identified with a finger and there was no objective measure of the trigger point itself. The fact that trigger points could only be identified by individual palpation and not by objective measures left open the significance, and even the reality of the trigger points. Hubbard and Berkoff placed needle electrodes in the trigger points of the subjects of their study. They also placed needle electrodes immediately beside the trigger point within the same muscle. They connected the needle electrodes to an electromyograph (EMG), which is a very sensitive machine for measuring electrical activity. Electrical activity in muscle is considered to be a measure of its level of activity.

Their results were remarkable because they found a sustained level of increased electrical activity in the trigger point, while there was no increased electrical activity found in the tissue immediately beside the trigger point. They theorized that this prolonged increase in electrical activity becomes painful by affecting the spindle capsule. (The spindle capsule is a microscopic part of the muscle tissue that the authors speculated was affected by the increased electrical activity and was the source of pain). This increased electrical activity was seen to be associated with the pain experienced subjectively, either when the trigger point is pressed on or even when it is not.

We have found the presence of trigger points in a large majority of our patients who have pelvic pain and dysfunction. We often (not always) are able to recreate the symptoms of patients we see when we press on these trigger points. We also find that when we complete a course of myofascial treatment, the trigger points usually disappear along with the pain and exquisite sensitivity. Furthermore, the reduction of trigger point sensitivity is often directly related to a subjective improvement in patient symptoms. The findings in this study, in confirming objective and measurable activity specifically within the trigger point, as well as our own clinical experience offer compelling evidence that the trigger points found in the pelvic floor are likely to have central significance to a person's experience of pain in other chronic pelvic pain syndromes.

Kruse and Christiansen examined the temperature of the skin in the area to which pain was referred after a trigger point was palpated. This study provides some objective basis for validating patients' reports of referred pain from a trigger point. They found that the area where a patient reported referred pain had a colder temperature than adjacent skin areas. It is assumed that the colder area is caused by a reduction in blood flow. Therefore, the area of referred pain being colder than the adjacent tissue supports the idea that ischemia (reduced blood flow) may be part of the pain and dysfunction we see in patients who have chronic pelvic pain syndrome.

In a conversation with Dr. Richard Gevirtz, who has done research in the relationship between trigger points and emotional reactivity, he shared with us that the impetus for the research that discovered increased electrical activity in trigger points in relationship to stress or anxiety originally came from Italian researchers and their work in the early and mid 1990s. They had claimed that the sympathetic nervous system activity directly affected skeletal muscle and particularly the spindle part of the muscle. Gevirtz and Hubbard showed in the mid 1990s that trigger point activity significantly increased when the subject experienced anxiety, and the trigger point activity decreased in the absence of emotional arousal. Needle electrodes monitored electrical activity in trigger points of subjects asked to do arithmetic calculations (a standard way in which researchers arouse anxiety). In considering the results of this study that connect anxiety and trigger point activity, we begin to make sense of the intimate relationship between stress and pelvic pain and dysfunction symptoms reported to us by many of our patients.

In our own work, we previously measured the level of muscle tension in the rectum and the vagina of patients who came to see us for pelvic pain and dysfunction. Men with prostatitis had an increased level of pelvic floor muscle tension. This level was reduced after they participated in the treatment program that has led to the current one. Dr. Howard Glazer at Cornell University in New York reported that men who had prostatodynia had higher than normal levels of rectal tension and that their resting level of tension was what he called "unstable" compared to normal subjects. Furthermore, he found that the level of strength in the contraction of those muscles of the prostatodynia patients was higher, but more unsteady than normal.

Glazer has also consistently seen increased levels of vaginal tension in women who have vulvar pain. He sees a weakness in the strength of contraction of these women when asked to do Kegel exercises monitored by an electromyograph. The focus of Glazer's successful approach with women with vulvar pain has been to help them relax, strengthen, and stabilize their pelvic muscles.

The *Wise-Anderson Protocol*

After many years of treating patients with CPPS utilizing both manual physical therapy as well as cognitive behavior relaxation training, we determined that intensive or immersion therapy over several days was an ideal method to break long-term pain cycles and teach patients to care for themselves. Patients are evaluated by a urologist and then immerse themselves into daily physical therapy and *Paradoxical Relaxation* training over a 6-day period. We have conducted over 80 monthly sessions of this type and several months of follow-up (3 to 24 months) has revealed significant benefit to a large proportion of patients.

We reported a case series study of self-referred men with long-standing CPPS and attempted to describe the relationship between the locations of myofascial trigger points (TrPs) or restrictive muscular tissue, both internal and external to the pelvis, and the sites of pain initially described by the patients at the time of their evaluation. We hypothesized that palpation of certain myofascial TrPs would reproduce the pain sensations experienced by the patients.

The same physical therapist performed manual myofascial tissue palpation on all subjects. A traditional palpation force of approximately for tender points (recommended for examination of fibromyalgia) was used for the assessment of pain. Pain was ranked as 0 (none) to 3+ (severe) for each area examined. Only categorical pain levels of 2+ or 3+ were counted as "Yes—pain is present," while scores of 0 or 1+ were counted as "No pain". Sets of muscles that typically reproduced pain sensation in specific locations referred from TrPs were chosen for the investigation.

The median age of the 72 men with CPPS in this analysis was 40 years (range 20-72; IQR = 32, 49) with a median duration of symptoms of 44 months (range 4 - 408 months). The severity of symptoms at the time of the initial examination was measured by the pain VAS score and NIH-CPSI score with higher scores representing greater severity. The median VAS score was 5 out of 10 (range 1-9). The median NIH-CPSI overall score was 27 (43 is the maximum possible) with a median pain domain score of 13 (possible maximum = 21), urinary complaints of 5 (possible maximum = 10) and quality of life score of 10.5 (possible maximum =12). The median total number of self-reported locations of pain was 4 out of a possible 7 pre-designated sites. There was no correlation between pain score and total number of painful locations. However, we did find that tenderness in the puborectalis and/or pubococcygeus muscles was associated with a higher pain score. For example, 90% of men stated that they felt pain associated with palpation of the puborectalis and/or pubococcygeus muscles. Palpation of the puborectalis and/or pubococcygeus muscles elicited pain in the penis in 93% of the patients. At least 2 of the 10 trigger points could elicit or refer pain to every one of the anatomical sites in a large number of patients and every trigger point was able to reproduce pain in at least one site. The most reactive muscles were the rectus abdominus and external obliques; palpation of TrPs in these muscles elicited pain in 4 of the 7 sites. Perineal pain was the most reproducible, being elicited by 8 out of 10 TrPs.

The frequency with which TrP palpation referred pain to a patient's self-reported chronic pain location was remarkable. The odds ratio implied that these patients were 32 times more likely to have penile pain reproduced by the pubococcygeus muscle palpation than patients without penile pain. These physical examination findings may lead to greater understanding of pathogenic mechanisms and lead to more focused therapy. No asymptomatic men were examined as control subjects, therefore we are unable to compare how patients without CPPS would respond to these palpations. However, the purpose of this study was to examine patients with CPPS rather than compare their responses to normal subjects. Finally, it is difficult to objectively measure pain and thus we relied on patients' self reported responses. If a painful location was not reported during the initial history, we could not account for it in our later analyses. We recognize that some individuals may be naturally more sensitive to muscle palpations and pressure that could cause pain in the pelvic region even though they do not suffer from CPPS.

The *Wise-Anderson* Internal Wand For Chronic Pelvic Pain

The ideal therapeutic provider combination for care of UCPPS should include a urologist evaluating the urologic signs and symptoms in a systematic fashion, a knowledgeable psychologist to provide psychosocial interpretation, psychological support and cognitive behavior training such as progressive relaxation therapy and possible medical hypnosis, and a skilled physiotherapist who understands myofascial trigger points, how to release them and how to teach the patient self care.

It is not always possible for patients to find follow-up physiotherapy from those who may be appropriately trained and skilled in the techniques required. We have introduced and taught patients self treatment utilizing a personal therapeutic wand that can be inserted into the rectum or vagina to seek and release TrPs (Figures 1). Previous self-treatment devices have been inadequate to reach appropriate trigger points accurately and safely. Patients are carefully instructed regarding the location of their

TrPs and then observed and guided to using the wand within specific pressure ranges to avoid any mucosal trauma or induction of internal tissue damage. These pressures have ranged between 2 to 6 pounds per square inch. Fibromyalgia tender point testing is typically performed at 4 kilograms per square centimeter. In some instances we have been able to train a spouse or significant other to assist in administering the therapeutic wand. Aside from one or two limited transient bleeding episodes, due to overly enthusiastic pressure used by the user of the wand, no significant adverse effects have been noted. Patients are currently enrolled in a clinical trial under Institutional Review Board approval and followed for a period of 6 months, evaluating safety and efficacy. The intention is to enroll and evaluate 100 patient subjects. To date 64 patients have finished their 6-month evaluation, but 26 patients dropped out for various reasons. The average pelvic muscle sensitivity using the wand decreased by 40% at 6 months and 85% of the patients felt that the wand was effective with virtually no concerns or complications. We intend to soon publish all of the details of this study in the medical literature.

Pudendal nerve entrapment

We should mention the concept of the pudendal nerves being compressed, stretched or entrapped in the pelvis as a potential cause of chronic pelvic pain. There are 5 essential diagnostic criteria some propose: (1) pain along the anatomical distribution of the pudendal nerve; (2) the pain aggravated by sitting; (3) the patient is not awakened at night by the pain; (4) there is no objective sensory loss on clinical examination; and (5) the pain is improved by an anesthetic pudendal nerve block. Neurophysiologic tests such as pudendal nerve motor latency test and EMG may serve as complementary diagnostic measures.

Surgical procedures, which are very controversial and have little convincing evidence as to efficacy, presumably release fascia and ligaments of the pelvis and transpose nerves away from these impinging structures. Patients thought to have this syndrome typically have considerable pain while sitting and then completely relieved when standing. It is also relieved by sitting on a toilet seat, although both of these criteria exist to some degree in PPS. There are theories that athletic endeavors may have caused distortion in the nerve pathway. Similarly, chronic constipation may contribute to the presumed condition.

While we rarely recommend pudendal nerve injections, nor do we recommend pudendal nerve surgery, several pudendal nerve injection studies to document the source and relief of pain have been proposed to be necessary before any surgery is undertaken. Certainly, any surgical approach to alleviate this condition must rely on documentation of nerve dysfunction as measured by nerve conduction studies. *It appears that less than 50% of patients experience any reduction of their pain with surgery.*

In our experience, most patients undergoing this procedure express regret at having undergone the surgery report less than satisfactory results and a high level of new symptoms and compromised pelvic floor stability. We have never seen a patient whose symptoms have resolved after pudendal nerve entrapment (PNE) surgery. We believe our protocol may provide significant relief and should be done before surgery is ever considered.

Isolated male orchalgia (pain in the testicles)

Chronic orchalgia or pain in the testis, vexes a lot of young men and they reluctantly bring this to the attention of their physician. Testicular pain occurs most commonly in young men in their 20's and 30's and requires careful history and physical examination, because this is also the age group where testicular cancer most commonly occurs. Usually the examination is negative, with a complaint of pain localization to one side or other, and when the head of the epididymis organ is squeezed, it reproduces the pain for the patient. Rarely does a vasectomy result in such tenderness or chronic orchalgia.

It is important to understand the nerve supply to the testis so that the diagnostic evaluation can make some functional sense. The pelvic nerve plexus supplies the input, and pain can arise from both the normal sensory nerves and the autonomic nerves. These fibers are carried in the branches of the genitofemoral and ilioinguinal nerves. Findings of fluid around the testicle, varicose veins, or sperm cysts (spermatocele), are usually coincidental and are never the cause of the chronic orchalgia. This pain is almost always spermatic cord/ epididymal nerve pain and not testicular pain.

Removal of the epididymis as an approach to treat chronic testes pain has met with failure. Slightly more successful when all else has failed has been cutting the nerves, using a microscopic method, to remove all nerve fibers from the spermatic cord arising from the testicular tissue or the scrotal contents. We always perform a selective anesthetic spermatic cord nerve block as a diagnostic and sometimes therapeutic procedure first, adding a cortisone solution to a long-acting anesthetic. Several of these nerve blocks at intervals can sometimes relieve the cyclical nature of this syndrome. A recent report by Dr. Magdy Hassouna from Canada proposes that sacral nerve root electrical stimulation may be beneficial in these patients, and in some cases, skin surface electrical stimulation has been helpful.

CHAPTER 11

HOW TO CONTACT US

The amelioration or resolution to the pelvic pain we treat has eluded the best medical minds for more than a century. Most people reading this book would not be reading it if they were able to find help within the context of conventional treatment. It is not uncommon for individuals with pelvic pain to either have it on a continual basis or to have it wax and wane for many years and to go from doctor to doctor receiving little help. To date, there is no simple solution to this problem and for the most part, there is very little that has helped. This is the context in which people with the kind of pelvic pain we treat find themselves.

Our book offers a new model or paradigm for this problem. We propose that instead of pelvic pain being the result of an infection, a trapped nerve, an autoimmune disorder, or degenerative disease, that the major contributing factor to the conditions we discuss centrally involves a chronically knotted up, contracted pelvis – a kind of ongoing pelvic charley horse. This chronic contraction is fed by anxiety, dysfunctional protective guarding and conditioning in a person's past that prompts him or her to tighten the pelvic muscles under stress. This is a new understanding of this problem and one that qualitatively departs from conventional medical models.

One of the major points of this book is that the treatment that we have found to be most effective, addresses very difficult and hard to treat sources of the problem. Namely these sources of the problem include: 1) pelvic pain coming from trigger points inside and outside pelvic floor muscles; 2) chronic elevated tone in the pelvic muscles that someone has become used to; 3) the often long conditioned tendency to tighten the pelvis under stress; 4) the instinctive protective guarding that occurs in response to pain; 5) the difficult issue of worrying and thinking anxious and often catastrophic thoughts in relationship to one's condition in particular and in relationship to one's life in general; 6) living in a world in which anxiety-producing information, time urgency and multitasking are the norm.

Dealing with these central aspects of pelvic pain is daunting in the most ideal of circumstances. With the best of treatment we can offer, resolving one's pelvic pain is a challenge and with some individuals beyond our ability to help, even though we help the large majority of those we treat. Nevertheless, this is the reality those with pelvic pain face.

Can reading this book enable one to do the *Wise-Anderson Protocol* on him or herself?

There are a few readers of our book who have reported that by reading this book they have significantly reduced their symptoms by reading about and then applying the methods we describe here. That being said, we cannot recommend doing the methods that we describe here on oneself or others without proper supervision from someone competent in the methods that we discuss.

We cannot endorse this book as a self-help book because we cannot know if a reader understands what we are saying in the way that we mean to communicate it. We don't know how a reader relates to his or her body and do not want to be responsible for actions individuals take, in relationship to themselves, that we cannot supervise and correct when necessary. Pressing on a trigger point for one individual may mean using too little pressure, for another just enough pressure or for another bruising pressure. Accepting and relaxing with tension, as we describe in *Paradoxical Relaxation* to one individual might result in a significant relaxation of tension and symptoms and in another individual, this instruction might be wholly misinterpreted and result in tension that increases and that sours him on using this method. There are often many variables involved in our treatment that are open for confusion without competent instruction.

Again, given all of this some readers have designed their own program using our model and have helped themselves. They have written to us with gratitude for our roadmap. Others have been less successful at doing this.

We sometimes receive calls from individuals who want to know if they can help themselves by just reading our book. In this section, we want to address this question.

The basic premise of the Wise-Anderson Protocol is that patients must learn the protocol and become responsible for their own treatment. The purpose of our protocol is to train patients to be able to treat themselves. We have found that weekly treatment by a professional tends to be a tepid kind of treatment without a committed daily program of pelvic floor relaxation, stretching, and effective physical therapy self-treatment. The *Wise-Anderson Protocol* sees the treatment of pelvic pain as an inside job. *The proactive, daily self-treatment, in all aspects of the protocol, of the patient is essential and in our experience, without it, treatment almost always fails.*

For understandable reasons relating to constraints of time in conventional treatment, training patients in self-treatment tends to be an afterthought in most treatments of pelvic pain. Lip service is given to patient daily self-treatment with little time for patient training or backup. The *Wise-Anderson Protocol* makes the training of the patients in doing their treatment its primary goal. Instead of being an afterthought, it is the main point. The question is to what extent someone can learn this self-treatment from a book or from a brief few minute's instruction at the end of a weekly or biweekly session of therapy. We strongly endorse any treatment offered for pelvic pain that takes this principle to heart.

Devoting a daily hour and a half or more of self-treatment to oneself is not easy

Most of us are resistant to changing our routine. It is our experience that taking at least an hour and a half or more a day to do one's home program for at least many months is the bare minimum for our protocol to be effective. Carving out an hour and a half or so from one's life for most people, bumps up against real barriers. These barriers include huge inertia of a routine shaped by the demands of work, family and the desire for down time that often makes one feel there is no room for any other activity.

In our experience, only the yearning to get out of pain and the related suffering of pelvic pain syndromes is a strong enough motivation for patients to accommodate the self-treatment requirements we describe. Our patients tend to stick to their home practice over the long term when they see that their symptoms are improving.

What does it take to learn the home self-treatment, essential to the success of any treatment of pelvic pain?

The question of what it takes to learn effective methods of self-treatment is a critical question we are discussing here. There is no uniform answer to this question. There are some individuals of strong drive and high discipline who have been able to help themselves with little help or professional instruction. They have been able to research our methodology carefully and have helped their symptoms.

The majority of individuals, in our experience, struggle in trying to learn our methodology simply from reading this book. The best scenario is to learn the methods we describe from someone competent in them.

The biggest contribution we have to offer is a new view of the problem of pelvic pain and a roadmap for its amelioration. If we have done this in writing this book, we have accomplished something huge. We want to be realistic about what is possible and not possible. *While many people report that their symptoms get better after reading our book, for most people (and not everyone) simply reading this book is not adequate to be able to do our protocol successfully.* However this book is used, we hope that the *Wise-Anderson Protocol* can shine a light on the path of resolving pelvic pain.

For inquires about the 6-day intensive clinic or regarding other questions:

Email: ahip@sonic.net

Telephone: (707) 874-2225
Toll free: (866) 874-2225

Website: www.pelvicpainhelp.com

Mail: National Center for Pelvic Pain
P.O. Box 54
Occidental, CA 95465

Disclaimer

Many readers have found that reading this book has helped them better deal with or reduce their symptoms. This book, however, is not intended as a self-help book and is not meant to be a substitute for competent medical or psychological or physical therapy, diagnosis, instruction or supervision in home self-treatment. The aim of the *Wise-Anderson Protocol* is to help patients become independent and to be able to reduce or resolve their symptoms themselves without reliance on others. This independence requires training with and consultation by those competent in *Paradoxical Relaxation* and *Trigger Point Release*. Our approach is used when medical evaluation has ruled out physical illness and pathology.

About the authors

David Wise, PhD, spent 8 years in the Department of Urology at Stanford University Medical Center as a Visiting Research Scholar in the development of a new treatment for prostatitis and chronic pelvic pain syndromes. He is a licensed psychologist in California and his research interests are in behavioral medicine and autonomic self-regulation. He enjoys playing the mandolin, watercolor painting, and carpentry. He has made 5 musical CD's and is currently writing a musical play.

Rodney U. Anderson, MD, FACS is Professor of Urology (Emeritus-active) at Stanford University School of Medicine. His sub-specialty clinical expertise is NeuroUrology and Female Urology. His focus has been on chronic pelvic pain syndromes, pelvic floor dysfunction, interstitial cystitis, benign prostatic hyperplasia, urinary incontinence, urinary retention, spinal cord injuries, spina bifida, multiple sclerosis, Parkinsonism and stroke. He has also directed a clinic devoted to the problem of Female Sexual Dysfunction. He continues to be actively engaged in clinical research at Stanford on the *Wise-Anderson Protocol* and other research. He is a classical pianist and enjoys painting and golf.

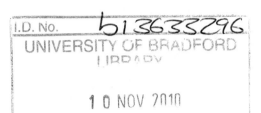